THE HUMAN NERVOUS SYSTEM

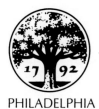

J.B. Lippincott Company

PHILADELPHIA
London   Mexico City   New York
St. Louis   São Paulo   Sydney

THE HUMAN NERVOUS SYSTEM

An Anatomical Viewpoint

FIFTH EDITION

Murray L. Barr, M.D., D.Sc., F.R.C.P.(C), F.R.S.

Emeritus Professor, Department of Anatomy
Health Sciences Centre
University of Western Ontario
London, Ontario, Canada

John A. Kiernan, M.B., Ch.B., Ph.D., D.Sc.

Professor, Department of Anatomy
Health Sciences Centre
University of Western Ontario
London, Ontario, Canada

Acquisitions Editor: Lisette Bralow
Developmental Editor: Richard Winters
Manuscript Editor: Elizabeth Galbraith
Indexer: Ann Cassar
Design Coordinator: Susan Hess Blaker
Designer: Rita Naughton
Cover Designer: Stephen Cymerman
Cover Photo: © Manfred Kage, Peter Arnold, Inc.
Production Manager: Carol A. Florence
Production Editor: Rosanne Hallowell
Production Coordinator: Charlene C. Squibb
Compositor: Ruttle, Shaw & Wetherill, Inc.
Text Printer/Binder: Kingsport Press
Cover Printer: New England Book Components

Fifth Edition

6   5   4   3

Library of Congress Cataloging-in-Publication Data

Barr, Murray Llewellyn, 1908–
   The human nervous system.

   Includes bibliographies and index.
   1. Neuroanatomy.   2. Anatomy, Human.   I. Kiernan,
J. A. (John Alan)   II. Title. [DNLM: 1. Nervous
System—anatomy & histology.   WL 101 B268h]
QM451.B27 1988   611'.8   87-17095
ISBN 0-397-50883-2

Preface

Knowledge of the nervous system is increasing so rapidly that a textbook for students is of necessity incomplete because of omissions and simplified explanations. In preparing this fifth edition, we have introduced new information when it helps to clarify the normal functional mechanisms or contributes to the understanding of how disease causes disordered function.

Most of the recently acquired neuroanatomical information relates to rodents and cats, whose systems of neuronal connections are not necessarily the same as those of the human nervous system. The use of primates in neuroanatomical research has declined in recent years, even though a system that is more important in the monkey than in the cat is likely to be more important still in man. Unfortunately, precise information about connectivity cannot be obtained from human material. We have therefore added only those data that certainly or probably apply to man, and we have removed some material that was included in earlier editions but which now seems to have little relevance to the human nervous system.

On the other hand, modern diagnostic techniques, especially computer assisted x-ray tomography, nuclear magnetic resonance imaging, regional blood-flow studies, and positron emission tomography, permit the accurate localization of destructive lesions and even of metabolic aberrations in the living human brain. These methods, which can be mentioned only briefly in this book, show promise of providing new insights into the functions of parts of the human central nervous system.

We are grateful to Dr. John Hore for helpful comments and suggestions concerning several physiological points, to Miss Deborah Allen for advice on the newer physical methods of imaging the brain, and to Miss Louise Gadbois for the new and revised illustrations. We also appreciate the work done by the staff of J.B. Lippincott, especially David Barnes, Richard Winters, Rosanne Hallowell, Charlene Squibb, and Susan Hess Blaker.

Murray L. Barr, M.D.,D.SC., F.R.C.P.(C), F.R.S.
John A. Kiernan, M.B., CH.B., PH.D., D.SC.

Preface
to the
First Edition

Because of the intricacies of neuronal connections and the necessity of being able to visualize structures three-dimensionally, the anatomy of the central nervous system offers a particular challenge to the student. It is only through an adequate understanding of the structure of the brain and spinal cord that concurrent studies along physiologic and clinical lines can progress. In particular, the interpretation of neurologic signs and symptoms must rest on a sound basis of neurologic anatomy. It is hoped that this textbook will provide such a basis for students in the health sciences and others studying the central nervous system of man. The book is written for those approaching the neurosciences for the first time; several excellent larger books on neurological anatomy are available to the advanced student.

The material has been arranged in four sections. The first section deals mainly with neurohistology. The second and largest section is concerned with the regional anatomy of the central nervous system, beginning with the spinal cord and then progressing to the highest levels of the brain. Although the sensory and motor systems are discussed regionally, experience in teaching has shown the necessity of reviewing these clinically important systems in their entirety, and this is done in the third section. The fourth section deals with the blood supply of the central nervous system, its meningeal coverings, and the cerebrospinal fluid.

Eponyms are used freely in neurology, in spite of attempts to eliminate them; they frequently offer welcome alternatives to the more formal, and sometimes formidable, anatomical terms. Some facts concerning individuals whose names are attached to structures are provided at the end of the book for students who are curious about the source of the eponyms. In addition, since many neurological terms are derived from Greek and Latin, a glossary is included for those students who have not received instruction in the classics.

It is a pleasure to acknowledge the valued assistance of several persons. A special note of appreciation goes to Mrs. Margaret Corrin for the preparation of the drawings, all of which are her own work. Illustrations of this type are of particular importance in a textbook of neurological anatomy. I also wish to thank Mrs. Aileen Densham, who carried out the secretarial work most efficiently. I am greatly indebted to Mr. J. E. Walker for the technical preparation of anatomical specimens for reproduction, to Mr. C. E. Jarvis for the photomicrographs, and to the staff of the Art Services Department of the Health Sciences Centre, University of Western Ontario, for their fine photography.

Several colleagues have given of their time to read drafts of all chapters and make valuable suggestions. They are Dr. H. W. K. Barr, of the Department of Clinical Neurological Sciences, and Drs. R. C. Buck, M. J. Hollenberg, and D. G. Montemurro, of the Department of Anatomy. I am also grateful for the many helpful discussions on specific topics with Dr. J. P. Girvin, of the Departments of Clinical Neurological Sciences and Physiology, and with Dr. A. Kertesz, of the Department of Clinical Neurological Sciences. Finally, I wish to express my appreciation to the staff of Harper & Row for their patience, advice, and assistance.

Murray L. Barr, M.D., D.SC., F.R.C.P.(C), F.R.S

Contents

THE HUMAN NERVOUS SYSTEM

INTRODUCTION AND NEUROHISTOLOGY

ONE

Development, Composition, and Evolution of the Nervous System

All living organisms respond to chemical and physical stimuli. The response may be a movement, or it may be the expulsion of biosynthetic products from cells. These receptive, motor, and secretory functions are all combined in a single cell in the most primitive animals, the protozoa. The simplest multicellular animals, the porifera (sponges), are colonies of cells having similar properties. Even adjacent cells of these creatures are not functionally connected with one another. In all other groups of animals, cells are able to communicate so that the reception of a stimulus by one cell may result in the motile or secretory activity of other cells. Specialized cells known as **neurons** exist to transfer information rapidly from one part of an animal's body to another. All the neurons of an organism, together with their supporting cells, constitute a **nervous system.**

In order to carry out its communicative function a neuron exhibits two different but coupled activities. These are **conduction of impulses** and **synaptic transmission.** An impulse is a wave of electrical depolarization that is propagated within the surface membrane of the neuron. A stimulus applied to one part of the neuron initiates an impulse that travels to all other parts of the cell. Neurons commonly have long cytoplasmic processes known as **neurites,** which end in close apposition to the surfaces of other cells. The ends of the neurites are called **synaptic terminals,** and the cell-to-cell contacts they make are known as **synapses.** The neurites in higher animals are usually specialized to form **dendrites** and **axons,** which conduct impulses toward and away from the cell body, respectively. The arrival of an impulse at a terminal triggers the process of synaptic transmission. This event usually involves the release of a chemical compound from

3

the neuronal cytoplasm, which evokes some type of response in the postsynaptic cell. At some synapses the two cells are electrically coupled. Another type of neuron exists that discharges its chemical products into the circulating blood, thereby influencing distant parts of the body. Neurons of the latter type are functionally related to endocrine gland cells, and are known as **neurosecretory cells.**

DEVELOPMENT OF THE NERVOUS SYSTEM

The nervous system develops from the dorsal ectoderm of the early embryo. Nerve cells, together with neuroglial or interstitial cells, are therefore derived from the outer ectodermal layer, similar to the cells of the epidermis covering the body surface. The first indication of the future nervous system is the neuroectoderm comprising the **neural plate,** which appears in the dorsal midline of the embryo at the 16th day of development. The neural plate changes 2 days later into a **neural groove** with a **neural fold** along each side; by the end of the third week the neural folds have begun to fuse with one another, thereby converting the neural groove into a **neural tube** (Fig. 1–1). The transformation proceeds rostrally and caudally, and the openings at each end (the rostral and caudal neuropores) close at about the 24th and 26th days, respectively. The neural tube is the forerunner of the brain and spinal cord.

Neuroectodermal cells not incorporated into the tube form **neural crests** running dorsolaterally along each side of the neural tube. From the neural crests are derived the dorsal root ganglia of spinal nerves, some of the neurons in sensory ganglia of cranial nerves, autonomic ganglia, the nonneuronal cells (neuroglia) of peripheral nerves, and secretory cells of the adrenal medulla. Thus, the cells of the neural crest are notable for their extensive migrations. Many of them even differen-

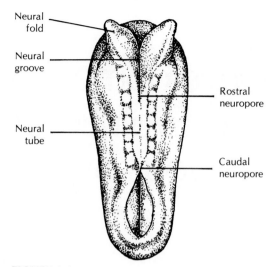

FIGURE 1-1.
Dorsal view of embryo at about 22 days.

tiate into cells of nonneural tissue, including the melanocytes of the skin and some of the bones, muscles, and other structures of the head that are generally of mesodermal origin.

A few nervous elements are also derived from **placodes,** which are thickened regions of the ectoderm of the surface of the head. Thus, the olfactory neurosensory cells, the sensory cells and associated ganglia of the inner ear, and some of the neurons in the sensory ganglia of cranial nerves are derived from placodes.

Growth and differentiation occur to the greatest extent in the rostral portion of the neural tube, from which the large and complex brain develops; the remainder of the neural tube becomes the spinal cord. As described conventionally, three **primary brain vesicles** appear at the end of the fourth week: the **prosencephalon** (forebrain), **mesencephalon** (midbrain), and **rhombencephalon** (hindbrain)—Fig. 1–2A. During the fifth week each of the first and third vesicles changes into two swellings so that there are five **secondary brain vesicles:** the **telencephalon, diencephalon, mesencephalon, metencephalon,** and

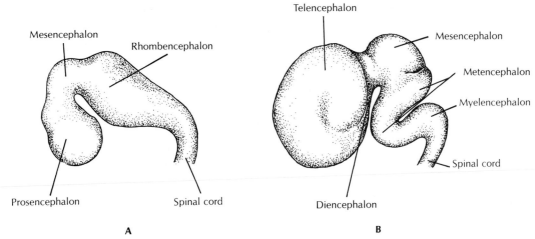

FIGURE 1-2.
(A) Primary brain vesicles (fifth week). **(B)** Secondary brain vesicles (seventh week). The diencephalon is partly hidden by the expanding telencephalon, which develops into the cerebral hemispheres.

myelencephalon (Fig. 1–2*B*).* As cellular proliferation and differentiation proceed in the spinal cord, a longitudinal groove called the **sulcus limitans** appears along the inner aspect of each lateral wall. The sulcus demarcates a dorsal **alar plate** from a ventral **basal plate;** they acquire afferent and efferent connections, respectively, and continue forward as far as the rostral end of the mesencephalon. The neural canal within the neural tube becomes the ventricles of the brain and the central canal of the spinal cord.

The first populations of cells produced in the neural tube are **neuroblasts,** the precursors of neurons. The number of neuroblasts formed in the neural tube exceeds the number of neurons in the adult brain and spinal cord. The large numbers of neuroblasts that fail to make synaptic connections die as part of the normal course of

development. This occurrence, known as **programmed cell death,** is seen in many embryonic systems throughout the animal kingdom.

Congenital malformations of the central nervous system include those that result from failure of the neural folds to fuse normally. In anencephaly the folds do not fuse at the rostral end of the developing neural tube so that forebrain derivatives are lacking and the concurrent absence of a cranial vault exposes the rudiment of the brain to the exterior. Anencephaly occurs once in about 1000 births and is incompatible with sustained life. In a rarer condition the neural folds fail to meet and fuse in the lumbar region. This error results in an especially severe form of spina bifida known as spina bifida with myeloschisis (cleft spinal cord).

DERIVATIVES OF THE BRAIN VESICLES

The regions of the brain that develop from the secondary brain vesicles acquire a distinctive structure, and some of the formal embryological names are replaced by others for common usage (Table 1–1 and

---

* The concept of brain vesicles is especially pertinent to the chick embryo, which is a favorite subject for embryological investigation. The same concept is used as a general convention, even though it provides a less satisfactory basis for the developing mammalian brain.

TABLE 1-1. Development of the Mature Brain from the Brain Vesicles

PRIMARY BRAIN VESICLES	SECONDARY BRAIN VESICLES	MATURE BRAIN
Rhomben- cephalon	Myelencephalon Metencephalon	Medulla oblongata Pons and cerebellum
Mesen- cephalon	Mesencephalon	Midbrain
Prosen- cephalon	Diencephalon	Thalamus, epithalamus, hypothal- amus, and subthalamus
	Telencephalon	Cerebral hemispheres, consisting of the olfactory system, corpus striatum, cortex, and medullary center

Fig. 1–3). The myelencephalon becomes the medulla oblongata, and the metencephalon develops into the pons and cerebellum. The mesencephalon of the mature brain is usually called the midbrain. The names diencephalon and telencephalon are retained because of the diverse nature of their derivatives. A large mass of gray matter, the thalamus, develops in the diencephalon. Adjacent regions are known as the epithalamus, hypothalamus, and subthalamus, each with distinctive structural and functional characteristics. The telencephalon undergoes the greatest development in the human brain, in respect both to other regions and to the telencephalon of other animals. It includes the olfactory system, the corpus striatum (a mass of gray matter with motor functions), an extensive surface layer of gray matter known as the cortex or pallium, and a medullary center of white matter.

The medulla, pons, and midbrain together make up the brain stem, to which the cerebellum is attached by three pairs of peduncles. The diencephalon and telencephalon constitute the cerebrum, of which the telencephalon is represented by two massive cerebral hemispheres. The lumen of the neural tube is converted into a lateral ventricle in each cerebral hemisphere, a third ventricle in the dienceph-

alon, and a fourth ventricle bounded by the medulla, pons, and cerebellum. The third and fourth ventricles are connected by a narrow channel or aqueduct through the midbrain.

SUMMARY OF MAIN REGIONS OF THE NERVOUS SYSTEM

Certain features of the main regions are noted in the following summary, by way of introduction and to provide a first acquaintance with some neurological terms.

Spinal Cord

The spinal cord is the least differentiated component of the central nervous system. The segmental nature of the spinal cord is reflected in a series of paired spinal nerves, each of which is attached to the cord by a dorsal sensory root and a ventral motor root. The central **gray matter,** in which nerve cell bodies are located, has a roughly H-shaped outline in transverse section. **White matter,** which consists of nerve fibers running longitudinally, occupies the periphery of the cord. The spinal cord includes neuronal connections that provide for spinal reflexes. There are also pathways conveying sensory data to the

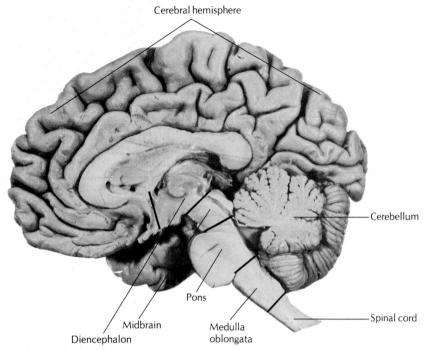

Cerebral hemisphere

Cerebellum

Pons

Spinal cord

Midbrain

Diencephalon

Medulla
oblongata

FIGURE 1-3.
Regions of the mature central nervous system, as seen in sagittal section. ($\times$ ½; courtesy of Dr. D. G. Montemurro)

brain and other pathways conducting impulses, mainly of motor significance, from the brain to the spinal cord.

Medulla Oblongata

The fiber tracts of the spinal cord are continued in the medulla, which also contains clusters of nerve cells called nuclei. The most prominent of these, the **inferior olivary nuclei,** send fibers to the cerebellum through the inferior cerebellar peduncles, which attach the cerebellum to the medulla oblongata. Of the smaller nuclei, some are components of cranial nerves.

Pons

The pons consists of two distinct parts. The dorsal portion has features shared with the rest of the brain stem. It therefore includes sensory and motor tracts, together with

some nuclei of cranial nerves. The basal (ventral) portion of the pons is special to this part of the brain stem. Its function is to provide for extensive connections between the cortex of a cerebral hemisphere and that of the contralateral cerebellar hemisphere. These connections contribute to maximal efficiency of motor activities. A pair of middle cerebellar peduncles attaches the cerebellum to the pons.

Midbrain

Like other parts of the brain stem, the midbrain contains sensory and motor pathways, together with nuclei for two cranial nerves. There is a dorsal region, the roof or **tectum,** which is concerned principally with the visual and auditory systems. The midbrain also includes two prominent motor nuclei, the **red nucleus** and the **substantia nigra.** The cerebellum is attached to the midbrain by the superior cerebellar peduncles.

Cerebellum

The cerebellum is especially large in the human brain. Receiving data from most of the sensory systems and the cerebral cortex, the cerebellum eventually influences motor neurons supplying the skeletal musculature. The function of the cerebellum is to produce changes in muscle tonus in relation to equilibrium, locomotion, and posture, as well as nonstereotyped movements based on individual experience. The cerebellum operates behind the scenes at a subconscious level.

Diencephalon

The diencephalon forms the central core of the cerebrum. The largest component of the diencephalon, the **thalamus,** consists of several regions or nuclei, some of which receive data from sensory systems and project to sensory areas of the cerebral cortex. Part of the thalamus has connections with cortical areas that are concerned with complex mental processes. Other regions participate in neural circuits related to emotions, and certain thalamic nuclei are incorporated into pathways from the cerebellum and corpus striatum to motor areas of the cerebral cortex. The **epithalamus** includes small tracts and nuclei, together with the pineal gland, an endocrine organ. The **hypothalamus** is the principal autonomic center of the brain and, as such, has an important controlling influence over the sympathetic and parasympathetic systems. In addition, neurosecretory cells in the hypothalamus synthesize hormones that reach the bloodstream by way of the neurohypophysis or influence the hormonal output of the adenohypophysis through a special portal system of blood vessels. The **subthalamus** includes sensory tracts proceeding to the thalamus, nerve fibers originating in the cerebellum

and corpus striatum, and the subthalamic nucleus (a motor nucleus). The retina is a derivative of the diencephalon; the optic nerve and the visual system are therefore intimately related to this part of the brain.

Telencephalon (Cerebral Hemispheres)

The telencephalon includes the cerebral cortex, corpus striatum, and medullary center. Small areas of **cerebral cortex** have an ancient lineage (paleocortex) and receive data from the olfactory system, which dominates the cerebrum of lower vertebrates. Certain areas of cortex, which likewise appeared early in vertebrate evolution, are called archicortex. They are included in the limbic system, which is involved with memory, emotions, and the influence of emotions on visceral function through the autonomic nervous system.

The appearance of neocortex in the reptilian brain was a most significant event, and the presence of substantial amounts of neocortex is a mammalian characteristic. The extent and volume have increased during the course of mammalian evolution, so that nine tenths of the human cerebral cortex is neocortex. This includes areas for all modalities of sensation (except smell), motor areas, and large expanses of association cortex, in which the highest levels of neural function presumably take place, including those inherent in intellectual activity.

The **corpus striatum** is a large mass of gray matter with motor functions, situated near the base of each hemisphere. It consists of caudate and lentiform nuclei, the latter being subdivided into a putamen and a globus pallidus. The **medullary center** of the hemisphere consists of fibers connecting cortical areas of the same hemisphere, fibers crossing the midline in a large commissure known as the corpus callosum to connect cortical areas of the two hemispheres, and fibers passing in both directions between cortex and subcortical centers. Fibers of the last category converge to form a compact internal capsule in the region of the thalamus and corpus striatum.

The weight of the mature brain varies according to age and body stature. The normal range in the adult man is 1100 to 1700 g (average 1360 g). The lower figures for the adult woman (1050–1550 g, average 1275 g) reflect the smaller stature of women in general, compared with men. There is no evidence of a relation between brain weight, within normal limits, and a person's level of intelligence.

EVOLUTION OF THE NERVOUS SYSTEM

The embryology and components of the human nervous system have been briefly discussed. It will be useful now to present some evolutionary background regarding the comparative anatomy of the invertebrate and vertebrate nervous systems.

Invertebrates

The simplest Coelenterata, such as the hydra, are branched tubular animals. A netlike arrangement of neurons, each with two or more processes, is interposed between the epithelium that covers the outside of the animal and the epithelium that lines the digestive cavity. A stimulus applied to any part of the animal causes the propagation of signals among the neurons of the nerve net, and results in contraction or bending of the tubular body and its tentacles. The site and intensity of the stimulus determine the strength and direction of the response. With this simple nerve net the hydra may move about, vary its length, and use its tentacles to push food particles into its mouth. Occasional strong contractions of the whole animal serve to expel indigestible material from the same orifice, which also serves as an anus.

In the higher Coelenterata, such as the jellyfish, and in all other invertebrate animals, the neurons are not uniformly distributed in the wall of the body, but instead are collected together in aggregates known as **ganglia.** In invertebrates, only the cytoplasmic processes (neurites) of the neurons are involved in synaptic contacts. The cell bodies usually lie in the outer rind of the ganglion. Many neurites synapse with one another in the central core, whereas others travel in bundles called **connectives** to other ganglia or in **nerves** to receptor and effector organs. Receptor cells are located mainly on the surface of the body, often in highly differentiated organs such as eyes. In bilaterally symmetrical animals, such as worms and arthropods, pairs of ganglia are arrayed along the length of the body, joined longitudinally and across the midline by connectives. In such creatures there is usually a distinct head that bears special sensory organs for the perception of light and chemical stimuli. This concentration of important functions in the head is associated with the presence there of ganglia larger and more complex than those in the more posterior parts of the body. Such ganglia may be said to constitute a **brain.**

Vertebrates

Vertebrates are thought by biologists to have evolved from simpler animals that lacked backbones. Their lowly ancestors may never be known, because they must be extinct, but they might have resembled the modern wormlike nemertea, or primitive chordata such as the amphioxus. These are all bilaterally symmetrical creatures with brains in their heads.

The nervous systems of all vertebrate animals—fishes, amphibians, reptiles, birds, and mammals—are of similar construction. The brain is a hollow structure that extends posteriorly toward the tail as a tubular spinal cord. The brain is encased in the skull, and the spinal cord is encircled intermittently by the vertebrae of the spinal column. Ganglia are associated with nerves connecting the spinal cord and the caudal parts of the brain with the skin, other sense organs, muscles, and viscera. A second system of neurons, which forms a plexus within the wall of the alimentary canal, is connected with the main nervous system but can also function independently. There is thus a **central nervous system** composed of the brain and spinal cord, a **peripheral nervous system** composed of the spinal and cranial nerves, and an **autonomic nervous system** that innervates smooth muscle and gland cells, together with cardiac muscle.

The structural plan of the spinal cord and of its associated nerves and ganglia is essentially the same in all vertebrates. The size, vascularity, variety of nonneuronal cells, and complexity of neuronal circuitry in the central nervous system all increase with the phylogenetic advance from the primitive fishes to the mammals. The most conspicuous differences among the nervous systems of vertebrates are found in the relative sizes of the various parts of the brain (Fig. 1–4).

The rhombencephalon and mesencephalon contain groups of neurons connected with most of the **cranial nerves.** These are similar to the spinal nerves, although their segmental organization is less obvious. The cranial nerves supply structures in the head, as well as large parts of the cardiopulmonary and alimentary systems. Fishes have 10 pairs of cranial nerves, numbered rostrocaudally. Two additional pairs of cranial nerves are found in amphibians and are also present in reptiles, birds, and mammals. In addition to the cranial nerve nuclei, the brain stem contains many groups of neurons whose synaptic connections are related to other parts of the central nervous system. These vary in size and complexity in the different vertebrate classes, generally becoming larger and more diverse as the phylogenetic scale is ascended.

The **cerebellum** in fishes receives most of its input from the vestibular and lateral line receptors, with smaller contributions from the optic system, the spinal cord, and some sensory nuclei of the cranial nerves. Spinal afferents are more numerous in reptiles and birds. In mammals there are also extensive indirect connections with the cerebral cortex, which attain their greatest development in humans. The increasing importance of the cerebellum is apparent from its greater size in the more advanced animals.

The dorsal part of the mesencephalon reaches its highest degree of development, relative to other parts of the brain, in bony fishes and in amphibians. In these forms the **optic tectum** is a many-layered structure of great synaptic complexity that forms prominent bilateral bulges on the dorsal surface of the brain. In addition to receiving most of the output of the retina, it is significantly involved in other modalities of sensation and in the control of movement. In mammals the relatively small tectum consists of a **superior** and an **inferior colliculus** on each side. The superior colliculus, homologous with the optic tectum, is an important visual center in lower mammals, such as rodents, but is of lesser importance in humans. The inferior colliculus is part of the polysynaptic pathway by which auditory sensation is relayed to the forebrain.

The diencephalon has four parts, all of which are present in all vertebrates. The **epithalamus** is the largest part in the most primitive fishes, in which, as in higher vertebrates, it forms a link between the telencephalon and the midbrain. The **hypothalamus** is the largest division of the diencephalon in both cartilaginous and bony fishes. It retains its functional importance in higher animals but is relatively smaller because of the increased size of the **thalamus** (the "dorsal thalamus" of comparative anatomists). The size and complexity of the thalamus increase in association with the evolution of the telen-

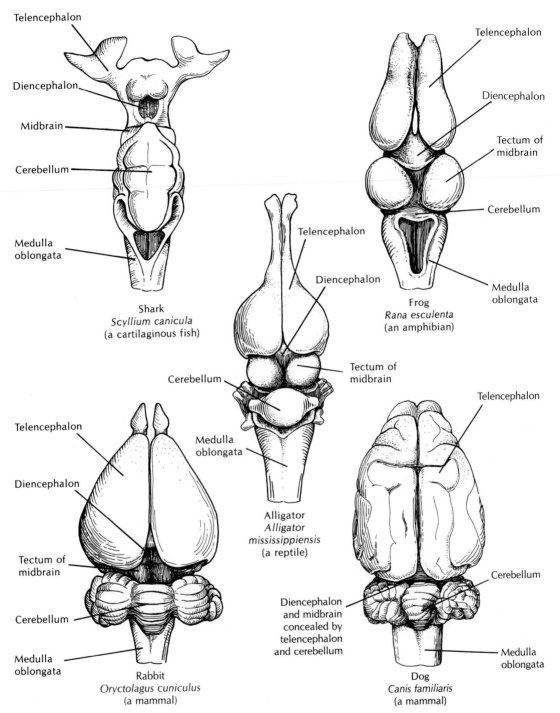

FIGURE 1-4.
Dorsal views of the brains of five vertebrate animals, showing the relative sizes of the main regions.

cephalon. The **subthalamus** (also known as the "ventral thalamus") is always the smallest part of the diencephalon.

The telencephalon consists of the two **cerebral hemispheres,** each containing a lateral ventricle, derived from the bifurcated neural tube. In fishes and amphibians the most rostral part of the hemisphere is the **olfactory lobe,** which receives the olfactory nerves. The olfactory lobe is joined to the diencephalon by a simple tubular structure in which the ventricular cavity is surrounded by gray matter, external to which is a layer of nerve fibers; this arrangement is similar to that of the spinal cord. The nervous tissue dorsal to the ventricle is the **pallium,** that ventrolateral to the ventricle is the **striatum,** and that ventromedial to the cavity is the **septum.** All these regions receive input from the olfactory lobe. In these lower vertebrates the telencephalon is implicated in decisive as distinct from purely reflex responses. Decisions and judgments in these animals are strongly influenced by olfactory stimuli and are important in relation to the recognition and treatment of potential food, mates, and enemies. In reptiles all parts of the telencephalon are larger than in amphibians, and the striatum is especially prominent. Reciprocal connections with the thalamus and with lower levels of the nervous system are also more developed.

In mammals the cerebral hemispheres are even larger. The olfactory bulb, equivalent to the olfactory lobe of lower vertebrates, projects mainly to the ventral and medial parts of the forebrain. The striatum forms a large mass of gray matter, the **corpus striatum,** inside each hemisphere, and the pallium forms an outer covering of gray matter, the **cerebral cortex.** The more complex behavioral patterns are observed in those mammals in which the area and therefore the volume of the cerebral cortex is greater. The increased area is accommodated by the development of convolutions in the surface of the cortex, which are most numerous in primates, including humans.

SUGGESTED READING

Hopkins WG, Brown MC: Development of Nerve Cells and Their Connections. Cambridge, Cambridge University Press, 1984

Korr H: Proliferation of different cell types in the brain. Adv Anat Embryol Cell Biol 61:1–72, 1980

LeDouarin NM: The Neural Crest. New York, Cambridge University Press, 1982

Lemire RJ, Loeser JD, Leech RW, Alvord EC: Normal and Abnormal Development of the Nervous System. Hagerstown, Harper & Row, 1975

Moore KL: The Developing Human: Clinically Oriented Embryology, 3rd ed. Philadelphia, WB Saunders, 1982

Müller F, O'Rahilly R: The first appearance of the major divisions of the human brain at stage 9. Anat Embryol 168:419–432, 1983

Northcutt RG: Evolution of the vertebrate central nervous system: Patterns and processes. Am Zool 24:701–716, 1984

Purves D, Lichtman JW: Principles of Neural Development. Sunderland, MA, Sinauer & Associates, 1985

Sarnat HB, Netsky MG: Evolution of the Nervous System, 2nd ed. New York, Oxford University Press, 1981

TWO

Cells of the Central Nervous System

There are two classes of cells in the central nervous system in addition to the usual cells found in walls of blood vessels. **Nerve cells** or **neurons** are specialized for excitation (or inhibition) and nerve impulse conduction, and are therefore responsible for most of the functional characteristics of nervous tissue. **Neuroglial cells,** collectively known as the **neuroglia** or simply as **glia,** have important ancillary functions.

The central nervous system consists of gray matter and white matter. **Gray matter** contains the cell bodies of neurons, each with a nucleus, embedded in a **neuropil** made up predominantly of delicate neuronal and glial processes. **White matter,** on the other hand, consists mainly of long processes of neurons, the majority being surrounded by myelin sheaths, and nerve cell bodies are lacking. Both the gray and the white matter contain large numbers of neuroglial cells and a network of blood capillaries. In some parts of the central nervous system, notably the brain stem (medulla, pons, and midbrain), there are regions that contain both nerve cell bodies and numerous myelinated fibers. These regions are therefore an admixture of gray matter and white matter.

THE NEURON

Neurons are structural and functional cellular units. They have special features for the reception of nerve impulses from other neurons, the effect of which may be either excitation or inhibition, and conduction of nerve impulses. The part of the cell that includes the nucleus is called the **cell body,** and its cytoplasm is known as the **perikaryon. Dendrites** are typically short branching processes that form a major part of the receptive area of the cell. Most neurons of the central nervous system have several dendrites and are therefore multipolar in shape. By reaching out in various directions, these processes increase the ability of a neuron to receive nerve impulses from diverse sources. Each cell has a single **axon.** This process, which varies greatly in length from one type of neuron to another, conducts impulses away from the cell body, usually to other neurons in the central nervous system. Some neurons have no axons, and their dendrites conduct impulses in both directions. Axons of efferent neurons in the spinal cord and brain stem are included in spinal and cranial nerves; they end on striated muscle fibers or on nerve cells of sympathetic or parasympathetic ganglia.

The fact that each neuron is a structural and functional unit is known as the **Neuron Theory,** proposed in the latter part of the 19th century in opposition to the then prevailing view that nerve cells form a continuous reticulum or syncytium. The unitary concept, conforming to the Cell Theory, was advanced by His on the basis of embryological studies, by Forel on the basis of the response of nerve cells to injury, and by Ramón y Cajal from his histological observations. The Neuron Theory was given wide distribution in a general review by Waldeyer of the whole subject of the individuality of nerve cells. Because of the special relationship between neurons at synapses, definite proof had to await the introduction of electron microscopy, which showed that the apposed surfaces of two neurons are in fact separated by a narrow interval known as a synaptic cleft.

Variations Among Neurons

Although all nerve cells conform to the general principles outlined above, there is a wide range of structural diversity. The size of the cell body varies from 5 μm for the smallest cells in complex circuits to 135 μm for large motor neurons. Dendritic

morphology, in particular the pattern of branching, varies greatly and is distinctive for neurons that constitute a specific cell group or nucleus. The axon of a minute neuron is a fraction of a millimeter in length, exceedingly fine, and devoid of a myelin covering. The axon of a large neuron, on the other hand, is nearly 1 meter long in extreme cases, has a substantial diameter, and is enclosed in a myelin sheath.

The large neurons of a nucleus or comparable region are called Golgi type I or principal cells because their axons carry the encoded output of information from the region containing their cell bodies to other parts of the nervous system. The dendrites of a principal cell are contacted by axonal terminals of several other neurons. These may include principal cells of other areas and nearby small neurons. The latter are known variously as Golgi type II, internuncial, or local circuit neurons or, more simply, as interneurons, and they greatly outnumber the principal cells.

Some examples of large and small neurons are illustrated in Figure 2–1, which shows the cells as they might appear in specimens stained by the Golgi method.

Neurocytological Techniques

The intrinsic structure of the neuron, although basically similar to that of other cells, has some specialized characteristics. Information about neurocytology has accumulated over many decades by the application of various staining methods for light microscopy and subsequently by the use of electron microscopy.

Routine staining methods, such as the hematoxylin and eosin stain used for most tissues, are of little value in the light microscopic study of the normal nervous system. Special techniques are used instead, of which the most important are the following.

Cationic dyes, such as cresyl violet, toluidine blue, and thionine, often called

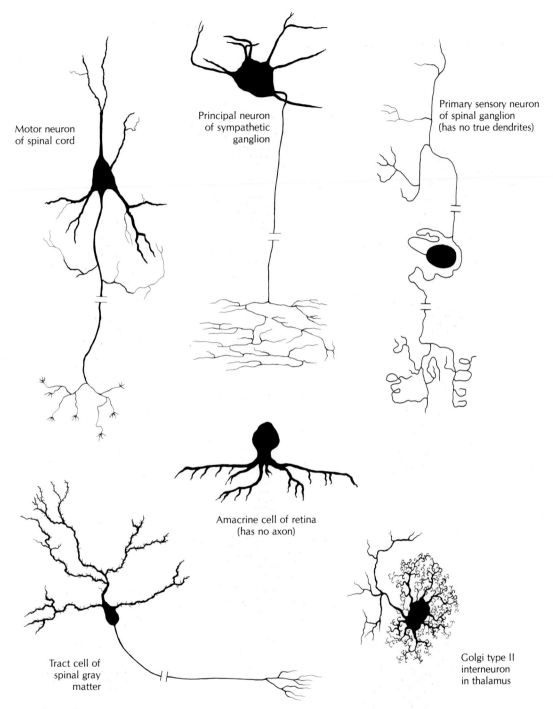

Motor neuron
of spinal cord

Principal neuron
of sympathetic
ganglion

Primary sensory neuron
of spinal ganglion
(has no true dendrites)

Amacrine cell of retina
(has no axon)

Tract cell of
spinal gray
matter

Golgi type II
interneuron
in thalamus

FIGURE 2-1.
Examples of neurons illustrating variations in size, shape, and branching of processes.

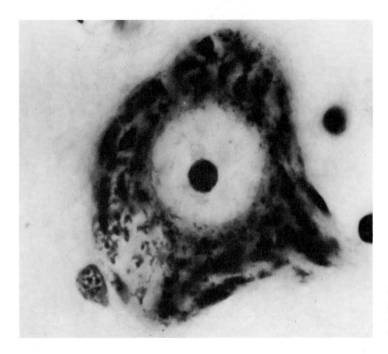

FIGURE 2-2.
Motor neuron in the spinal cord. (Stained with cresyl violet, × 1000)

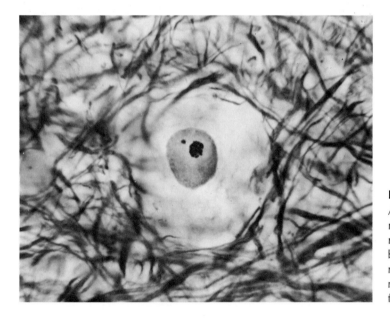

FIGURE 2-3.
A nerve cell surrounded by neuropil. In addition to the nucleolus, the small accessory body of Cajal is seen in the nucleus. (Cajal's silver nitrate method after chloral hydrate fixation, × 1200)

"Nissl stains," bind to nucleic acids (Fig. 2–2). They therefore demonstrate nuclei and nucleoli, and also the cytoplasmic Nissl substance of neurons.

Reduced silver methods produce dark deposits of colloidal silver in various structures (Fig. 2–3). The most widely used techniques are those of Ramón y Cajal, Bielschowsky, Bodian, and Holmes (for axons). Other methods, especially those of Ramón y Cajal, del Rio Hortega, and Penfield, are available for the selective demonstration of different types of neuroglial cell.

Stains for myelin reveal the major tracts of fibers other than those few that consist entirely of unmyelinated axons. Some of the illustrations in this book (*e.g.*, in Chap. 7) are of sections stained by Weigert's method. At low magnification the myelinated tracts are shown in blue-black whereas cellular areas such as nuclei are usually colorless. Combined myelin and Nissl stains are commonly used in research and in neuropathology.

The Golgi method, which has many variations, is valuable for the study of neuronal morphology, especially of dendrites (Fig. 2–4). In the original method, pieces of tissue are treated sequentially with solutions containing potassium dichromate and silver nitrate, after which sections 100 μm to 200 μm thick are prepared. Some of the neurons, including the finest branches of their dendrites, stand out in brown or black against a clear background. Occasional neuroglial cells are similarly displayed but axons are generally unstained. An important feature of these methods is the staining of only a small proportion of the cells; if all were blackened it would be impossible to resolve the structural detail.

Histochemical and immunocytochemical methods are available for localizing substances contained in specific populations of neurons. These substances include putative neurotransmitters (*e.g.*, norepinephrine, dopamine, serotonin, and various peptides) and enzymes involved in the synthesis or degradation of neurotransmitters (*e.g.*, dopamine β-hydroxylase, choline acetyltransferase, and acetylcholinesterase). Several previously unrecognized systems of neurons have been identified by the use of these methods in laboratory animals, and it is reasonable to surmise that equivalent systems exist also in humans.

Electron microscopy reveals the detailed internal structure of neurons and the specializations existing at synaptic junctions. However, the necessity of using ultrathin sections makes it difficult to re-

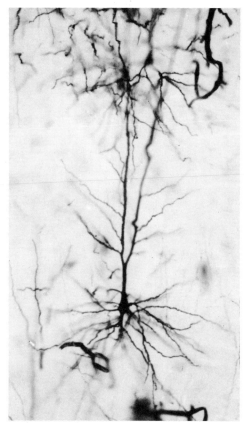

FIGURE 2-4.
Pyramidal cell in the cerebral cortex. (Golgi technique, × 90; courtesy of Dr. E. G. Bertram)

construct in three dimensions. A combination of light and electron microscopy provides a comprehensive view of neuronal and neuroglial structure. The diversity of nerve cells makes the "typical neuron" an abstraction, but Figure 2–5 is a simplified diagrammatic representation of the principal features common to most neurons.

Cytology of the Neuron

Cell Surface

The surface or limiting membrane of the neuron assumes special importance because of its role in the initiation and transmission of nerve impulses. The plasma membrane or plasmalemma is a double

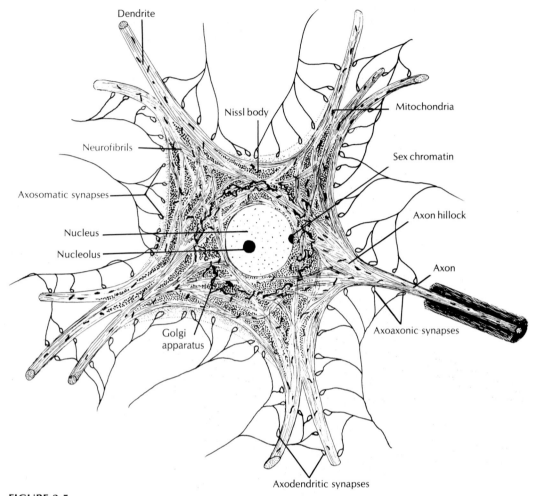

FIGURE 2-5.
Semidiagrammatic representation of the constituents of a nerve cell.

layer of phospholipid molecules whose hydrophobic hydrocarbon chains are all directed toward the middle of the membrane. Embedded in this structure are protein molecules, many of which pass through the whole thickness. These provide hydrophilic **channels** through which inorganic ions may enter and leave the cell. Each of the common ions (Na^+, K^+, Ca^{2+}, Cl^-) has its own specific type of molecular channel. The channels are **voltage gated,** which means that they open and close in response to changes in the electrical potential across the membrane,

which will be mentioned presently. Other protein molecules have side chains bearing carbohydrate groups that form, on the external surface, the outermost layer of the cell membrane, known as the glycocalyx or cell coat. Nerve impulses are propagated along the cell membrane of the neuronal surface. A simplified account of this process follows.

Conduction

Extracellular fluid has a high concentration of sodium ions (Na^+) and a low concentration of potassium ions (K^+), whereas in neuronal cytoplasm there is a high concentration of K^+ and a low concentration of Na^+. In the resting state, K^+ ions can leave the cell by diffusion through their channels in the membrane. Only small numbers of Na^+ ions diffuse in through the membrane, which, at rest, is only slightly permeable to these ions. Larger quantities of sodium enter when impulses are being conducted. The entry of Na^+ and the loss of intracellular K^+ are opposed by another membrane protein, the **sodium pump.** A pump is a molecule that uses energy (from ATP) to move ions through a membrane against a concentration gradient. Thus, the ionic concentrations in the cytoplasm are maintained, with expenditure of energy, largely as a consequence of the activity of the sodium pump. The resulting differences in concentrations of ions impart to the membrane a **resting potential,** with the inside of the cell at about -70 mV with respect to the outside.

During excitation, which may be due to any of a variety of chemical or physical stimuli, there is a reduction of the membrane potential, and the membrane is said to be **depolarized.** The reduction of potential spreads laterally in the plane of the membrane, declining in magnitude with distance from its site of initiation. This graded potential change is the only type of signaling in the dendrites and cell body. However, stimuli of sufficient number and intensity may reduce the membrane potential of the initial segment of the axon by as much as 10 to 15 mV. This is a threshold value, and it triggers the opening of the voltage-gated sodium channels of the axonal membrane. Na^+ ions surge locally from the outer to the inner surface, moving down a concentration gradient and also attracted by the excess of negative electrical charge in the axoplasm. The inside of the axon is transiently some $+40$ mV with respect to the outside. This change is called an **action potential.** Once generated, the action potential is self-propagated along the membrane by local circuits of electric current, which open the nearby Na^+ channels. The traveling action potential is also called a **nerve impulse,** and it can be recorded from the outer surface of the nerve fiber as a wave of negative potential.

Stimuli that depolarize the neuronal membrane are said to be excitatory, because sufficient numbers of them will initiate an action potential. Some stimuli have the opposite effect of **hyperpolarization,** in which the membrane potential exceeds its resting value of -70 mV. Stimuli that cause hyperpolarization inhibit the generation of action potentials, because they oppose the effects of depolarizing stimuli.

Nucleus

The spherical nucleus of the neuron is usually situated centrally in the cell body. It is vesicular in large neurons (*i.e.,* the chromatin is finely dispersed), whereas in most small neurons the chromatin is in coarse clumps. There are a few binucleate nerve cells in sympathetic ganglia. The **nuclear membrane** has the usual double-layered ultrastructure with numerous pores. There is usually a single prominent **nucleolus.** In females one of the two X chromosomes of the interphase nucleus is compact (heterochromatic) rather than elongated (euchromatic) like the remaining 45 chromosomes of the complement. The compact X chromosome is evident as a mass of **sex chromatin,** which is usually situated at the inner surface of the nuclear membrane. A small spherical intranuclear structure of unknown significance, called the **accessory body of Cajal,** is seen in sections stained by silver methods (see Fig. 2–3).

Cytoplasmic Organelles

Neurofibrils, Neurofilaments, Microtubules, and Microfilaments.   When certain silver stains are used, the cytoplasm is seen by light microscopy to contain neurofibrils, sometimes grouped into bundles, that run through the perikaryon and into the cell processes. In electron micrographs of nerve cells, the cytoplasm contains neurofilaments, 7.5 to 10 nm in thickness. The neurofilaments are made of structural proteins similar to those of the intermediate filaments of other types of cell. They are probably responsible for the neurofibrils of light microscopy. Electron microscopy also shows microtubules about 25 nm in external diameter, similar to those of other types of cell. These are involved in the rapid transport of protein molecules and small particles in both directions along axons and dendrites. Microfilaments (4 nm) are molecules of the contractile protein actin. They occur on the inside of the plasmalemma and are particularly numerous in the tips of growing neurites.

Nissl Substance.   When nervous tissue is stained with a cationic dye, such as cresyl violet or thionine, clumps of basophilic material are seen in most nerve cells. These are known as Nissl bodies, after Franz Nissl (1860–1919), a Heidelberg neurologist. The amount of Nissl material increases with the size of the neuron, and its arrangement varies from one type of nerve cell to another. For example, the clumps are coarse in motor neurons (see Fig. 2–2), whereas in sensory neurons the basophilic material is more finely distributed. The Nissl substance extends into dendritic processes but is lacking in both the axon hillock (*i.e.*, the peripheral zone of the perikaryon where the axon emerges) and the axon itself. Nissl material is the same as the basophilic substance, sometimes called ergastoplasm or chromidial substance, in the cytoplasm of secretory cells.

The Nissl substance is seen by electron microscopy to consist of orderly arrays of **granular endoplasmic reticulum** (Fig. 2–6). This is a system of flattened cisternae or vesicles bearing ribosomal particles on their outer surfaces, and with polyribosomes in the adjacent cytoplasmic matrix. The ribosomes contain ribonucleic acid (RNA), which accounts for the basophilia. They participate in the synthesis of structural and enzymatic proteins, accounting for the abundance of Nissl material in large neurons that have considerable cytoplasm to maintain in long processes. It has been shown by several methods, including autoradiography following the administration of radioactively labeled amino acids, that the proteins of nerve cells are synthesized predominantly in the perikaryon.

Golgi Apparatus, Smooth Endoplasmic Reticulum, and Lysosomes.   The Golgi apparatus (complex) is a universal cytoplasmic organelle with special historical interest in relation to neurons, having been first demonstrated in these cells by the Italian histologist Camillo Golgi (1843–1926). With staining methods for light microscopy, the Golgi apparatus appears as a dark irregular network, often disposed around the nucleus. The Golgi apparatus appears in electron micrographs as clusters of closely apposed, flattened cisternae, arranged in stacks and surrounded by many small vesicles. This membranous system is continuous with agranular or smooth-surfaced endoplasmic reticulum, and the latter is continuous with granular endoplasmic reticulum. The Golgi area is the site of addition of carbohydrates to some proteins, which thus become glycoproteins. These substances are packed into several types of membrane-bound vesicles for transport distally along the cytoplasmic processes. The vesicles are used for the renewal of synaptic vesicles in axonal endings and for the renewal of the cell membrane.

Lysosomes, which are derived from the smooth endoplasmic reticulum and the Golgi apparatus, are large membrane-bound vesicles containing enzymes that catalyze the breakdown of unwanted large

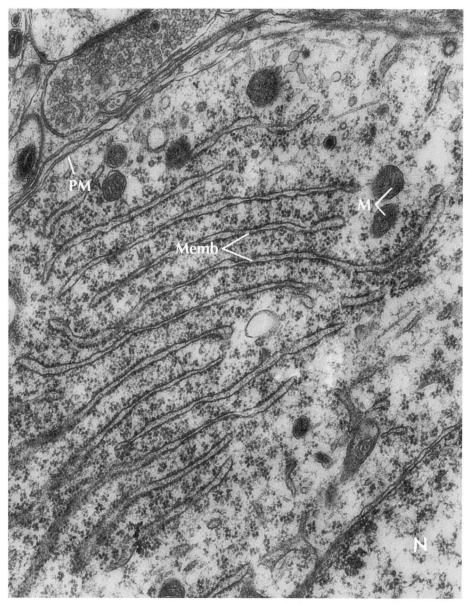

FIGURE 2-6.
Electron micrograph of a portion of a neuron in the preoptic area of a rabbit's brain. The series of membranes, together with the free polyribosomes between the membranes, constitute the Nissl material of light microscopy. **(M)** Mitochrondria. **(Memb)** Membranes of endoplasmic reticulum. **(N)** Nucleus. **(PM)** Plasma membrane. (× 36,000; courtesy of Dr. R. Clattenburg)

molecules. Lysosomes are seen occasionally in normal neurons; they are more numerous and conspicuous in injured or diseased cells.

Mitochondria.   Mitochondria are cytoplasmic organelles scattered throughout the perikaryon, dendrites, and axon. They are spherical, rod-shaped, or filamentous, measuring from 0.2 to 1.0 μm by about 0.2 μm. The mitochondria of nerve cells show the surface double membrane and internal folds or cristae that are present in mitochondria of cells generally. Mitochondria are the repository of enzymes involved in several aspects of cell metabolism, including respiration and phosphorylation. They are the site of the energy-producing reactions of cellular physiology.

Pigment Material

The perikaryon may contain cytoplasmic inclusions (deposits of nonliving material, as opposed to organelles), of which the most conspicuous are pigment granules. **Lipofuscin** (lipochrome) pigment occurs as clumps of yellowish brown granules. Traces of this pigment appear in neurons of the spinal cord and medulla at about the eighth year of life, and in cells of spinal and sympathetic ganglia at about the same time. The amount of the pigment increases with age. The significance of lipofuscin is unknown, except that it is related to the aging process, and it is found at other sites, including cardiac muscle fibers. Some types of neuron, of which Purkinje cells in the cerebellar cortex are an example, do not accumulate lipofuscin, even in old age.

The presence of dark **melanin** pigment in the cytoplasm is restricted to a few cell groups, the largest being the substantia nigra in the midbrain and the locus ceruleus in the pons. The metabolic precursor of this pigment is dihydroxyphenylalanine (DOPA), which is converted to melanin by a series of oxidations followed by polymerization. DOPA is also a precursor of dopamine, a neurotransmitter used by the pigmented neurons of the substantia nigra, and of norepinephrine, which is used by the cells of the locus ceruleus. Melanin may accumulate as a by-product of the synthesis of dopamine and norepinephrine. The pigment in the substantia nigra appears at the end of the first year, increases

until puberty, and normally remains constant thereafter.

Processes of the Nerve Cell

Dendrites taper from the cell body and branch in its immediate environs; the branching may be exceedingly profuse and intricate. The cytoplasm of dendrites resembles that of the perikaryon, with granular endoplasmic reticulum (Nissl substance) in their proximal trunks and at points of branching. In some neurons the smaller branches bear large numbers of minute projections, called **dendritic spines** or **gemmules,** which participate in synapses. The surface of the cell body is also usually included in the receptive field of the neuron. In motor neurons of the spinal cord, for example, large numbers of axonal endings are in synaptic relationship with the cell body, as well as with the dendrites (Fig. 2–7).

The single **axon** of a nerve cell has a uniform diameter throughout its length. In interneurons it is a short delicate process, branching terminally to establish synaptic contact with one or more adjacent neurons. Some interneurons have no axon, so they can conduct only graded changes of membrane potential. In principal cells the diameter of the axon increases in proportion to its length. Collateral branches may be given off at right angles to the axon. The terminal branches are known as **telodendria;** they end typically as swellings or synaptic end bulbs. The cytoplasm of the axon is called **axoplasm,** and the surface membrane is known as the **axolemma.** The axoplasm includes neurofilaments and microtubules, scattered mitochondria, and patches of smooth endoplasmic reticulum.

The axon of a principal cell is usually surrounded by a myelin sheath, which begins near the origin of the axon and ends short of its terminal branching. Within the central nervous system the myelin is laid down by oligodendrocytes and consists of

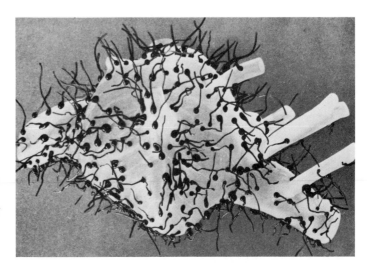

FIGURE 2-7.
Model of a nerve cell with apposed synaptic end bulbs in the spinal cord, prepared from thin sections stained by the Cajal silver nitrate method. (Haggar RA, Barr ML: J Comp Neurol 93:17–36, 1950)

closely apposed layers of their plasma membranes. The sheath therefore has a lipoprotein composition. Interruptions called **nodes of Ranvier** indicate those points at which regions formed by different oligodendrocytes adjoin. Voltage-gated sodium channels are present only at the nodes of a myelinated axon, so the ionic movements of impulse conduction occur only at these sites. The sheath insulates the axon between nodes, and thus there is almost instantaneous conduction of the action potential from one node to the next. This **saltatory conduction** permits much faster signaling in a myelinated than in an unmyelinated axon. The thickness of the myelin sheath and the distance between nodes are directly proportional to the diameter and length of the axon. The greater the diameter of the nerve fiber, the faster is the conduction of the nerve impulse. (A nerve "fiber" in the central nervous system consists of the axon and the surrounding myelin sheath, or of the axon only in the case of unmyelinated fibers.) The formation and structure of the myelin sheath are discussed in Chapter 3 in the context of peripheral nerve fibers, in which these aspects of the myelin are studied in greater detail.

Synapses

A neuron influences other neurons at junctional points, or synapses. The term *synapse*, meaning a conjunction or connection, was introduced by Sherrington in 1897. A nerve impulse can be propagated in any direction on the surface of a neuron. However, the direction it follows under physiological conditions is determined by a consistent polarity at most synapses, where transmission is from the axon of one neuron to the surface of another neuron. Most synaptic junctions are of the type known as **chemical synapses,** in which a substance, the **neurotransmitter,** diffuses across the narrow space between the two cells and becomes bound to **receptors,** which are special protein molecules that reside in the postsynaptic membrane. The nature of the neurotransmitter and the receptor molecule determines whether the effect produced will be excitation or inhibition of the postsynaptic cell. Some synapses are therefore excitatory whereas others are inhibitory. As soon as the neurotransmitter has accomplished its purpose, it is released from the receptors and is immediately inactivated. Inactivation may be effected either by chemical degradation catalyzed by an enzyme present at the synapse, or by reabsorption of the neurotransmitter into the presynaptic terminal.

In only a handful of instances is the identity of a synaptic transmitter known beyond reasonable doubt. Among the first transmitters to be recognized were acetylcholine at the neuromuscular junction and in the autonomic nervous system (Chap. 24) and norepinephrine, used by most neurons of the sympathetic division of the autonomic system. However, there are many other putative neurotransmitters, including other amines, amino acids, and many peptides. Some of these substances may be **neuromodulators** rather than classical transmitters. The modulatory action consists of making the postsynaptic membranes more or less susceptible to the action of the chief transmitter. Immunohistochemical studies show that probably all neurons, even those with well-known classical transmitters, secrete two or more substances that might be neurotransmitters or neuromodulators, and it is not yet known if and how all these substances act in concert upon the postsynaptic cells.

The arrival of an impulse at an excitatory synapse locally depolarizes the postsynaptic membrane, whereas an impulse arriving at an inhibitory synapse causes local hyperpolarization. These changes in the membrane potential are additive over the whole receptive surface of the postsynaptic neuron. If the net electrical change is one of depolarization, an action potential will be initiated at the axon hillock and will travel along the axon. Thus, the sum of the postsynaptic responses in the receptive field of a neuron determines whether or not, at any given moment, an impulse will be sent along the axon.

Several types of chemical synapse can be recognized at the ultrastructural level. In all of them the pre- and postsynaptic cell membranes are separated by a synaptic cleft about 20 nm wide. The presynaptic terminal contains many small vesicles, usually clustered beneath the site of the functional contact, and several mitochondria. The **synaptic vesicles** contain the neurotransmitter substances. They probably discharge their contents into the synaptic cleft by fusing with the presynaptic axolemma, a process of exocytosis. The presynaptic endings of axons are commonly enlarged to form structures known as **end bulbs** (of Held–Auerbach) or **boutons terminaux,** visible by light microscopy (see Fig. 2–7). At other sites the presynaptic elements are not at the ends of telodendria, so the axons make synaptic contacts *en passant.*

The most abundant types of synapse are those designated as **Gray's type I** (asymmetrical) and **Gray's type II** (symmetrical). In Gray's type I synapses the vesicles are spherical, 40 nm in diameter, and the postsynaptic membrane is thickened by a deposition of electron-dense material on its cytoplasmic surface (Fig. 2–8). In Gray's type II synapses the vesicles are of similar size but are ellipsoidal in shape, and there are thickenings of both the presynaptic and postsynaptic membranes. The small synaptic vesicles in types I and II synaptic boutons contain various putative neurotransmitters, including acetylcholine, γ-aminobutyric acid, glycine, and glutamic and aspartic acids. It is not possible, however, to identify the transmitter from the ultrastructural appearance of the vesicles in a presynaptic terminal. Another common type of synapse, usually with asymmetrical membrane thickenings, is one in which spherical synaptic vesicles are about 50 nm in diameter and have electron-dense cores. In these the neurotransmitters are believed to be the monoamines—norepinephrine, dopamine, and serotonin. Even larger (80–100 nm) dense-cored synaptic vesicles may contain peptide neurotransmitters. There are also synapses with mixed granular and agranular vesicles, and it is suspected that some neu-

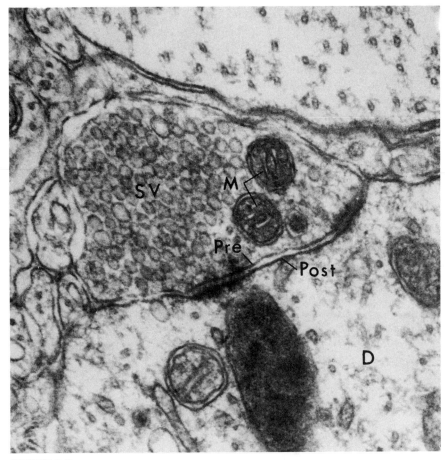

FIGURE 2-8.
Electron micrograph of an axodendritic Gray's type I synapse in the suprachiasmatic nucleus of the rabbit's hypothalamus. **(D)** Dendrite. **(M)** Mitochondria. **(Pre)** Presynaptic membrane. **(Post)** Postsynaptic membrane. **(SV)** Synaptic vesicles. (× 82,000; courtesy of Dr. R. Clattenburg)

rotransmitters may be released by diffusion from the axoplasmic cytosol, rather than by exocytosis of vesicles.

Synapses are also classified according to the parts of the neurons that form the presynaptic and postsynaptic components. **Axodendritic** and **axosomatic** synapses are the most abundant, but **axoaxonal** and **dendrodendritic** contacts are also present in many parts of the nervous system. Furthermore, an axonal terminal or dendritic branchlet commonly engages several other axons or dendrites to form a **synaptic com-** **plex.** Some of the common types of synapse and synaptic complex are illustrated in Figure 2–9. The transmitter is released by the arrival of an action potential at an axonal terminal. In the case of a dendrodendritic synapse, the quantity of transmitter released varies with fluctuations in membrane potential of the presynaptic dendrite.

Electrical synapses, as opposed to the chemical synapses already described, are common in invertebrates and lower vertebrates, and they have been observed at

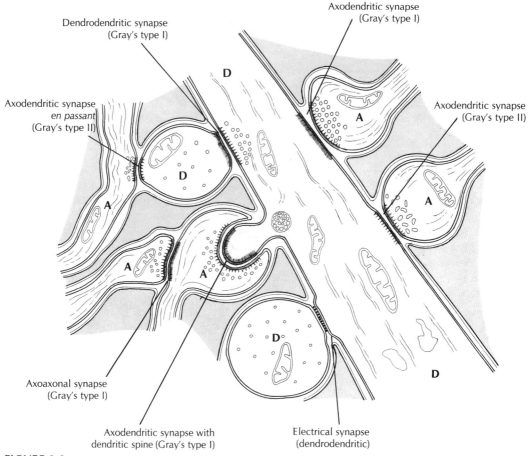

FIGURE 2-9.
Ultrastructure of various types of synapse. **(A)** Axons. **(D)** Dendrites. The shaded areas represent the cytoplasmic processes of astrocytes.

a few sites in the mammalian nervous system. They consist essentially of a close apposition (2 nm) of presynaptic and postsynaptic membranes, across which the cytoplasms of the two cells are joined by tubular protein molecules, through which water and small ions and molecules move freely. Electrical synapses offer a low resistance pathway between neurons, and there is no delay because a chemical mediator is not involved. Unlike most chemical synapses, electrical synapses are not polarized, and the direction of transmission fluctuates with the membrane potentials of the connected cells.

Axonal Transport

Proteins, including enzymes, membrane lipoproteins, and cytoplasmic structural proteins, are transported distally within axons from their sites of synthesis in the perikaryon. Two major rates of transport have been identified by studying the distribution of proteins labeled by incorporation of radioactive amino acids. Most of the protein moves distally at a rate of about 1 mm per day. This component consists largely of structural proteins, including the subunits of neurofilaments and microtubules. A smaller proportion is transported much more rapidly, at a mean velocity of 300 mm per day. Transport also occurs simultaneously in the reverse direction, from the synaptic terminals to the cell body. The retrogradely transported material includes proteins imbibed from the extracellular fluid by axonal terminals, as well as proteins that reach the axon terminals by fast anterograde transport and are returned to the perikaryon. The rate of retrograde transport is variable, but most of the material moves at about two thirds the speed of the fast component of the anterograde transport.

The mechanisms of axonal transport are only partially understood. The rapid components in both directions involve predominantly particle-bound substances, and require the integrity of the microtubules of the axoplasm. Particles probably move along the outside of the tubules. It is an amazing feat of biological engineering that different substances can move at different rates and in different directions at the same time within a tube as thin as an axon.

NEUROGLIAL CELLS

Although neuroglial cells are not primarily involved with excitation, inhibition, and propagation of the nerve impulse, they have their own ancillary roles. It has also become evident that certain of these cells have an intimate relationship with nerve cells, leading to a high degree of interdependence. The term *neuroglia* originally referred only to these cells in the central nervous system. However, it is now applied also to the nonneuronal cells that are intimately related to neurons and their processes in peripheral ganglia and nerves. The central neuroglia will now be discussed. Peripheral neuroglial cells are considered in Chapter 3.

Types

The neuroglial cells of the normal adult brain and spinal cord are probably all derived from the ectoderm of the neural tube. It was once thought that resting microglial cells migrated into the nervous system from mesodermal tissue in the embryonic stage, but there is no experimental evidence to support this contention. The nomenclature of neuroglial cells is summarized in Table 2–1, and the principal structural features of each type are shown in Figure 2–10.

Astroglia

Astrocytes are variable cells with medium-sized spherical or ellipsoidal nuclei, often with deep indentations, having moderately dispersed chromatin. The cytoplasm has numerous processes and contains the characteristic organelles of these cells, the **gliofilaments,** which are slightly finer than neurofilaments and are gathered into bundles. The filaments are made of a substance known as glial fibrillary acidic protein (GFAP). Mitochondria interspersed among the bundles probably correspond to the "gliosomes" seen by light microscopy. The cytoplasm also contains numerous inclusions, 20 to 40 nm in diameter, which are composed of glycogen. Many astrocytic processes are closely applied to capillary blood vessels, where they are

TABLE 2-1. Classification of Neuroglial Cell Types in the Central Nervous System of the Normal Adult

Astroglia	Fibrous astrocytes Protoplasmic (velate) astrocytes
Oligodendroglia	Interfascicular oligodendrocytes Satellite oligodendrocytes
Microglia	Resting microglial cells
Ependyma	Ependymocytes Tanycytes Choroidal epithelial cells

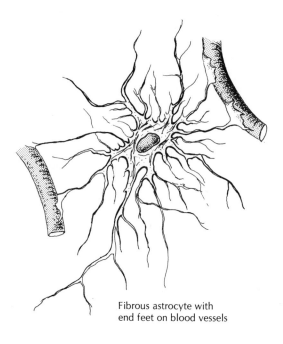

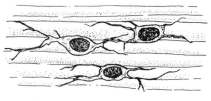

Interfascicular oligodendrocytes

Fibrous astrocyte with
end feet on blood vessels

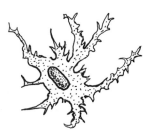

Resting microglial cell
in gray matter

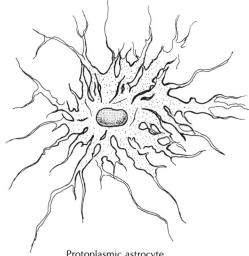

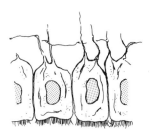

Ependymal cells

Protoplasmic astrocyte

FIGURE 2-10.
Neuroglial cells of the central nervous system.

known as perivascular end feet or foot plates. They cover about 80% of the external surface area of each capillary. Other end feet are applied to the pia mater at the external surface of the central nervous system (including the outer surfaces of the perivascular spaces around larger blood vessels), forming the **external glial limiting membrane.** Astrocytic end feet form the **internal glial limiting membrane** beneath the single layer of ependymocytes lining the ventricular system.

Two types of astrocyte are recognized, although intermediate forms are commonly encountered. **Fibrous astrocytes** occur in white matter. They have long processes with coarse bundles of gliofilaments. **Protoplasmic** or **velate astrocytes** are found in gray matter. Their processes are greatly branched, and are flattened to form delicate lamellae around the terminal branches of axons, dendrites, and synaptic complexes. Müller cells (in the retina) and pituicytes (in the neurohypophysis) are morphologically distinct varieties of protoplasmic astrocytes.

Oligodendroglia

The nuclei of oligodendrocytes are small and spherical, with dense chromatin. A thin rim of cytoplasm surrounds the nucleus and produces a few long thin processes. The cytoplasm is conspicuous because of its high electron density and because it contains much granular endoplasmic reticulum and many polyribosomes. Gliofilaments and glycogen are absent, but there are numerous microtubules in the processes. **Interfascicular oligodendrocytes** occur in rows among myelinated axons, where their cytoplasmic processes form and remain continuous with the myelin sheaths. One cell is connected to several myelinated nerve fibers. **Satellite oligodendrocytes** are closely associated with the cell bodies of large neurons. However, astrocytes and resting microglial cells also occur as perineuronal satellites.

Microglia

About 5% of the total neuroglial population is composed of **resting microglial cells**. These have small elongated nuclei with dense but patchy chromatin. The cytoplasm is scanty, with several short branched processes. Resting microglial cells occur in gray and white matter, and are most often seen as perineuronal satellites and among the astrocytic processes that form the internal and external glial limiting membranes.

Ependyma

The ependyma is the simple cuboidal to columnar epithelium that lines the ventricular system. Three cell types are recognized in the ependyma. **Ependymocytes** constitute the great majority of ependymal cells. Their cytoplasm contains all the usual organelles, as well as many filaments similar to those found in astrocytes. Most ependymocytes bear cilia and microvilli on their free or apical surfaces (Fig. 2–11). The bases of the cells lie on the astrocytic end feet of the internal glial limiting membrane. **Tanycytes** differ from ependymocytes in having long basal processes. Most of these cells are found in the floor of the third ventricle. Their basal processes end on the pia mater and on blood vessels in the median eminence of the hypothalamus (see Fig. 11–17). **Choroidal epithelial cells** cover the surfaces of the choroid plexuses. They have microvilli at their apical surfaces and invaginations at their basal surfaces, which rest on a basement membrane. Adjacent choroidal epithelial cells are joined by tight junctional complexes.

Functions

Astroglia

Astrocytes, similar to other glial cells, fill in the spaces that would otherwise exist among the neurons and their processes. The gliofilaments may confer some rigidity upon the cytoplasm of astrocytes, thereby providing physical support for the other cellular elements of the nervous system. The disposition of astrocytic processes with their perivascular end feet, together with the apparent lack of extracellular space in the central nervous system, suggest that these cells may be involved in the exchange of metabolites

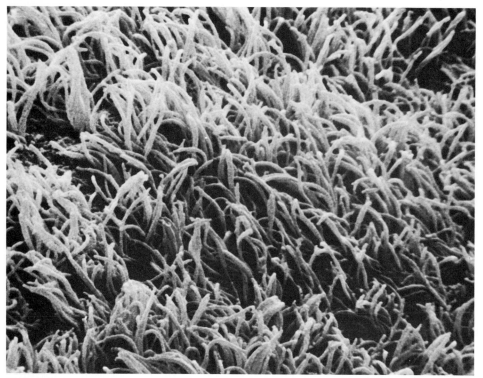

FIGURE 2-11.
Scanning electron micrograph showing the surface of the third ventricle in the rabbit, representing an area in which the ependymal lining is heavily ciliated. (× 2880; courtesy of Dr. J. E. Bruni and Dr. D. G. Montemurro)

between neurons and the blood. However, it is possible that the extracellular space is considerably larger *in vivo* than is apparent in electron micrographs of conventionally fixed tissue.

Synapses and synaptic complexes are surrounded by the lamellar cytoplasmic processes of protoplasmic astrocytes. This may serve to restrain the diffusion of neurotransmitters and the spread of electrical disturbances through the neuropil.

When the brain or spinal cord is injured, the astrocytes near the lesion undergo hypertrophy. The cytoplasmic processes become more numerous and are densely packed with gliofilaments. There may also be a small increase in the number of the cells caused by mitosis of mature astrocytes. These changes, known as **gliosis**, occur in many pathological conditions, and the reactive astrocytes sometimes acquire phagocytic properties.

Oligodendroglia

Interfascicular oligodendrocytes are responsible for producing and maintaining the myelin sheaths of axons in the central nervous system. The concentrically organized membrane of the myelin is continuous with the plasmalemma of the oligodendrocyte. This function is equivalent to that of the Schwann cell in peripheral nerves. One cytoplasmic process of an oligodendrocyte provides the myelin of one internode (the myelinated interval between two nodes of Ranvier) of one axon. The fact that each oligodendrocytic process is attached to a different axon indicates that the layers of the myelin sheath could not possibly have been formed by a rotational movement of the cell around the axon.

Satellite oligodendrocytes are in contact with some neuronal cell bodies. Astrocytes and resting microglial cells are also often closely associated with neuronal cell bodies. These cells are presumably equivalent to the satellite cells of peripheral ganglia. It is thought that neuroglial cells provide essential metabolic support for the adjacent neurons, but the nature of this symbiotic relationship has not yet been determined.

Microglia

The functions of resting microglial cells are still unknown. Cells with similar structure and staining properties appear in large numbers at the sites of injury or inflammatory disease in the central nervous system. Experimental evidence indicates that these pathological cells, known as **reactive microglial cells,** arise from monocytes that enter the nervous system by immigrating from the lumina of abnormal blood vessels. The immunocytochemical properties of reactive microglial cells are different from those of resting microglial cells, which are now thought to be of neuroectodermal origin. The reactive microglial cells have a phagocytic function equivalent to that of macrophages in other parts of the body.

Ependyma

Ependymocytes line the ventricular system and are thus in contact with the cerebrospinal fluid (CSF). Movements of their cilia may assist in a chemical exchange between the fluid and neural tissue.

It has been suggested that the tanycytes of the ventral hypothalamic region respond to changing levels of blood-derived hormones in the CSF by discharging secretory products into the capillary vessels of the median eminence. Such activity

may be involved in the control of the endocrine system by the anterior lobe of the pituitary gland (see Chap. 11).

The choroidal epithelial cells are joined together by tight junctions, thus preventing the passive movement of plasma proteins into the CSF. The cells are also metabolically active in controlling the chemical composition of the fluid, which is secreted by the choroid plexuses into the cerebral ventricles.

DEVELOPMENT OF NEURONS AND NEUROGLIAL CELLS

The cells lining the lumen of the neural tube of the embryo are known as neuroepithelial cells, and they constitute the ventricular zone. The first daughter cells produced in this zone are **early neuroblasts,** which migrate outward and differentiate into neurons. Other neuroepithelial cells become radial neuroglial cells, with long processes crossing the whole thickness of the wall of the neural tube. These processes evidently provide directional guidance for the outwardly migrating neuroblasts.

At a later stage the neuroepithelium produces a population of cells in the subventricular zone in which further mitoses occur, with the formation of **late neuroblasts** and **early glioblasts.** The former differentiate into neurons and the latter into astroglia, oligodendroglia, and resting microglia. The radial neuroglial cells persist into adult life in lower vertebrates, but in mammals they almost all disappear as the central nervous system grows. Ependymocytes and choroidal epithelial cells are derived directly from the neuroepithelium of the ventricular zone, although some may be radial neuroglial cells that have retracted their cytoplasmic processes.

SUGGESTED READING

Barr ML: The significance of the sex chromatin. Int Rev Cytol 19:35–95, 1966
Bunge RP: Glial cells and the central myelin sheath. Physiol Rev 48:197–251, 1968

Chan-Palay V, Engel EG, Wu JY, Palay SL: Coexistence in human and primate neuromuscular junctions of enzymes synthesizing acetylcholine, catecholamine, taurine and γ-aminobutyric acid. Proc Natl Acad Sci USA 79:7027–7030, 1982

Cuello AC, Priestley JV, Sofroniew MV: Immunocytochemistry and neurobiology. J Exp Physiol 68:545–578, 1983

Fujita S, Kitamura T: Origin of brain macrophages and the nature of the microglia. In Zimmermann HM (ed): Progress in Neuropathology, Vol III, Chap 1. New York, Grune & Stratton, 1976

Grafstein B, Forman DS: Intracellular transport in neurons. Physiol Rev 60:1167–1283, 1980

Lund RD: Development and Plasticity of the Brain. New York, Oxford University Press, 1978

Oehmichen M: Mononuclear phagocytes in the central nervous system. Clarkson MM (trans): Berlin, Springer-Verlag, 1978

Osborne NN: Communication between neurones: Current concepts. Neurochem Int 3:3–16, 1981

Peters A, Palay SL, Webster H de F: The Fine Structure of the Nervous System: The Neurons and Supporting Cells. Philadelphia, WB Saunders, 1976

Shepherd GM: The Synaptic Organization of the Brain, 2nd ed. New York, Oxford University Press, 1979

Shepherd GM: Neurobiology. New York, Oxford University Press, 1983

Stevens CF: The neuron. Sci Am 241:54–65, 1979

Varon SS, Somjen GG (eds): Neuron–glia interactions. Neurosci Res Program Bull 17:1–239, 1979

THREE

Peripheral Nervous System

Certain aspects of the peripheral nervous system are especially pertinent to a study of the brain and spinal cord. These include the sensory receptors, motor endings, histology of peripheral nerves, and structure of ganglia. The following introductory comments refer to all spinal nerves and to those cranial nerves that are not restricted to the special senses. The structures discussed in this chapter are shown in Figure 3–1, which represents a spinal nerve in the thoracic and upper lumbar regions in which neurons for visceral innervation are included.

The general sensory endings are scattered profusely throughout the body. They are biological transducers, in which physical or chemical stimuli create action potentials in nerve endings. The resulting nerve impulses, on reaching the central nervous system, produce reflex responses, awareness of the stimuli, or both. Sensory endings that are superficially located, such as those in the skin, are called **exteroceptors**; they respond to stimuli for pain, temperature, touch, and pressure. **Proprioceptors** in muscles, tendons, and joints provide data for reflex adjustments of muscle action and for awareness of position and movement.

Nerve impulses from exteroceptors and proprioceptors are conducted centrally by primary sensory neurons, whose cell bodies are located in dorsal root ganglia (or in a cranial nerve ganglion). On entering the spinal cord, the dorsal root fibers divide into ascending and descending branches; these are distributed as necessary for reflex responses and for transmission of sensory data to the brain.

There is a third class of sensory endings, known as **interoceptors**, in the viscera. Central conduction occurs through primary sensory neurons such as those al-

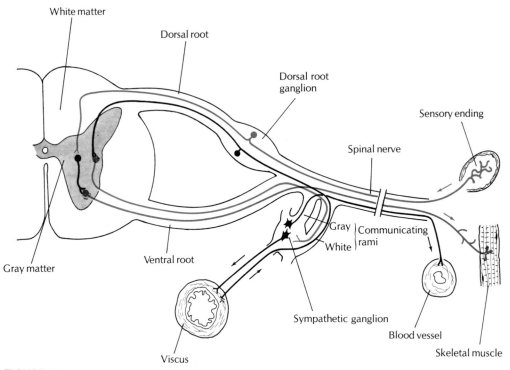

FIGURE 3-1.

Components of a spinal nerve between the first thoracic and second lumbar segments.

ready noted, except that the peripheral process follows a different route. The fiber reaches the sympathetic trunk through a white communicating ramus and continues to a viscus in a nerve arising from the sympathetic trunk. The spinal connections of these neurons are those required for visceral reflex responses and for transmission of data of visceral origin to the brain. There are therefore two broad categories of sensory endings and afferent neurons: **somatic afferents** for the body (soma) generally and **visceral afferents.**

There are also two categories of efferent or motor neurons. The cell bodies of **somatic efferent** neurons are situated in the ventral gray horns of the spinal cord and motor nuclei of cranial nerves. The axons of ventral horn cells traverse the ventral roots and spinal nerves, and terminate in motor end plates on skeletal muscle fibers. The **visceral efferent** or autonomic system has a special feature in that at least two neurons participate in transmission from the central nervous system to the viscera. In the sympathetic division of the autonomic system, for example, the cell bodies of preganglionic neurons are located in the thoracic and upper lumbar segments of the spinal cord. The axons traverse the corresponding ventral roots and white communicating rami, ending either in ganglia of the sympathetic trunk or in prevertebral ganglia such as those found in the celiac and superior mesenteric plexuses of the abdomen. Axons of postganglionic neurons in these locations proceed to smooth muscle and secretory cells of some viscera, to the heart, and to neurons of the enteric plexuses in the alimentary canal. Axons from some of the cells in ganglia of the sympathetic trunk enter spinal nerves through gray communicating rami for distribution to blood vessels, sweat glands, and arrector pili muscles of hairs.

Results of recent studies have shown that a substantial number of unmyelinated fibers in the ventral roots originate in dorsal root ganglia. These sensory fibers approach the cord, but do not enter it: they turn abruptly back and then join the mixed spinal nerve.

SENSORY ENDINGS

The sensory endings are supplied by nerve fibers that differ in size and other characteristics. This is a matter of some interest because there is a correlation between fiber diameter and the rate of conduction of the nerve impulse, and because different sensory endings tend to be supplied by fibers of specific sizes.

A commonly used classification of peripheral nerve fibers is given in Table 3–1, which includes the sensory modalities and efferent neurons associated with the three main categories. The diameters of group A and group B fibers include the thickness of the myelin sheaths. Group A is further subdivided into alpha, beta, gamma, and delta fibers in decreasing order of size. There is some overlapping of the diameters of the A, B, and C groups because physiological properties, especially the form of the spike potential and the afterpotential, are taken into consideration when defining the groups. In brief, the smallest fibers (group C) are unmyelinated and have the slowest conduction rate, whereas the myelinated fibers of group B and group A exhibit rates of conduction that progressively increase with increasing fiber size.

A second classification of nerve fibers applies specifically to somatic afferent fibers of the dorsal roots. Table 3–2 lists some of the receptors from which impulses traverse each of the four categories in the numerical system, together with their equivalents in the alternative classification.

On a structural basis two classes of sensory endings are recognized. **Nonencapsulated endings** are terminal arborizations of the nerve that may be closely applied to cells or may lie freely in the extracellular spaces of connective tissue. **Encapsulated endings** have distinctive arrangements of nonneuronal cells that completely enclose the terminal parts of the

TABLE 3-1. Classification of Fibers in Peripheral Nerves

	GROUP	DIAMETER (μm)	SPEED OF IMPULSE CONDUCTION (m/sec)	FUNCTION
Myelinated	A (α, β, γ, δ)	1–20	5–120	Afferent fibers for proprioception, vibration, touch, pressure, pain, and temperature; somatic efferent fibers
Myelinated	B	1–3	3–15	Visceral afferent fibers; preganglionic visceral efferent fibers
Unmyelinated	C	0.5–1.5	0.6–2.0	Afferent fibers for pain and temperature; postganglionic visceral efferent fibers

TABLE 3-2.   Classification of Somatic Dorsal Root Fibers

NUMBER	EXAMPLES OF RECEPTORS	LETTER EQUIVALENT
Ia	Annulospiral ending of neuromuscular spindle	Aα
b	Neurotendinous spindle	
II	Flower spray ending of neuromuscular spindle; touch and pressure receptors	Aβ and γ
III	Pain and temperature receptors	Aδ
IV	Pain and temperature receptors	C

axons. In the following account the receptors are described according to location, with exteroceptors and some proprioceptors being illustrated in Figures 3–2 and 3–3, respectively.

Cutaneous Sensory Endings

Most of the skin bears hairs that vary greatly in length, thickness, and abundance from one part of the body to another. Glabrous skin, which is smooth and lacks hairs, is present on the palmar surfaces of the hands and fingers, the soles of the feet, and parts of the face and external genitalia. There are different patterns of innervation in hairy and glabrous skin.

Histology of Cutaneous Innervation

The skin is supplied by cutaneous branches of the spinal and cranial nerves. The terminal branches of these nerves pass through the subcutaneous connective tissue into the dermis. The axons spread out horizontally to form three plexuses, which lie in the plane of the surface of the skin. The **subcutaneous plexus** lies in the loose connective tissue deep to the skin, the **dermal plexus** is within the densely collagenous reticular layer that constitutes the deeper part of the dermis, and the **papillary plexus** lies in the papillary layer of the dermis, which is immediately beneath the epidermis. The axons of each plexus send branches into the adjacent tissues.

The density of cutaneous innervation varies considerably from one region to another. For example, the face and limbs are more richly innervated than is the dorsal aspect of the trunk.

Free nerve endings occur in the subcutaneous tissue and dermis, and occasionally extend among the cells of the epidermis. They are the terminal branches of group C fibers and the unmyelinated terminal branches of group A fibers, and are receptive to all modalities of cutaneous sensation. Although they are called "free endings," these axons are always invested with Schwann cells (the neuroglia of peripheral nerves) and do not contact the extracellular fluid directly. Indeed, it is impossible to identify the exact point of termination of an axon within the skin. The existence of free nerve endings is inferred from the functional sensitivity of regions of skin in which no other types of sensory ending can be recognized.

Merkel endings are found in the germinal layer (stratum basale) of the epidermis. Axonal branches end as flattened expansions that contain mitochondria and small, electron-lucent vesicles. Each axonal terminal is closely applied to a **Merkel cell**. This small cell differs from the other epidermal cells in having an indented nucleus and electron-dense cytoplasmic granules 80 nm in diameter. Merkel cells are found in glabrous skin and in the outer root sheaths of hairs. Another type of Merkel ending in hairy skin

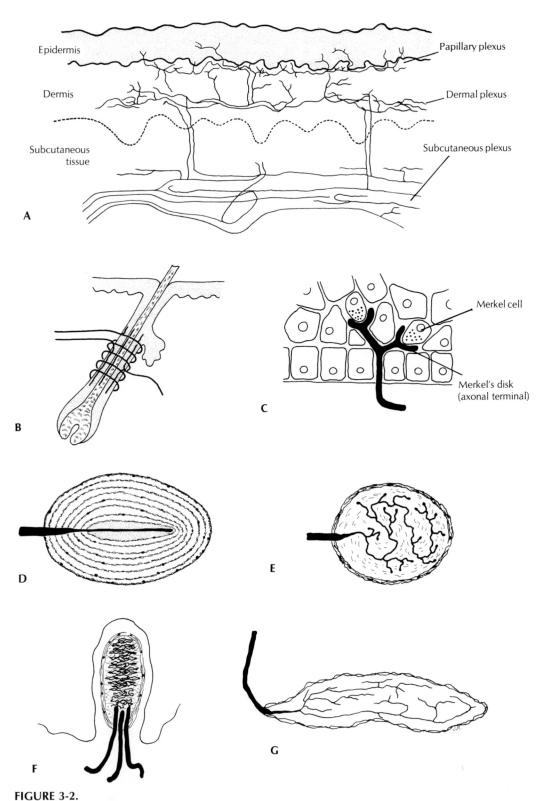

FIGURE 3-2.
Sensory innervation of skin. **(A)** Plexuses. **(B)** Peritrichial ending. **(C)** Merkel ending in epidermis. **(D)** Pacinian corpuscle. **(E)** End bulb. **(F)** Meissner's corpuscle. **(G)** Ruffini ending.

Epidermis

Papillary plexus

Dermis

Dermal plexus

Subcutaneous tissue

Subcutaneous plexus

A

B

C

Merkel cell

Merkel's disk (axonal terminal)

D

E

F

G

is the *Haarscheibe,* a domelike elevation about 0.2 mm in diameter that contains many Merkel cells supplied by branches of a single myelinated axon. The Haarscheiben are about 1 cm apart in human skin but are more abundant in furry animals.

Peritrichial nerve endings are cagelike formations of axons that surround hair follicles. By extensive branching a single axon in an overlapping arrangement supplies many hair follicles, and each follicle is supplied by from two to twenty different axons. The axons approach the follicle deep to its sebaceous gland and branch in the connective tissue outside the outer root sheath. Some branches encircle the follicle, and others run parallel to its long axis. Expanded axonal terminals are applied to Merkel cells in the outer root sheath.

Several types of encapsulated ending are involved in cutaneous innervation. The **Ruffini ending,** typically about 1 mm long and 20 μm to 30 μm wide, is a greatly branched array of expanded terminal branches of a myelinated axon, surrounded by capsular cells. The **pacinian corpuscle** (or corpuscle of Vater–Pacini) consists of a single axon that loses its myelin sheath on entering the corpuscle and is encapsulated by several layers of flattened cells with greatly attenuated cytoplasm. The whole corpuscle is ellipsoidal, with an average length of 1 mm and a diameter of 0.7 mm. Ruffini endings and pacinian corpuscles are present in the subcutaneous tissue and dermis of both hairy and glabrous skin. **Meissner's tactile corpuscles** are present in large numbers in the dermal papillary ridges of the fingertips, and are less abundant in other hairless regions. Each corpuscle is supplied by three or four myelinated axons whose terminal branches form a complicated knot that is infiltrated with modified Schwann cells and enclosed in a cellular, collagenous capsule. Meissner's corpuscles are

about 80 μm × 30 μm in size and are oriented with their long axes perpendicular to the surface of the skin. **End bulbs** vary in size and shape, and several types have been described (*e.g.*, end bulbs of Krause, Golgi–Mazzoni endings, genital corpuscles, mucocutaneous endings), although all may be variants of the same structure. They are commonly spherical, about 50 μm across, with each containing a coiled, branching axonal terminal surrounded by a thin cellular capsule. End bulbs occur mainly in mucous membranes (mouth, conjunctiva, anal canal) and in the dermis of glabrous skin close to orifices (lips, external genitalia).

Physiological Correlates

The types of sensation that are consciously perceived from the skin are known as **modalities.** The different sensations are not always clearcut, but in medical practice it is customary to recognize five modalities that are easily tested by clinical examination. These are fine (discriminative) touch, vibration, light touch, temperature (warmth or cold), and pain. The central pathways that process these sensations are fairly well known, but for other modalities (*e.g.*, itch, tickle, rubbing, firm pressure) they are only poorly understood. Careful testing has revealed that the human skin is a mosaic of spots, each of which responds selectively to only one of the four elementary sensations of touch, warmth, cold, or pain. The response of any one of these spots is always the same, whatever the nature of the stimulus. For example, a feeling of coldness will be experienced from a "cold spot" even if it is heated or injured.

Several attempts have been made to correlate the modalities of sensation in humans with the distribution of morphologically identified nerve endings, but the results have been inconclusive. Each modality-specific spot is supplied by several axons, and the qualities of the sensation perceived cannot be correlated with the distribution of microscopically identifiable nerve endings. However, results of electrophysiological studies in animals have shown that, although no cutaneous receptors have an absolute specificity, there is a high degree of selectivity for certain end organs. Merkel endings and Meissner's corpuscles respond preferentially to tactile stimuli, and pacinian corpuscles initiate nerve impulses when they are deformed, with a special sensitivity to vibration. Ruffini endings also respond to mechanical stimuli, including pressure upon and stretching of the skin. Peritrichial endings respond to mechanical displacement of the hair shaft, so that hair follicles serve as receptor organs for light touch. For some sensations, such as warmth and cold, no sensory endings have been identified. It is presumed that these modalities are transduced into nerve impulses by free nerve endings derived from the dermal and papillary plexuses. Painful sensations are also received by free nerve endings, termed nociceptors, which are stimulated by various substances released from damaged cells.

Sensory Endings in Joints, Muscles, and Tendons

Proprioceptors in the capsules of joints, in muscles, and in tendons furnish the central nervous system with information required for the performance of properly coordinated movements through reflex action. In addition, proprioceptive information reaches consciousness so that there is awareness of the position of body parts and of their movements (kinesthetic sense). Pain arising in muscles, tendons, ligaments, and bones is probably detected by free nerve endings in connective tissue. These nociceptive endings respond to physical injury and to local chemical changes, such as those that may be caused by ischemia.

Joints

Four types of sensory ending, each having a distinctive morphology and physiological responsiveness, are recognized within and around the capsules of synovial joints. Encapsulated formations very similar to the Ruffini cutaneous endings are present in the capsules of joints; these are derived from group A myelinated afferent fibers. Small pacinian corpuscles in the connective tissue outside the articular capsule are also supplied by group A fibers. They respond to the initiation and cessation of movement (*i.e.*, to acceleration and deceleration). The articular ligaments contain receptors identical to Golgi tendon organs that are supplied by group A axons. These receptors mediate reflex inhibition of the adjacent musculature when excessive strain is placed on the joint. The importance of articular innervation is highlighted by Hilton's Law, which states that every peripheral nerve supplying a muscle sends a branch to the joint moved by the muscle and to the skin overlying the joint.

Free nerve endings are abundant in the synovial membrane, capsule, and periarticular connective tissues. They are believed to respond to potentially injurious mechanical stresses and to mediate the pain that arises in diseased or injured joints.

Muscles

The proprioceptive organs contained in skeletal muscles are the neuromuscular spindles. In addition to functioning as a sensory receptor, the neuromuscular spindle has a significant motor role because it is a component of the gamma reflex loop.

These slender spindles are a fraction of a millimeter wide and up to 6 mm long. They lie in the long axis of the muscle, and their collagenous capsules are continuous with the fibrous septa that separate the muscle fibers. The fibrous septa are in mechanical continuity with the skeletal attachments of the muscle so that the spindles are lengthened whenever the muscle is passively stretched. Spindles are generally located near the tendinous insertions of muscles and are especially numerous in muscles that perform highly skilled movements, such as those of the hand.

Each spindle consists of a fusiform capsule of connective tissue, with from 2 to 14 intrafusal muscle fibers. The latter differ in several respects from the main or extrafusal fibers of the muscle. Intrafusal fibers are considerably smaller than the extrafusal; the equatorial region lacks cross striations and contains many nuclei that are not in the subsarcolemmal position characteristic of mature striated muscle. The equatorial region is expanded in some intrafusal fibers (**nuclear bag fibers**) and in others it is not (**nuclear chain fibers**). Nuclear bag fibers project from the capsular investment of the spindle poles before inserting onto the extrafusal connective tissue or tendon.

Each neuromuscular spindle is supplied by two afferent nerve fibers. One of these is an Aα or Ia fiber; the myelin cov-

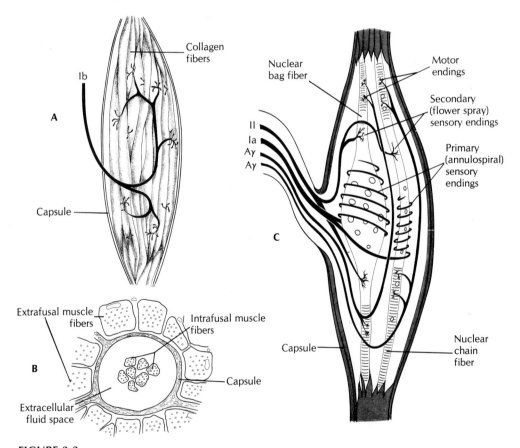

FIGURE 3-3.
Specialized sensory endings in skeletal muscle and in tendon. **(A)** Golgi tendon organ.
(B) Neuromuscular spindle (transverse section). **(C)** Sensory and motor innervation of neuromuscular spindle.

ering ends as the fiber pierces the capsule, and the terminal portion of the fiber winds spirally around the midportion of the intrafusal muscle fibers in the form of an **annulospiral ending.** The second, slightly smaller, afferent fiber (Aβ or II) branches terminally and ends as varicosities on the intrafusal muscle fibers some distance from the midregion. The latter terminals are called **flower spray endings.** The annulospiral and flower spray terminals are also known as **primary** and **secondary sensory endings** of the spindle.

The neuromuscular spindles also have an efferent or motor innervation. The extrafusal fibers composing the main mass of a muscle are innervated by large motor cells (alpha motor neurons), whose axons are of alpha size in the A group. Smaller motor cells (gamma motor neurons), with axons of gamma size in the A group, supply the intrafusal muscle fibers of the spindle. There are motor end plates in the midpolar region on both sides of the specialized equatorial zone of the intrafusal muscle fibers.

Neuromuscular spindles contribute to muscular function in several ways, the simplest role being that of a receptor for the stretch or extensor reflex. Slight stretching of a muscle lengthens the intrafusal muscle fibers; the sensory endings are stimulated and nerve impulses pass to alpha motor neurons that supply the main mass of the muscle. The latter thereupon contracts, in response to stretch, through a two-neuron reflex arc. Stimulation of the spindles ceases when the muscle contracts because the spindle fibers, in parallel with the other muscle fibers, return to their original lengths. The stretch reflex is in constant use in the adjustment of muscle tonus. It also forms the basis of tests for tendon reflexes, such as the knee jerk test (extension at the knee on tapping the patellar tendon), which are standard items in a clinical examination.

The spindles also have an important role in muscle action that results from neurological processes in the brain. A considerable proportion of the motor fibers that originate in the brain and descend in the white matter of the spinal cord influence gamma motor neurons in the ventral gray horns, either by synapsing with them directly or through the mediation of interneurons. Contraction of the intrafusal muscle fibers in response to stimulation by gamma motor neurons causes firing of the sensory nerve terminals, resulting in contraction of the regular muscle fibers through reflex stimulation of alpha motor neurons. The **gamma reflex loop** consists of the gamma motor neuron, neuromuscular spindle, afferent or sensory neuron, and alpha motor neuron supplying extrafusal muscle fibers. It is an important adjunct to the more direct control of muscular activity by means of descending fibers from the brain that control the alpha motor neurons, both directly and through local circuit neurons.

Tendons

Neurotendinous spindles, also known as **Golgi tendon organs,** are most numerous near the attachment of tendons to muscles. Each receptor consists only of a thin capsule of connective tissue that encloses a few collagenous fibers of the tendon on which a nerve fiber ends. It is an Aα or Ib fiber (there may be more than one) that enters the spindle and breaks up into branches ending as varicosities on the intrafusal tendon fibers. These sensory endings are stimulated by tension on the tendon, with greater tension required than for excitation of neuromuscular spindles by stretch. The afferent impulses reach interneurons in the spinal cord. These have an inhibitory effect on alpha motor neurons, causing relaxation of the muscle to which the particular tendon is attached. The opposing functions of the neuromuscular spindles (excitatory) and the neurotendinous spindles (inhibitory) are in balance in the total integration of spinal reflex activity. By acting as constant monitors of tension, the inhibitory effect of neurotendinous spindles also provides protection against damage to muscle or tendon because of excessive tension.

Conscious Proprioception

As already noted, the various types of proprioceptor provide essential information for neuromuscular control at the subconscious level. This includes reflexes that involve the spinal cord and brain stem, provision of proprioceptive data required by the cerebellum, and sensorimotor integration in the cerebral cortex. The role of specific proprioceptors in conscious proprioception (kinesthesia) is still debated. For many years, awareness of position and movement was attributed mainly to receptors in joints, especially to the Ruffinilike endings in joint capsules. More recent assessment of the available evidence has identified the neuromuscular spindles as the principal receptors for kinesthesia, with other sensory endings playing an important but subsidiary role.

Sensory Endings in Viscera

Except for pacinian corpuscles, most of which are in mesenteries, the sensory endings in viscera consist mainly of nonencapsulated terminal branches of nerve fibers, some of which are quite complicated. In general, visceral afferents function in physiological visceral reflexes, in the sensations of fullness of the stomach, rectum, and bladder, and in pain caused by visceral dysfunction or disease.

EFFECTOR ENDINGS

The nervous system acts upon muscle fibers and upon secretory cells. Control of these nonneural cells is effected by a mechanism similar to that of chemical synaptic transmission between neurons. At the neuroeffector endings, axons terminate in relation to skeletal, cardiac, and smooth muscle fibers and to the cells of exocrine and endocrine glands. When the response to a neural signal must be rapid (as in the case of contraction of skeletal muscles or secretion from the cells of the adrenal medulla), the axon terminals are closely applied to the effector cells. The distance between the two elements is often greater in viscera and in exocrine glands, in which responses are somewhat slower. Many endocrine organs are controlled, directly or indirectly, by hypothalamic neurosecretory neurons that discharge their products into blood vessels for subsequent delivery to the target cells. The nerve endings in skeletal muscles, viscera, and glands will now be described.

Motor End Plates

The **motor end plates** or **myoneural junctions** on extrafusal and intrafusal fibers of skeletal striated muscles are synapselike structures with two components: the ending of a motor nerve fiber and the subjacent part of the muscle fiber. In regard specifically to the extrafusal fibers, the axon of an alpha motor neuron divides terminally to supply variable numbers of muscle fibers. A **motor unit** consists of a motor neuron and the muscle fibers that it innervates. The number of muscle fibers in a motor unit varies from fewer than ten to several hundred, depending on the size and function of the muscle. A large motor unit, in which a single neuron supplies many muscle fibers, is adequate for the functions of muscles such as those of the trunk and proximal portions of the limbs. However, in small muscles such as the extraocular and intrinsic hand muscles, which must function with precision, the motor units include only a few muscle fibers. Such an anatomical arrangement provides for intricate control of muscle action.

Each branch of the nerve fiber gives up its myelin sheath on approaching a muscle fiber and ends as several branchlets that

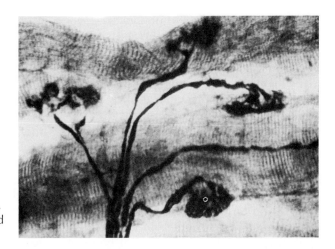

FIGURE 3-4.
Motor end plates. (Gold chloride stain,
× 800; courtesy of Dr. R. Mitchell and
Dr. A. S. Wilson)

constitute the neural component of the end plate (Fig. 3–4). The end plate is typically 40 to 60 μm in diameter, and is usually located midway along the length of the muscle fiber. Each peripheral nerve fiber is surrounded by two sheaths external to the myelin sheath. The neurolemmal sheath consists of the nucleated cytoplasmic portion of Schwann cells, whose cell membrane wraps around the axon or axis cylinder to form the myelin sheath. The neurolemmal sheath continues around the terminal branches of the motor fiber after the Schwann cells cease to form a myelin sheath, but it does not intervene between the nerve ending and the muscle fiber. The nerve fiber is surrounded outside the neurolemma by a delicate endoneurial sheath of connective tissue. The endoneurium is continuous at the motor end plate with the thin endomysium or connective tissue sheath of the muscle fiber, forming a "tent" over the myoneural junction.

The ultrastructure of the axonal endings within the end plate is similar to that of a synaptic end bulb. They contain small, spherical synaptic vesicles and mitochondria. The surface of the muscle fiber is slightly elevated at the myoneural junction. The accumulation of sarcoplasm at this site constitutes the sole plate, in which there are nuclei of the muscle fiber

and mitochondria. Each axonal branchlet occupies a groove or "synaptic gutter" on the surface of the sole plate; there is an interval of 20 to 50 nm, constituting a synaptic cleft between the surface of the nerve terminal and that of the muscle fiber. The plasma membrane and associated basement membrane, which together constitute the sarcolemma of the muscle fiber, have a wavy outline where they appose the nerve terminal, with the irregularities being known as junctional folds. The folded region of the sarcolemma, the **subneural apparatus,** is demonstrable histochemically by its content of acetylcholinesterase, the enzyme that inactivates acetylcholine.

Acetylcholine released from the synaptic vesicles by nerve impulses that travel along the axon reduces the membrane potential of the sarcolemma, as it does in postsynaptic neuronal membranes. The resulting action potential propagates along the sarcolemma and is carried into the muscle fiber to the contractile myofibrils by an ultramicroscopic membrane system in the form of tubules (transverse tubular system).

Postganglionic Autonomic Endings

The effector nerve endings on smooth muscle and secretory cells are also similar to those of synapses. The presynaptic terminals are swellings along the courses and at the tips of the fine axons. These swellings contain accumulations of mitochondria, together with clusters of synaptic vesicles. The terminals are applied to the effector cells, but not as closely as they are in skeletal muscle, and there are no obvious postsynaptic structural specializations. Noradrenergic terminals of the sympathetic nervous system contain electron-dense synaptic vesicles, whereas cholinergic terminals (mostly parasympathetic) contain small electron-lucent vesicles. Terminals that contain other types of synaptic vesicles are commonly seen in the alimentary canal; some of them are thought to use peptide neurotransmitters.

GANGLIA

The **spinal ganglia** are swellings on the dorsal roots of spinal nerves situated in the intervertebral foramina, just proximal to the union of dorsal and ventral roots to form the spinal nerves. These ganglia contain the cell bodies of primary sensory neurons, mainly in a large peripheral zone. The center of the ganglion is occupied by nerve fibers, which are the proximal portions of peripheral and central processes of the nerve cells. Dorsal root ganglia and ganglia of cranial nerves involved with general sensation have the same histological structure.

These sensory neurons develop from the embryonic neural crests, which consist of neuroectodermal cells and lie along the dorsolateral borders of the neural tube. (Some of the neurons in the sensory ganglia of cranial nerves originate from placodes, which are thickened regions of the ectoderm of the surface of the head.) The cells are at first bipolar, but the two processes soon unite to form the single process of this unipolar type of neuron. The processes that arise from the smaller cell bodies are short and straight, whereas those given off by larger cells often wind at first around the parent cell body. In both the fiber divides into peripheral and central branches or processes; the former terminates in a sensory ending, and the latter enters the spinal cord through a dorsal root. The nerve impulse passes directly from the peripheral to the central process, thereby bypassing the cell body. Both processes have the structural and electrophysiological characteristics of axons, although the peripheral process resembles a dendrite in the sense of conduction toward the cell body.

The spherical cell bodies vary from 20 to 100 μm in diameter; their processes are similarly of graded size, ranging from small unmyelinated fibers of the C group to the largest myelinated fibers in the A group. The large neurons are for proprioception and discriminative touch; those of intermediate size are concerned with light touch, pressure, pain, and temperature; the smallest neurons transmit impulses for pain and temperature. Each cell body is closely invested with a capsule consisting of two types of cell. An inner layer of satellite cells is continuous with the Schwann cell sheath surrounding the processes. External to this are cells supported by connective tissue fibers that form a layer of the capsule continuous with the endoneurial connective tissue of the peripheral nerve.

The electron microscope reveals synaptic boutons in contact with the neuronal cell bodies in dorsal root ganglia of laboratory animals. The presynaptic axons have been shown to be collateral branches of the axons of motor neurons. The functions of these connections are not yet known.

One of the most common disorders involving spinal or cranial nerve ganglia is herpes zoster (shingles), in which a viral infection of the ganglion causes pain and other sensory disturbances in the cutaneous area of distribution of the affected nerve.

Autonomic ganglia include those of the

sympathetic trunks along the sides of the vertebral bodies, collateral or prevertebral ganglia in plexuses of the thorax and abdomen (*e.g.*, the cardiac, celiac, and mesenteric plexuses), and certain ganglia near viscera. The multipolar nerve cells of autonomic ganglia are 20 to 45 μm in diameter. The nucleus is often eccentric, and binucleate cells are occasionally encountered. The cell body is surrounded by satellite cells similar to those that compose the inner capsular layer around the nerve cells of spinal ganglia. The dendrites, of which there are several, branch externally to the capsule and are in synaptic contact with terminals of preganglionic fibers. The thin unmyelinated axon (group C fiber) takes the most convenient route to smooth muscle and gland cells in some viscera, to the heart, to the enteric plexus, to blood vessels throughout the body, and to sweat glands and arrector pili muscles in the skin.

In addition to their principal cells, autonomic ganglia also contain interneurons, which are small cells with no axons. Their short dendrites are postsynaptic to the axons that innervate the ganglion and presynaptic to the dendrites of the principal cells.

PERIPHERAL NERVES

The constituent fibers of all but the smallest peripheral nerves are arranged in bundles or fasciculi, and three connective tissue sheaths are recognized. The entire nerve is surrounded by an **epineurium,** the sheath enclosing a bundle of fibers is known as the **perineurium,** and individual nerve fibers have a delicate covering of connective tissue constituting the **endoneurium,** or sheath of Henle.

Nerve Fibers

A nerve fiber consists of the axon or axis cylinder, the myelin sheath of fibers belonging to groups A and B, and the neurolemmal sheath (of Schwann). The **axis cylinder** has no features that are not shared with long axons in the central nervous system. Its cytoplasm (**axoplasm**) contains neurofilaments, microtubules, patches of smooth-surfaced endoplasmic reticulum, and mitochondria. The plasma membrane is called the **axolemma.**

The **neurolemma** (also spelled neurilemma) and the **myelin sheath** have several points of interest, centering around the fact that both are components of Schwann cells. The myelin has no significant intrinsic structure at the level of light microscopy (Fig. 3–5A). That it contains lipids has been obvious because the myelin is partially dissolved by lipid solvents and is stained black by osmium tetroxide, which reacts with lipids. Proteins were also known to be present in myelin; they remain as fibrillar material ("neurokeratin") after the lipids have been dissolved. The detailed chemistry of myelin became known subsequently through the results of biochemical studies.

The myelin sheath is interrupted at intervals by **nodes of Ranvier;** the length of an internode varies from 100 μm to about 1 mm, depending on the length and thickness of the fiber. Funnel-shaped clefts, called the **incisures of Schmidt–Lanterman,** are clearly visible in the myelin sheath in longitudinal sections of a nerve stained with osmium tetroxide. (Demonstration of these incisures in the central nervous system has been difficult, but they have been seen in large myelinated fibers in electron micrographs.) Using light microscopy, the neurolemmal sheath is seen as a series of **Schwann cells,** one for each internode. Most of the cytoplasm is in the region of the ellipsoidal nucleus, but traces of cytoplasm and the plasma membrane closely surround the myelin sheath from one node of Ranvier to the next.

Observations on the growth of nerve fibers in embryos and in tissue cultures, and on regeneration of fibers following

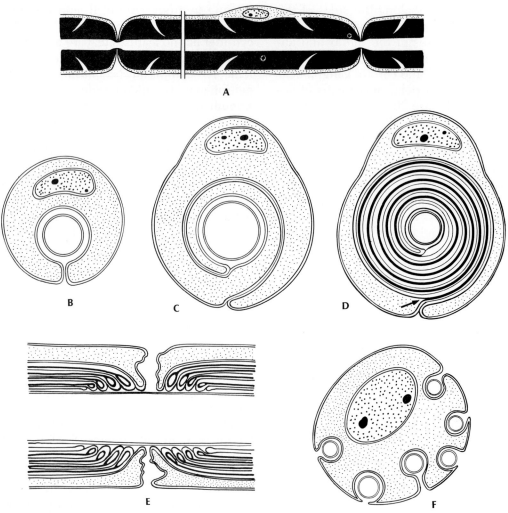

FIGURE 3-5.
(A) The myelin sheath and Schwann cell, as seen by light microscopy. **(B, C, D)** Successive stages in the development of the myelin sheath from the plasma membrane of a Schwann cell.
(E) Ultrastructure of a node of Ranvier. **(F)** Relation of a Schwann cell to several unmyelinated fibers.

trauma to a peripheral nerve, have established that Schwann cells are responsible for laying down the myelin sheath around the axis cylinder. Use of electron microscopy has established that the myelin is not only formed by the Schwann cell but in fact consists of its plasma membrane wrapped around the axis cylinder. The term *neurolemmal sheath* or *sheath of Schwann* is used to distinguish the nu-

cleated cytoplasmic layer from the layer of myelin. In fact, the Schwann cell is included in both sheaths, with the cytoplasmic portion forming the neurolemma and an extensive proliferation of the plasma membrane constituting the myelin. The Schwann cells are contiguous with satellite cells that surround nerve cell bodies in cerebrospinal and autonomic ganglia. The cellular layer that is in such intimate relationship with all nerve fibers and ganglion cells of the peripheral nervous system originates mainly from cells of the embryonic neural crest, with the addition of some cells that migrate from the neural tube along with growing motor fibers. Oligodendrocytes are the comparable cells in the central nervous system, with the transition between oligodendrocytes and Schwann cells occurring at the junction of the nerve roots and spinal cord (or brain stem).

Myelin sheaths are laid down during the later part of fetal development and during the first year postnatally in the manner shown in Figure 3–5B, C, and D. The ultrastructure of the sheath is seen in Figure 3–6. In order to explain the alternating layers of electron-dense and less-dense material, it is necessary to show the plasma membrane as a double line that represents the outer and inner, electron-dense protein layers separated by an electron-lucent interval composed of lipids.

The axon is first surrounded by the Schwann cell; the external plasma membrane is continuous with the membrane immediately around the axon through a mesaxon. By a mechanism that has not yet been elucidated, the plasma membrane then forms layers around the axon, with the direction of the spiral being clockwise in some internodes and counterclockwise in others. The cytoplasm between the layers of cell membrane gradually disappears, except for surface cytoplasm that is most abundant in the region of the nucleus. The thickness of the myelin sheath of the mature nerve fiber, which is determined by the number of turns of membrane, varies in direct proportion to the diameter and length of the axon. The major dense line, 2.5 nm in thickness, consists of two inner protein layers of the plasma membrane that fuse along a line indicated by the arrow in Figure 3–5D. The less dense layer, about 10 nm wide, consists of a double thickness of the lipid layer of the cell membrane. The fused outer protein layers of the membrane become exceedingly thin, forming an inconspicuous intraperiod line in the middle of the lighter lipid layer (see Fig. 3–6).

The node of Ranvier is the interval between the plasma membrane systems of two Schwann cells (Fig. 3–5E). The neurolemmal sheath portion of the adjoining Schwann cells has an irregular edge at the

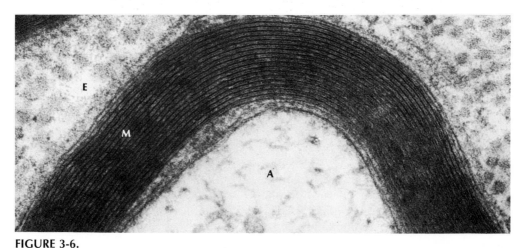

FIGURE 3-6.
Ultrastructure of the myelin sheath **(M)** consisting of alternating dense and less dense layers; the latter includes a thin intraperiod line. **(A)** Axoplasm. **(E)** Collagen fibers of the endoneurium. (× 107,500; courtesy of Dr. R. C. Buck)

node, and there is a narrow space between the Schwann cells through which the axolemma at the node is bathed by tissue fluid. Voltage-gated sodium channels are present in the axolemma only at nodes. Consequently, the action potential skips electrically from node to node, and the transmission of a nerve impulse along a myelinated fiber is called saltatory conduction (from the Latin *saltare*, to jump). This type of conduction depends on adequate electrical insulation, namely the myelin sheath, between the internodal axoplasm and the extracellular fluid. The length of internodes therefore has a bearing on the conduction rate of the nerve impulse, and the internodes are longer, up to a maximum of about 1 mm, the thicker and longer the nerve fiber. The Schmidt–Lanterman incisures are formed by a loosening of the plasma membrane layers of the sheath with retention of cytoplasm between the membranes. These incisures may aid the passage of materials through the myelin sheath to the axon.

With respect to unmyelinated fibers, a Schwann cell envelops several (up to 15) thin axons, as shown in Figure 3–5*F*. The axon is surrounded by a single layer of the Schwann cell's plasma membrane; it is therefore unmyelinated and there are no nodes of Ranvier. The nerve impulse is a self-propagating action potential along the axolemma, without the accelerating factor of node-to-node or saltatory conduction. This accounts for the slow rate of conduction that is characteristic of unmyelinated fibers.

Disorders

The peripheral nervous system is subject to various disorders. Peripheral neuropathy (neuritis) is the most common of these, consisting of degenerative changes in peripheral nerves that produce sensory loss and motor weakness. Distal portions of nerves are affected first, with symptoms in the hands and feet. There are multiple causes of peripheral neuropathy, including nutritional deficiencies, toxins of various kinds, and metabolic disorders, such as diabetes.

Damage to a peripheral nerve by a penetrating wound may result in an incapacitating disorder known as causalgia. There is severe pain in the affected limb, together with trophic changes in the skin. A nerve may be pressed upon where it passes through a restricted aperture; for example, the ulnar nerve is subject to pressure at the elbow and the median nerve in the carpal tunnel at the wrist. The resulting "entrapment syndrome" includes motor and sensory disturbances in the area of distribution of the nerve. The major plexuses, especially the brachial plexus, may be involved in a traumatic lesion, or there may be compression of major bundles of a plexus (as in crutch palsy). The nerve roots are involved in a variety of disorders (radiculopathy), causing motor and sensory disturbances. The latter may include pain in cutaneous areas and in muscles supplied by the affected nerve roots.

SUGGESTED READING

Boyd IA: The structure and innervation of the nuclear bag muscle fibre system and the nuclear chain muscle fibre system in mammalian muscle spindles. Phil Trans R Soc Lond [Biol] 245:81–136, 1962

Bridgman CF: Comparisons in structure of tendon organs in the rat, cat and man. J Comp Neurol 138:369–372, 1970

Ferrell WR, Gandevia SC, McCloskey DI: The role of joint receptors in human kinaesthesia when intramuscular receptors cannot contribute. J Physiol (Lond) 386:63–71, 1987

Iggo A, Andres KH: Morphology of cutaneous receptors. Annu Rev Neurosci 5:1–31, 1982

Kayahara T, Sakashita S, Takimoto T: Evidence for spinal origin of neurons synapsing with dorsal root ganglion cells of the cat. Brain Res 293:225–230, 1984

Kennedy WR: Innervation of normal human muscle spindles. Neurology 20:463–475, 1970

Landon DN (ed): The Peripheral Nerve. New York, John Wiley & Sons, 1976

Matthews PBC: Where does Sherrington's muscular sense originate? Annu Rev Neurosci 5:189–218, 1982

McCloskey DI: Kinesthetic sensibility. Physiol Rev 58:763–820, 1978

Munger BL: Neural–epithelial interactions in sensory receptors. J Invest Dermatol 69:27–40, 1977

Nishi K, Oura C, Pallie W: Fine structure of Pacinian corpuscles in the mesentery of the cat. J Cell Biol 43:539–552, 1969

Risling M, Dalsgaard C-J, Cukierman A, Cuello AC: Electron microscopic and immunohistochemical evidence that unmyelinated ventral root axons make U-turns or enter the spinal pia mater. J Comp Neurol 225:53–63, 1984

Saurat JH, Didierjean L: The epidermal Merkel cell is an epithelial cell. Dermatologica 169:117–120, 1984

Sinclair D: Mechanisms of Cutaneous Sensation. Oxford, Oxford University Press, 1981

Swash M, Fox KP: Muscle spindle innervation in man. J Anat 112:61–80, 1972

FOUR

Response of Nerve Cells to Injury; Nerve Fiber Regeneration; Neuroanatomical Research Methods

Neurons may be injured by physical trauma or by involvement in pathological processes, such as infarction due to vascular occlusion. Small interneurons are likely to suffer total destruction, whereas injury to large neurons may result either in destruction of the cell body or in transection of the axon, with preservation of the cell body. The best known change proximal to the site of axonal transection is the **axon reaction,** which may be displayed in the cell body. When the cell body of a neuron is destroyed, the axon is isolated from the synthetic machinery of the cell and soon breaks up into fragments, which are eventually phagocytosed. Similar changes occur distal to the site of an axonal injury. The degeneration of an axon that has been detached from the remainder of the cell is called **wallerian degeneration.** The process affects not only the axon but also its myelin sheath, even though the

latter is derived from cells other than the injured neuron.

AXON REACTION

Changes in the proximal portion of a neuron subsequent to axonal transection vary according to neuron type. Cells in some locations undergo progressive degeneration and ultimately disappear. Conversely, the proximal portion of the neuron may not be significantly altered by axon section. The cytological details of the classical axon reaction are best seen in large neurons of motor type, such as those supplying skeletal muscle, which contain coarse clumps of Nissl material. The following account includes the more typical aspects of this response to injury in such cells.

The nerve fiber between the cell body and the lesion is not altered appreciably. The cell body, in sections stained by a cat-

50

ionic dye (the Nissl method), first shows signs of reaction 24 to 48 hours after interruption of the axon. The coarse clumps of Nissl substance are changed to a finely granular dispersion; this change, known as **chromatolysis,** occurs first between the axon hillock and the nucleus, gradually spreading throughout the perikaryon (Fig. 4–1). The nucleus assumes an eccentric position, away from the axon hillock, and the cell body swells. This aspect of the reaction reaches a maximum 10 to 20 days after axon injury, and is more severe the closer the injury to the cell body. Electron microscopy shows disorder of the granular endoplasmic reticulum and an increase in the number of polyribosomes in the cytoplasmic matrix.

There are signs of recovery from the early effects of trauma to the axon even while these changes are occurring. The nucleolus enlarges, and dense basophilic caps are often seen on the cytoplasmic side of the nuclear membrane. Both the nucleolar enlargement and the nuclear caps are evidence of accelerated RNA and protein synthesis, which would favor regeneration of the axon when conditions make regeneration possible. Recovery often takes several months, and the cell body is eventually smaller than normal if the axon does not regenerate.

In cells confined to the central nervous system, the axon reaction is conspicuous only in some large neurons. Changes in smaller neurons that have little Nissl substance are not detectable by light microscopy, and large cells may exhibit no axon reaction when collateral axonal branches that arise close to the cell body are spared.

The axon reaction has been exploited in the past as a means of identifying the cells of origin of fibers in nerves and the sources of some central tracts. As a research method it has been supplanted by more informative procedures, which are discussed further on.

WALLERIAN DEGENERATION IN PERIPHERAL NERVES

The nucleus is essential for the synthesis of cytoplasmic proteins, which are carried distally by axoplasmic flow and replace proteins that have been degraded as part of the metabolic activity of the cell. The axon therefore does not survive for long when separated from the cell body. Simultaneously throughout its length, that part of the axon distal to the lesion becomes

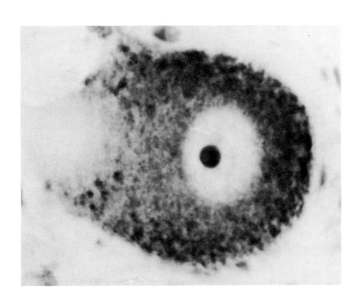

FIGURE 4-1.
Motor neuron undergoing axon reaction 6 days after transection of its axon. (Stained with cresyl violet, × 800)

slightly swollen and irregular within the first day and breaks up into fragments by the third to the fifth day. Muscular contraction on electrical stimulation of a degenerating motor nerve ceases 2 to 3 days after the nerve is interrupted. The degeneration includes the neural components of the sensory and motor endings.

The myelin sheath is converted into short ellipsoidal segments during the first few days after interruption of the fiber, and gradually undergoes complete disintegration. Meanwhile, the Schwann cells proliferate and fill the cylindrical space within the endoneurium. The remains of the axon and its myelin sheath, or the axon only in the case of unmyelinated fibers, are phagocytosed. Thus, the distal stump of a degenerated nerve contains tubular formations derived from the endoneurial sheaths, each containing a column of Schwann cells. These structures are known as the **bands of von Büngner.**

AXONAL REGENERATION IN PERIPHERAL NERVES

If a neuron is envisaged as a spherical cell body 15 μm in diameter, with an axon 10 cm long and 2 μm in diameter, a calculation shows that 99.4% of the protoplasm is in the axon. If the axon of this hypothetical neuron were severed halfway along its length the cell would lose 49.7% of its volume. This lost part of the neuron can be regrown when the injury occurs within the territory of the peripheral nervous system, a reparative process known as axonal regeneration. It is important to distinguish between this use of the word "regeneration" and its more usual connotation, which is the replacement of lost cells by mitosis and reorganization of tissue.

If a nerve has been severed, the regeneration of its axons requires apposition of the cut ends by placement of sutures through the epineurium. If only the axons have been transected, as after a crushing injury that leaves the connective tissues of the nerve intact, no surgical intervention is needed. The following description applies to nerves that have been cleanly cut through and repaired.

Axonal Growth

During the first few days, proliferating Schwann cells fill the interval between the apposed nerve ends. Regenerating fibers begin to invade the region by about the fourth day, with each fiber dividing into numerous branches having bulbous tips that grow along the clefts between Schwann cells. The rate of growth is slow at first; 2 to 3 weeks may elapse before the fibers traverse the region of the lesion. The fine branches may then find their way into endoneurial tubes of the distal segments, these tubes now being the bands of von Büngner. Several filaments enter each tube, and the invasion of a particular endoneurial tube leading to a specific type of end organ appears to be determined only by chance. Many filaments fail to enter an endoneurial tube and grow into adjacent tissue. This is the fate of all regenerating axons if the severed ends are too widely separated or if connective tissue or extraneous material intervenes. Such fibers often form complicated whorls (spirals of Perroncito), producing a swelling or neuroma that may be a source of spontaneous pain. At the other extreme is the almost perfect regeneration of the nerve through the growth of each fiber along its original endoneurial tube. This type of regeneration may occur if the nerve is crushed just enough to interrupt axons without disruption of the connective tissue sheaths.

After crossing the region of the lesion, the axonal filaments grow along the clefts between the columns of Schwann cells and the surrounding endoneurium. The regenerating fibers eventually reach motor and sensory endings; the proportion of endings that are reinnervated depends on conditions at the site of the original injury.

The rate of growth is approximately 2 mm to 4 mm daily. The amount of time that elapses between nerve suture and the beginning of functional return may be estimated on the basis of a regeneration rate of 1.5 mm daily. This value takes into account the time required for the fibers to traverse the lesion and for the peripheral endings to be reinnervated.

Maturation of Nerve Fibers

Meanwhile, changes occur along the course of the fibers. Each axon becomes surrounded by the cytoplasm of the Schwann cells. For axons that are to be myelinated, myelin sheaths are laid down by Schwann cells, with the mechanism being similar to that described in Chapter 3 for myelination that occurs in primary development. Myelination begins near the lesion and proceeds in a proximodistal direction. Although the myelin sheath is formed by the Schwann cells, its development is determined by the type of axon; all Schwann cells have the potential to produce or not to produce myelin, irrespective of the nature of the axons with which they have previously been associated.

Only one of the several axons growing in an endoneurial tube matures fully; the others gradually regress and disappear. The branching of axons as they begin to regenerate, the entry of branches from a single axon into a number of endoneurial tubes, and the presence of branches from several neurons in an individual endoneurial tube all improve a neuron's chance of reconnecting with a suitable sensory or motor ending. The appropriate fiber for the ending persists, whereas others in the endoneurial tube regress. A regenerated fiber tends to have a diameter, internodal length, and conduction velocity that are about 80% of the corresponding values for the original fiber. The motor unit for a regenerated fiber is larger, as compared with the pre-existing motor unit; that is, the

axon supplies more muscle fibers than it formerly did. This contributes to a less precise functioning of the reinnervated muscle. Taking all these factors into consideration, it is understandable that there are limitations to functional recovery after peripheral nerve injuries.

AXONAL DEGENERATION AND REGENERATION IN THE CENTRAL NERVOUS SYSTEM

The simplest lesion to visualize, although rather rare in clinical practice, is a clean incised wound. The space made by the instrument that causes such a wound fills with blood and later with collagenous connective tissue, which is continuous with the pia mater. The astrocytes in the nervous tissue on each side of the collagenous scar acquire longer and more numerous cytoplasmic processes, which form a tangled mass. The number of astrocytes in the region does not increase appreciably but there is a large increase in the total cell population, caused mainly by the emigration of monocytes from blood vessels to form phagocytic cells known as reactive microglia. The resting microglia that had been present in the central nervous tissue may also become phagocytes, but the great majority of such cells are derived from the blood. Reactive microglia also appear in parts of the central nervous system remote from the lesion, but occupied by axons that are degenerating in consequence of having been severed from their cell bodies. The process of wallerian degeneration is similar to that described for peripheral nerves, although the degradation and phagocytosis of debris is carried out much more slowly in the central nervous system. Degenerating fragments of myelinated axons are often still recognizable several months after the original injury.

A fundamental difference between the consequences of injuries to the peripheral and central nervous systems, and one that has an important bearing on clinical medicine, concerns the regeneration of axons. The proximal stumps of axons transected within the brain or spinal cord begin to regenerate, sending sprouts into the region of the lesion, but this growth ceases after about 2 weeks. Abortive regeneration of this type occurs in the central nervous systems of mammals, birds, and reptiles. Axonal regeneration in fishes and amphibia occurs efficiently in the central nervous system, with accurate restoration of synaptic connections.

The reasons for the failure of axonal regeneration in the central nervous systems of higher animals are unknown. Current hypotheses are concerned with axonal growth-promoting substances, perhaps derived from the blood or from the neuroglia, which are absent from or unable to act in the adult mammalian central nervous system. Earlier hypotheses, such as the lack of Schwann cells in the brain and spinal cord, and the obstruction of growing axons by scar tissue or cyst formation, although perhaps somewhat valid, fail to explain all the available experimental data.

There are a few circumstances in which axons do regenerate successfully within the mammalian brain. For example, the neurosecretory axons of the pituitary stalk and some monoamine-containing fibers in the brain stem regenerate effectively. However, the failure of most axons to regenerate means that permanent disability is likely to follow destruction of any tract that cannot be bypassed by redistribution of function to alternative pathways.

In rodents, axons will grow into and form synapses in tiny fragments of embryonic or fetal central nervous tissue transplanted into certain parts of the adult brain. Central axons can also grow from the brain, spinal cord, or optic nerve into transplanted pieces of peripheral nerve, and even into some nonneural tissues. Such experiments are contributing importantly to knowledge of axonal growth-promoting factors that are lost with the maturation of the central nervous system.

Transplantation into the brain or spinal cord is unlikely to acquire therapeutic significance, because the grafts are unrealistically small in relation to the parts of the recipient brain, and axons fail to grow out of the grafts into the adult central nervous tissue.

PLASTICITY OF NEURAL CONNECTIONS

Although axonal regeneration in the central nervous system occurs only negligibly, considerable functional recovery commonly follows traumatic or pathological damage in many regions, especially when the lesion is not large. For example, destruction of a small area of cerebral cortex having a well-defined motor or sensory function is followed by paralysis or loss of sensation, with recovery after several weeks. Similar recovery occurs after transection of tracts of fibers, provided that the lesions are not too large. Recovery from paralysis caused by occlusion of blood vessels in the cerebral hemispheres ("stroke") is commonly seen in clinical practice, and functional recovery may even follow partial transverse lesions of the spinal cord.

Functional recovery involves the taking over of the functions of the damaged region of the nervous system by other regions that remain intact. The reorganization of connections within the brain is known as plasticity. This may be an extension of a normally present adaptability used in the learning of often repeated tasks.

Structural changes accompany the functional plasticity that follows nervous system injury. Thus, when a group of neurons is deprived of part of its afferent input, the surviving preterminal axons, which may come from quite different places, commonly grow new branches that then form synapses at the sites denervated by the original lesion, an event known as axonal sprouting. This may occur over short distances within a small group of neurons or over greater distances, as when the axons of intact dorsal root ganglion cells extend their axons for three or four segments up and down the spinal cord after transection of neighboring dorsal roots. Axonal sprouting also occurs in the periphery; the anesthetic area of skin resulting from a peripheral nerve injury becomes smaller over several weeks, even if the severed nerve does not regenerate. The change is considered to be caused by sprouting of the axons of other cutaneous nerves within the skin. Axonal sprouting involves intact axons and should not be confused with the regeneration of transected axons. It is probable that axonal sprouting accounts for functional plasticity and recovery following lesions in the central nervous system, but a causal relationship has not yet been conclusively proved.

TRACING PATHWAYS IN THE CENTRAL NERVOUS SYSTEM

In histological material from normal animals it is rarely possible to follow a tract of axons from its cell bodies of origin to the end bulbs or boutons with which it terminates at some distant site. The small diameters and curved trajectories of axons, together with the fact that different pathways commonly occupy the same territory, make the tracing of connections impossible. It is therefore necessary to use experimental methods to determine the connections of the many groups of neurons in the brain and spinal cord. The results of investigations of the connections in laboratory animals, especially the cat and monkey, may be applicable to the human brain. This transfer of data from animals to humans is usually justifiable when there are no major differences between the connections found in taxonomically diverse groups of animals; a pathway present in rats, dogs, and monkeys is also likely to occur in humans. When variation among species is found, it is hoped that neuroan-

atomical information gained from primate studies, such as from monkeys, will be helpful with respect to the human brain. To a limited extent, the natural experiments produced by injury and disease in the human nervous system can also be used as sources of information about normal human neuroanatomy.

Neuroanatomical Methods Based on Degeneration

Until the introduction of methods based on axoplasmic transport, fiber tracts were traced by staining fibers undergoing wallerian degeneration following the placement of a destructive lesion at a selected site in the central nervous system of an animal. Although now largely of historical interest, such methods have contributed importantly to neuroanatomical knowledge.

The **Marchi technique,** which is still used on human postmortem material, depends on the staining of particles of degenerating myelin with osmium tetroxide in the presence of an oxidizing agent. The latter suppresses the staining of normal myelin, so that degenerating fibers appear as lines of black dots on a lighter background. The course of a tract can be followed in sections taken at appropriate intervals (Fig. 4–2). **Silver methods** for showing degenerating unmyelinated axons and synaptic boutons were not applicable to the human nervous system, but were much used for experimental animals.

Degenerating boutons can also be recognized in electron micrographs. When the general area of projection of a group of neurons or of a tract is known from light microscopy, the exact mode of termination of the fibers on the dendrites, somata, or axons of the postsynaptic cells may be determined. As with silver degeneration methods, electron microscopy cannot usually be applied to human material because the time of survival and the conditions of fixation of the tissue are critical.

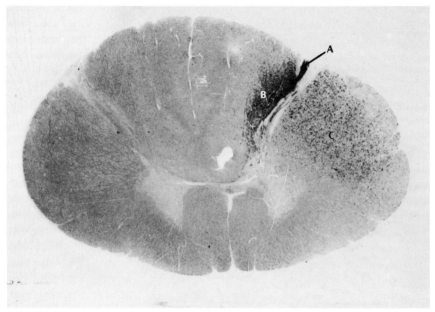

FIGURE 4-2.
Section of human spinal cord at the level of the third cervical segment. The patient succumbed 9 days after a traumatic lesion involved the dorsal roots of the second, third, and fourth cervical nerves on the right side, together with the dorsal portion of the lateral white funiculus in the second cervical segment. The following are the areas of Marchi degeneration: **(A)** Entering fibers of the third cervical dorsal root. **(B)** Ascending branches of fibers that entered the spinal cord in the third and fourth cervical dorsal roots (branches of these fibers are seen entering the gray matter). **(C)** Descending corticospinal fibers in the lateral white funiculus. (Marchi preparation, × 10)

Neuroanatomical Methods Based on Axoplasmic Transport

Research methods based on degenerating axons have been replaced by much more sensitive techniques that reveal both the cells of origin and the sites of termination of axons. The results of the extensive use of methods based on axoplasmic transport have currently necessitated a substantial revision of earlier accounts of neuronal connections in the central nervous system.

In the autoradiographic method a small volume of a radioactively labeled amino acid solution, commonly ^{3}H-leucine, is injected into the region containing the cell bodies of the neurons being investigated. The amino acid is taken up by the neurons and is incorporated into proteins, which are transported distally along the axons to the presynaptic boutons. The animal is killed 24 to 48 hours later and the appropriate parts of the nervous system are chemically fixed to immobilize the labeled proteins. Sections are cut and autoradiographs are prepared in the usual way. High concentrations of silver grains, indicating the presence of tritium in the tissue, are seen over the site of injection, over the terminal field of projection of the neurons, and often over the axons between these two regions.

With this technique it has been possible to trace connections previously undetectable by the use of degeneration methods. It also has the important advantage that the labeled amino acid enters only the cell bodies and dendrites of neurons. Axons that happen to be passing through the site of injection do not take up the tracer, thus avoiding confusion in interpreting the observed areas of terminal degeneration.

Research methods using the axon reaction and staining degenerating fibers have been replaced especially by techniques that take advantage of the uptake and transport of proteins and other substances. A histochemically detectable protein or a suitable fluorescent dye is injected into the region concerned. The foreign molecules are imbibed by presynaptic boutons in the region and transported retrogradely to their neuronal perikarya. The process takes 6 to 48 hours, according to the lengths of the axons. The animal is then killed and the tissue is removed and appropriately fixed and sectioned. A protein tracer is localized by histochemical means, thus revealing the neuronal cell bodies that innervated the site of the injection (Fig. 4–3). A fluorescent tracer is observed directly by fluorescence microscopy.

The first protein to be used extensively as a tracer in this way was the enzyme peroxidase, extracted from the root of the horseradish plant. In recent years, however, the method has been made even more sensitive by the use of lectins, which are carbohydrate-binding proteins of plant origin. Lectins bind strongly to cell surfaces, including those of axonal terminals, and are then taken up into the cytoplasm and transported. The lectin is rendered histochemically detectable by its covalent conjugation with an enzyme, usually horseradish peroxidase. Many neurons in the brain have axons that send branches to widely separated places. It is possible to demonstrate such branching by injecting a different tracer into each suspected terminal field. Dyes that fluoresce in different colors are most often used for this purpose. If both tracers are present in a single cell body, that neuron had axonal branches that went to both sites of injection.

Proteins and dyes are also taken up and transported retrogradely by injured axons

of passage, so care must be taken not to cause undue physical damage when injecting into an area containing nerve endings whose cells of origin are to be identified. Uptake by injured axons may, however, be deliberately studied by applying protein tracers at the sites of transection of tracts or to cut peripheral nerves.

With the development of increased sensitivity in methods for the histochemical detection of peroxidase, it has become possible to study the anterograde as well as the retrograde transport of tracer proteins. The amount of protein taken up by cell bodies and dendrites is less than that absorbed by presynaptic boutons. However, an appreciable amount does enter the cell bodies and is transported orthogradely in the rapid component of the axoplasmic transport system. The protein is detected histochemically in presynaptic boutons, which have an appearance quite different from that of labeled perikarya. The method therefore provides, for a smaller investment of time and effort, results comparable to those obtained by the autoradiographic method.

Deoxyglucose Method

The sugar 2-deoxy-D-glucose is an analogue of ordinary D-glucose. It enters cells in the same way as glucose but cannot be metabolized. When cells are active their glucose uptake increases so, if an active cell is supplied with 2-deoxyglucose, this sugar will accumulate in the cytoplasm. An experimental animal may be given an intravenous infusion of radioactively labeled 2-deoxyglucose while part of its nervous system is made highly active; for example, its visual system may be stimulated by light or its auditory system by sound. The radioactive sugar accumulates in all the neurons in the active system and may be detected there autoradiographically. In the visual system, for example, activity is detected in the retina and in certain layers of cells in the lateral geniculate nucleus

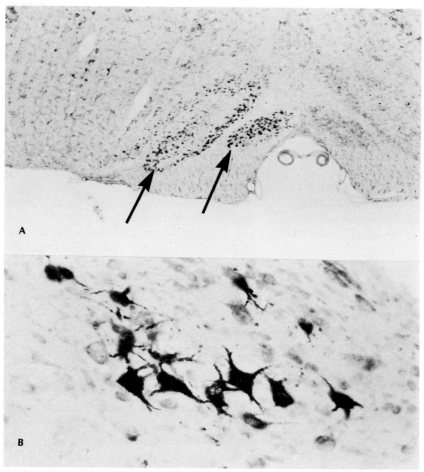

FIGURE 4-3.

Transverse section through the ventral part of the medulla of a rat in which horseradish peroxidase was injected into the cortex of one cerebellar hemisphere 24 hours before the animal was killed. The section was treated for histochemical detection of peroxidase activity, revealed as a dark blue deposit that appears black in these photomicrographs. **(A)** Labeled cell bodies in the inferior olivary complex of nuclei (*arrows*), contralateral to the site of injection ($\times$ 30). **(B)** Some of the labeled neurons at higher magnification ($\times$ 150). Other neurons appear gray because they were lightly counterstained with neutral red, a cationic dye. (Courtesy of Dr. B. A. Flumerfelt)

and in the calcarine cortex (see Chapter 20 for an explanation of the significance of these regions).

The deoxyglucose method can reveal those structures in the brain that are active when a particular system of pathways is in use. It may thus be possible to determine which of a multitude of connections demonstrated by neuroanatomical tracing methods are the most important in relation to function.

Regional Cerebral Blood Flow

In humans, it is possible to monitor blood flow in the cerebral cortex by computing regional variations in the gamma radiation detected around the head after injection of a suitable radioactive tracer. Sudden increases in blood flow are associated with activity in the underlying cortex. In clinical neurology, the technique is used to identify abnormally high or low blood flow due to disease.

Physiological and Pharmacological Methods

Nicotine was first used nearly a century ago by Langley to block synapses and thus establish their location, especially in autonomic ganglia. Anatomical studies of neuronal pathways have also been supplemented by stimulating neurons and observing the destination of nerve impulses by recording the potentials evoked elsewhere. The accurate measurement of the time elapsed between stimulation and recording provides information that may help determine the number of neurons, or synaptic delays, that are included in the pathway. This procedure is called "physiological neuronography."

Several toxic substances are used in experimental animals as adjuncts to the study of neuroanatomy. For example, local injection of kainic acid, an analogue of glutamic acid, causes death of many types of neurons without causing transection of passing fibers. This substance may kill cells by overstimulating them, mimicking the action of glutamate as an excitatory transmitter. The result is a lesion more selective than that which can be produced by physical methods. Cells that use mono-amines as synaptic transmitters are selectively intoxicated by analogues of these substances. Thus, neurons that make use of dopamine or norepinephrine are intoxicated by 6-hydroxydopamine, and serotonin cells are similarly sensitive to 5,6-dihydroxytryptamine.

SUGGESTED READING

Berry M: Regeneration of axons in the central nervous system. In Navaratnam V, Harrison RJ (eds): Progress in Anatomy, Vol 3, Chap 9, pp 213–233. Cambridge, Cambridge University Press, 1983

Björklund A, Stenevi U: Intracerebral neural implants: Neuronal replacement and reconstruction of damaged circuitries. Annu Rev Neurosci 7:239–308, 1984

Contestabile A, Mignani P, Poli A, Villani L: Recent advances in the use of selective neuron-destroying agents for neurobiological research. Experientia 40:524–534, 1984

Cotman CW, Nieto-Sampedro M, Harris EW: Synapse replacement in the nervous system of adult vertebrates. Physiol Rev 61:684–784, 1981

Jones EG, Hartman BK: Recent advances in neuroanatomical methodology. Annu Rev Neurosci 1:215–296, 1978

Kiernan JA: Hypotheses concerned with axonal regeneration in the mammalian nervous system. Biol Rev 54:155–197, 1979

Lund RD: Development and Plasticity of the Brain. New York, Oxford University Press, 1978

Plum F, Gjedde A, Samson FE: Neuroanatomical functional mapping by the radioactive 2-deoxy-D-glucose method. Neurosci Res Progr Bull 14:455–518, 1976

Seil FJ (ed): Nerve, Organ and Tissue Regeneration: Research Perspectives. New York, Academic Press, 1983

Sunderland S: Nerves and Nerve Injuries, 2nd ed. Edinburgh, Churchill-Livingstone, 1978

REGIONAL ANATOMY OF THE CENTRAL NERVOUS SYSTEM

FIVE

Spinal Cord

The spinal cord and dorsal root ganglia are directly responsible for innervation of the body, excluding most of the head. Afferent or sensory fibers enter the spinal cord through the dorsal roots of spinal nerves, and efferent or motor fibers leave by way of the ventral roots (the Bell-Magendie Law). In addition to initiating spinal reflex responses, data originating in sensory endings are relayed to the brain stem and cerebellum where they are used in various circuits, including those that influence motor performance. Sensory information is also transmitted to the thalamus and then to the cerebral cortex, where it becomes part of conscious experience and may elicit immediate or delayed behavioral responses. Motor neurons in the spinal cord are excited or inhibited by impulses originating at various levels of the brain, from the medulla to the cerebral cortex. The

spinal cord therefore has a complex internal structure.

As the tracts of the spinal cord are identified there will be references to components of the brain that are discussed in subsequent chapters. When the central nervous system is described by regions, it is necessary to probe ahead of the region under immediate consideration. An appreciation of the major systems is thus acquired step by step. The general sensory and motor systems are reviewed in Chapters 19 and 23, respectively.

GROSS FEATURES OF THE SPINAL CORD AND NERVE ROOTS

The spinal cord is a cylindrical structure, slightly flattened dorsoventrally, located in the spinal canal of the vertebral column. Protection for the cord is provided not only by the vertebrae and their ligaments but also by the meninges and a cushion of cerebrospinal fluid. The innermost meningeal layer of pia mater adheres to the surface of the spinal cord. The outermost layer of thick dura mater forms a tube that extends from the level of the second sacral vertebra to the foramen magnum at the base of the skull, where it is continuous with the dura mater around the brain. The arachnoid lies against the inner surface of the dura mater, forming the outer boundary of the fluid-filled subarachnoid space. The spinal cord is suspended in the dural sheath by a **denticulate ligament** on each side. This ligament is in the form of a ribbon, which is attached along the lateral surface of the cord midway between the dorsal and ventral roots (Fig. 5–1). The lateral edge of the denticulate ligament is serrated. Twenty-one points or processes are attached to the dural sheath at intervals between the foramen magnum and the level at which the dura mater is pierced by the roots of the first lumbar spinal nerve. An epidural space, filled with fatty tissue containing a venous plexus, occupies the interval between the dural sheath and the wall of the spinal canal.

The segmental nature of the spinal cord is demonstrated by the presence of 31 pairs of spinal nerves, but there is little indication of segmentation in its internal structure. Each dorsal root is broken up into a series of rootlets that are attached to the cord along the corresponding segment (Fig. 5–1). The ventral root arises similarly as a series of rootlets. The spinal nerves are distributed as follows: cervical, eight; thoracic, twelve; lumbar, five; sacral, five; coccygeal, one. The first cervical nerves lack dorsal roots in 50% of people, and the coccygeal nerves may be absent.

Segments of the neural tube (neuromeres) correspond in position with segments of the vertebral column (scleromeres) until the third month of fetal development. The vertebral column elongates more rapidly than the spinal

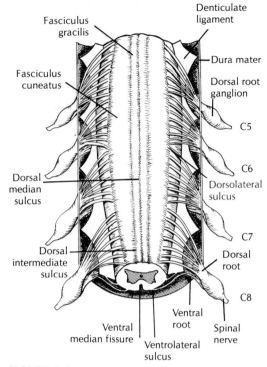

FIGURE 5-1.
Dorsal view of the cervical enlargement of the spinal cord and the corresponding roots of spinal nerves.

cord during the remainder of fetal life. The cord, which is fixed at its rostral end, gradually advances; by the time of birth the caudal end is opposite the disk between the second and third lumbar vertebrae. A slight difference in growth rate continues during childhood, bringing the caudal end of the cord in the adult opposite the disk between the first and second lumbar vertebrae (Fig. 5–2). This is an average level because the length of the spinal cord varies less than the length of the vertebral column. Thus the caudal end of the cord may be as high as the twelfth thoracic vertebral body or as low as the third lumbar vertebra.

The rostral shift of the cord during development determines the direction of spinal nerve roots in the subarachnoid space. As shown in Figure 5–2, spinal

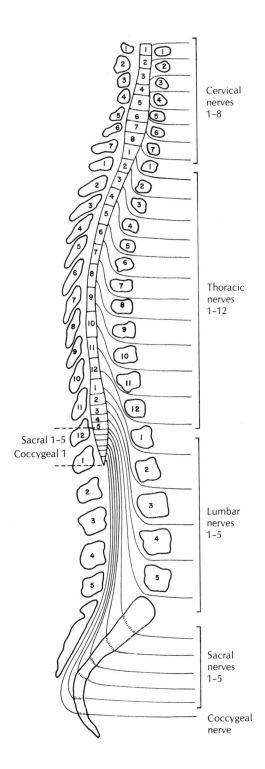

Cervical nerves 1-8

Thoracic nerves 1-12

Sacral 1-5
Coccygeal 1

Lumbar nerves 1-5

Sacral nerves 1-5

Coccygeal nerve

FIGURE 5-2.
Relation of segments of the spinal cord and spinal nerves to the vertebral column.

nerves from C1 through C7 leave the spinal canal through the intervertebral foramina above the corresponding vertebrae. (The first and second cervical nerves lie on the vertebral arches of the atlas and axis, respectively.) The eighth cervical nerve passes through the foramen between the seventh cervical and first thoracic vertebrae because there are eight cervical cord segments and seven cervical vertebrae. From that point caudally, the spinal nerves leave the canal through foramina immediately below the pedicles of the corresponding vertebrae. All intervertebral foramina are slightly rostral to the levels of the intervertebral disks.

The dorsal and ventral roots traverse the subarachnoid space and pierce the arachnoid and dura mater. At this point the dura becomes continuous with the epineurium. After a short course in the epidural space the roots reach the intervertebral foramina, where the dorsal root ganglia are located. The dorsal and ventral roots join immediately distal to the ganglion to form the spinal nerve. The length and obliquity of the roots increase progressively in a rostrocaudal direction because of the increasing distance between cord segments and the corresponding vertebral segments (Fig. 5–2). The lumbosacral roots are therefore the longest, and constitute the **cauda equina** in the lower part of the subarachnoid space. The cord tapers into a slender filament called the **filum terminale,** which lies in the midst of the cauda equina and has a distinctive bluish white color. The filum terminale picks up a dural investment opposite the second segment of the sacrum, and the resulting **coccygeal ligament** attaches to the dorsum of the coccyx. The filum terminale consists of pia mater and neuroglial elements; it is a vestige of the spinal cord of the embryonic tail, but in the adult it has no functional significance.

It may be necessary to insert a needle into the subarachnoid space to obtain a sample of cerebrospinal fluid for analysis

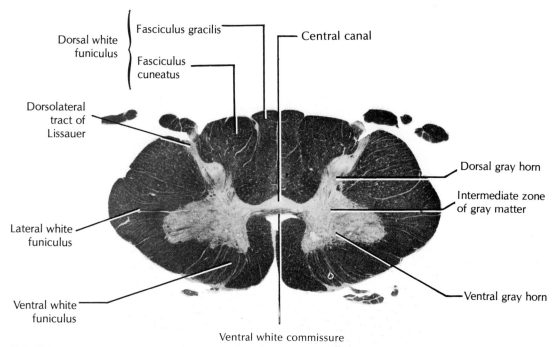

Dorsal white funiculus { Fasciculus gracilis

Fasciculus cuneatus

Central canal

Dorsolateral tract of Lissauer

Dorsal gray horn

Intermediate zone of gray matter

Lateral white funiculus

Ventral white funiculus

Ventral gray horn

Ventral white commissure

FIGURE 5-3.

Seventh cervical segment. (Weigert stain, × 6¼)

or for other reasons. A spinal lumbar puncture is the preferred method: the needle is inserted between the arches of the third and fourth lumbar vertebrae to avoid any damage to the spinal cord. It is helpful when examining a patient with a possible spinal cord or nerve root lesion to determine the location of the cord segments in relation to vertebral spines or bodies; these are shown for reference in Figure 5–2.

The spinal cord is enlarged in two regions for innervation of the limbs. The cervical enlargement extends from C4 through T1 segments, with most of the corresponding spinal nerves forming the brachial plexuses for the nerve supply of the upper limbs. Segments L2 through S3 are included in the lumbosacral enlargement, and the corresponding nerves constitute most of the lumbosacral plexuses for the innervation of the lower limbs. Individual segments are longest in the thoracic region

and shortest in the lower lumbar and sacral regions. The caudal end of the cord tapers rather abruptly and forms the **conus medullaris,** from which the filum terminale arises.

The surface of the spinal cord is marked off into dorsal, lateral, and ventral areas by longitudinal furrows. The deep **ventral median fissure** contains connective tissue of the pia mater and branches of the anterior spinal artery. The **dorsal median sulcus** is a shallow midline furrow. The **dorsal septum,** composed of pial tissue, extends from the base of this sulcus almost to the gray matter. The **ventrolateral sulcus** is indistinct, but its position is indicated by the zone of attachment of the ventral roots. The **dorsolateral sulcus** marks the line of attachment of the dorsal roots. The dorsal area on each side is divided above the midthoracic level into a medial part that contains the **fasciculus gracilis** and a lateral part that contains the **fasciculus cu-**

neatus. The intervening groove is called the **dorsal intermediate sulcus** (see Fig. 5–1).

GRAY MATTER AND WHITE MATTER

As seen in transverse section, the gray matter has a roughly H-shaped or butterfly outline (Figs. 5–3, 5–4, and 5–5). The small central canal is lined by ependymal epithelium, and the lumen may be obliterated in places. The gray matter on each side consists of **dorsal** and **ventral horns** and an **intermediate zone.** A small **lateral horn,** containing sympathetic efferent neurons, is added in the thoracic and upper lumbar segments.

There are three main categories of neuron in the spinal gray matter. The smallest cells involved in local circuitry are the internuncial neurons, or **interneurons. Motor cells** of the ventral horn supply the skeletal musculature and consist of alpha and gamma motor neurons. The cells of the lateral horn and the sacral autonomic nucleus are preganglionic neurons of the sympathetic and parasympathetic divisions of the autonomic system, respectively. The cell bodies of **tract cells,** whose axons constitute the ascending fasciculi of the white matter, are located mainly in the dorsal horn.

The white matter consists of three funiculi (Figs. 5–3, 5–4, and 5–5). (These are often called "columns," but this word is more appropriate for longitudinally aligned arrays of neuronal cell bodies in the gray matter.) The **dorsal funiculus,** bounded by the dorsal septum and the dorsal gray horn, consists of a medial **fasciculus gracilis** and a lateral **fasciculus cuneatus** above the midthoracic level, with the former corresponding with the entire dorsal funiculus caudal to the midthoracic region. The remainder of the white matter consists of **lateral** and **ventral**

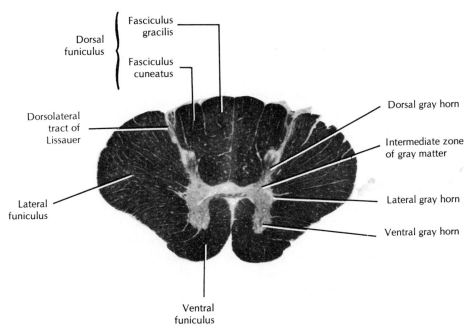

FIGURE 5-4.
Second thoracic segment. (Weigert stain, × 7)

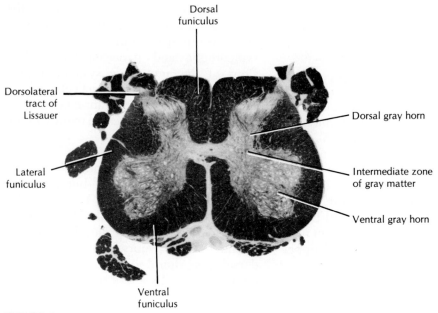

Dorsal
funiculus

Dorsolateral
tract of
Lissauer

Lateral
funiculus

Dorsal gray horn

Intermediate zone
of gray matter

Ventral gray horn

Ventral
funiculus

FIGURE 5-5.
First sacral segment. (Weigert stain, × 7)

funiculi, between which there is no anatomical demarcation. The distribution of tracts in the lateral white matter justifies subdivision into dorsolateral and ventrolateral funiculi, separated by a plane that passes through the central canal and the denticulate ligament. Nerve fibers decussate in the **ventral white commissure.** The **dorsolateral tract** (of Lissauer) occupies the interval between the apex of the dorsal horn and the surface of the cord. The white matter consists of partially overlapping fiber bundles (tracts or fasciculi), as will be described presently.

Although the general pattern of gray matter and white matter is the same throughout the spinal cord, regional differences are apparent in the photographs of transverse sections (Figs. 5–3, 5–4, and 5–5). For example, the amount of white matter increases in a caudal-to-rostral direction because fibers are added to ascending tracts and fibers leave descending tracts to terminate in the gray matter. The main variation in the gray matter is its

increased volume in the cervical and lumbosacral enlargements for innervation of the limbs. The small lateral horn of gray matter is characteristic of the thoracic and upper lumbar segments.

Neuronal Architecture of Spinal Gray Matter

As with other parts of the central nervous system, the spinal gray matter is composed of several different neuron populations. The cell types are classified according to their appearances in Nissl-stained sections, and it has been found that cells of the same type are usually clustered together into groups. Because the architecture of the spinal gray matter is essentially the same along the length of the cord, the populations of similar neurons occur in long columns. When viewed in transverse sections of the cord many of the cell columns appear as layers, especially within the dorsal horn. Ten layers of neurons are recognized, known as the **laminae of**

Rexed. Before the laminae were described in 1952 names were given to many of the cell columns, with all but a few of these names now having fallen into disuse. They were used differently by different authors, and confusing synonyms existed. The laminar scheme agrees well with the known sites of origin and termination of efferent and afferent fiber tracts, so it is possible to ascribe functions to at least some of the neuron groups in the cord. The few unambiguous names still in use for cell columns will be mentioned in association with the laminae in which they occur.

Laminar Organization

The laminae of Rexed are numbered consecutively by Roman numerals, starting at the tip of the dorsal horn and moving ventrally into the ventral horn (Fig. 5–6).

Lamina I receives some of the incoming dorsal root fibers. It is a thin layer of neurons that cap the dorsal horn. The larger neurons contribute a small proportion of the axons of the contralateral spinothalamic tract.

Lamina II, also known as the **substantia gelatinosa** (of Rolando), consists of small, densely packed neurons (gelatinosa cells) that have numerous, richly branched dendrites. Its afferent fibers are collateral branches of incoming dorsal root axons, together with descending fibers, many of which come from the reticular formation of the medulla.* The unmyelinated axons of the gelatinosa cells ascend or descend for up to four segments of the cord in the dorsolateral tract and in the adjacent white matter of the lateral funiculus. Their many branches establish synaptic contact with cells in laminae I, II, III, and IV at all these levels. The physiology of the substantia gelatinosa is not yet fully under-

---

* The reticular formation, described in Chapter 9, is a collection of groups of neurons that serve important functions in the medulla, pons, and midbrain.

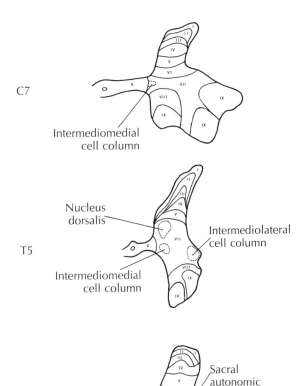

FIGURE 5-6.
Positions of cytoarchitectonic laminae of Rexed in the gray matter of the human spinal cord at three levels: the cervical enlargement, the thoracic region, and the lumbosacral enlargement. Note that lamina VI is present only in limb enlargements.

stood but this lamina is believed to be important for the editing of sensory input to the spinal cord, with the effect of determining which patterns of incoming impulses will produce sensations that will be interpreted by the brain as being painful.

Lamina III contains cells similar to those of lamina II, but receives larger numbers of fibers from the dorsal roots. It is penetrated by the dendrites of the larger neurons in laminae IV, V, and VI. Laminae I through VI all receive input from the dorsal roots, although this is densest in **lamina IV.** At the extreme rostral end of the spinal cord laminae I, II, III, and IV become continuous with the caudal end of the spinal trigeminal nucleus.

Lamina V contains many large neurons. It receives some primary afferent fibers and many descending fibers from the brain, especially corticospinal fibers, most of which end in laminae V, VI, and VII. Many of the cells in lamina V have axons that cross the midline and ascend in the contralateral spinothalamic tract. Most of the spinothalamic fibers originate in lamina V, although some come from lamina I, and a few arise in laminae VII and VIII.

Lamina VI is present only in the limb enlargements. Results of electrophysiological studies have shown that this lamina may be especially concerned with sensory data that originate in deep structures such as muscles, whereas the more superficial laminae deal predominantly with cutaneous sensory information.

Lamina VII is the largest cytoarchitectonic region of the spinal gray matter, occupying the intermediate zone between the dorsal and ventral horns as well as much of the space within the ventral horn. Its shape and position vary along the length of the cord, as do the shape and position of lamina VIII. Lamina VII contains many cells that function as interneurons, although most of these have long axons that run in the spinal white matter to the gray matter of other segments of the cord. The local circuitry is completed by collateral branches of the proximal parts of the axons of these cells. Three clearly delineated cell columns are recognized within lamina VII. The **intermediolateral cell column** occupies the lateral horn of the cord in segments T1 through L2 or L3. This column consists of the cell bodies of the preganglionic neurons of the sympathetic nervous system. The **intermediomedial cell column** is present just lateral to lamina X throughout the length of the

cord. It receives primary afferent fibers and may be involved in visceral reflexes. The **nucleus dorsalis** (nucleus thoracicus, or Clarke's column) is present on the medial aspect of the dorsal horn in segments C8 through L3. This cell column is composed of large neurons whose axons form the dorsal spinocerebellar tract. In addition to these three, the **sacral autonomic nucleus** is an inconspicuous column of cells in the lateral part of lamina VII in segments S2, S3, and S4. It consists of the cell bodies of the preganglionic neurons of the sacral division of the parasympathetic nervous system.

Lamina VIII in the ventral horn is a site of termination of some descending fibers, including many of those of the vestibulospinal and reticulospinal tracts. The neurons project both ipsilaterally and contralaterally, at the same and nearby segmental levels, to laminae VII and IX. Those axons that cross the midline do so ventral to the central canal.

Lamina IX takes the form of columns of neurons embedded in either lamina VII or lamina VIII. The cells in lamina IX include motor neurons, whose axons leave the spinal cord in the ventral roots to supply striated skeletal muscle fibers. The sizes of the cell bodies of motor neurons vary; those giving rise to long axons are among the largest of neurons, while those with shorter axons, and also those giving rise to the gamma efferent fibers to muscle spindles, are much smaller. In addition, lamina IX contains small neurons, greatly outnumbering the motor neurons, whose axons extend for considerable distances up and down the spinal cord in the fasciculus proprius adjacent to the gray matter. By virtue of collateral axonal branches that arise near the cell body, these cells also serve as local circuit neurons in the ventral horn.

Lamina X, which surrounds the central canal, is composed of decussating axons, neuroglia, and some cells that have the physiological properties of interneurons. A few dorsal root afferent fibers terminate in this area.

Outside the gray matter an isolated group of neurons is present in the lateral funiculus, adjacent to the tip of the dorsal horn. This is the **lateral cervical nucleus.** It is found in segments C1 and C2 but it is rarely conspicuous. Indeed, this nucleus is absent in about 50% of humans. In cats and monkeys the lateral cervical nucleus forms an essential part of the spinocervicothalamic sensory pathway, but its importance in humans is not yet known. It is possible that the human lateral cervical nucleus is commonly merged into the nearby reflection of lamina I overlying the lateral aspect of the tip of the dorsal horn. Rostrally the lateral cervical nucleus (in animals, and in humans when present) continues into the caudal third of the medulla.

In summary, the spinal gray matter is organized in the following way. Dorsal root afferents terminate in all laminae, but predominantly in those composing the dorsal horn. Impulses concerned with pain, temperature, and touch reach the tract cells from which the spinothalamic tract originates, most of which have their cell bodies in lamina V. The sensory information transmitted to the brain, especially for pain, is subject to modification (editing) by impulses for other modalities of sensation and by impulses that reach the dorsal horn by way of various descending pathways. Lamina II (the substantia gelatinosa) is thought to have a prominent role in modifying the perception of pain. Motor neurons in lamina IX supply the skeletal musculature. Usually with the intervention of interneurons, the motor neurons come under the influence of dorsal root afferents for spinal reflexes and of several descending tracts for the control of motor activity by the brain. Of the cell columns that constitute lamina IX, those consisting of neurons supplying axial musculature

are in the medial part of the ventral horn and those supplying the limbs are located more laterally. Distinct cell columns within laminae include two in lamina VII—namely, the nucleus dorsalis, which gives rise to the dorsal spinocerebellar tract, and the intermediolateral cell column, which consists of preganglionic sympathetic neurons.

Dorsal Root Entry Zone

Each dorsal root branches into six to eight rootlets as it approaches the spinal cord, and the axons become segregated into two divisions within each rootlet (Fig. 5–7). The lateral division contains most of the unmyelinated or group C axons and some thin group A myelinated axons. These axons enter the **dorsolateral tract** (of Lissauer) where they divide into ascending and descending branches, each giving off collaterals that enter the dorsal horn. Some of these fibers extend as far as four segments rostral or caudal to the segment at which they entered the cord, but most terminate in their own or in immediately adjacent segments. These fine caliber fibers, which are for pain and temperature, terminate mainly in laminae I, II, and V of the gray matter.

The medial division of dorsal root afferents, for modalities of sensation other than pain and temperature, consists largely of myelinated axons, including all the large caliber, rapidly conducting sensory fibers. These fibers enter the spinal white matter medial to the dorsal horn where, like those of the lateral division, they divide into ascending and descending branches. The descending branches run caudally within the dorsal funiculi for varying distances, some to nearby segments and others almost the whole length of the cord, to terminate eventually in the dorsal horn. Some of the long descending primary afferent fibers of the dorsal funiculi are collected into distinct bundles, the

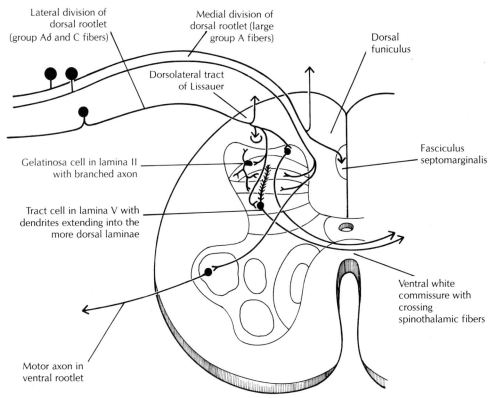

FIGURE 5-7.
Neuronal circuitry of the dorsal horn of spinal gray matter.

fasciculus septomarginalis adjacent to the dorsal septum, and the **fasciculus interfascicularis** between the fasciculi gracilis and cuneatus. The ascending branches of afferent fibers entering the dorsal funiculus are also of differing lengths, with many even reaching the medulla. At the other extreme some dorsal root fibers enter the gray matter at their own segmental levels. Axons from the medial division of the dorsal root end in all the laminae of Rexed, but with the highest concentration of synaptic boutons in laminae III and IV. Some of these primary afferent axons, conveying impulses from muscle spindles, have branches that terminate upon the motor neurons of lamina IX and are involved in the stretch reflex. Some synaptic arrangements in the dorsal gray horn are summarized in Figure 5–7.

Ventral Horn

As discussed previously, lamina IX contains motor neurons of two types, named after the diameters and therefore the conduction velocities of their axons. The alpha motor neurons supply the ordinary (extrafusal) fibers of striated skeletal muscles. The smaller gamma motor neurons are less numerous; they supply the intrafusal fibers of the neuromuscular spindles. The surfaces of both motor neuron types are densely covered with presynaptic boutons, which release either excitatory or inhibitory transmitter substances. Each alpha motor neuron receives approximately 20,000 synaptic contacts. The sources of the boutons are numerous; some are derived from descending tracts of the spinal cord while others are branches of axons of primary afferent neurons that receive input from neuromuscular spindles. The greatest numbers, however, are from intrinsic cells of the spinal gray matter, which behave physiologically as interneurons. The interneurons are located mainly in lamina VII. They receive their afferents from one another, from descending tracts, and from primary afferent neurons that are concerned with all modalities of sensation.

A special type of interneuron from the physiological standpoint is the **Renshaw cell,** which receives excitatory synaptic input from collateral branches of the axons of nearby motor neurons. The branched axon of the Renshaw cell forms inhibitory synaptic junctions upon motor neurons, including the same ones that are presynaptic

to the Renshaw cell itself. The Renshaw cells, which are in laminae VII and VIII, are also pre- and postsynaptic to other intraspinal neurons. The circuitry of the ventral horn is summarized in Figure 5–8.

The individual groups of cells constituting lamina IX are known as **somatic motor cell columns. A medial cell column** is present throughout the spinal cord for innervation of the muscles of the neck and trunk—that is, muscles attached to the axial skeleton together with intercostal and abdominal muscles. A **lateral cell column** innervates the muscles of the limbs and is therefore present in the cervical and lumbosacral enlargements.

There are two additional motor nuclei in the cervical cord, one for the phrenic

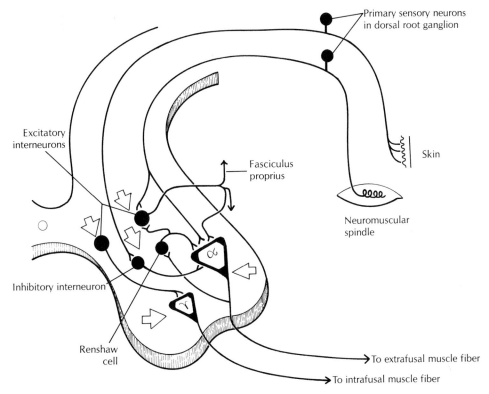

FIGURE 5-8.
Neuronal circuitry of the ventral horn of the spinal gray matter, showing afferents to the alpha (α) and gamma (γ) motor neurons. Many interneurons have long axons that travel in the fasciculus proprius. Large arrows point to the sites of termination of axons of descending tracts from the brain.

nerve and the other for the spinal root of the accessory nerve. The diaphragm develops from cervical myotomes and, although it migrates caudally during embryonic development, the origin of the diaphragm is reflected in its nerve supply. The **phrenic nucleus** is responsible for an enlargement of the medial group of ventral horn cells in segments C3 through C5, most prominently in C4. The **spinal accessory nucleus** consists of motor cells in the lateral region of the ventral horn in segments C1 through C5. The axons emerge in a series of rootlets along the lateral aspect of the spinal cord, just behind the denticulate ligament. The rootlets converge to form the spinal root of the accessory nerve, which ascends along the side of the cord in the subarachnoid space and enters the posterior cranial fossa through the foramen magnum. The spinal root joins the cranial (medullary) root along the side of the medulla. The accessory nerve then leaves the posterior cranial fossa through the jugular foramen and the spinal component supplies the sternocleidomastoid and trapezius muscles.

Tracts of Ascending and Descending Fibers

The spinal white matter is divided into three longitudinally aligned funiculi, whose positions have already been described. Each funiculus contains tracts of ascending and descending fibers. The positions of the tracts have been approximately determined from clinical and pathological studies and from comparison of clinical data with the more exact information obtained from animal studies. Most neuroanatomy and neurology textbooks contain diagrams such as Figure 5–9, showing the positions of the major tracts. It is important to realize, however, that the precise positions of some tracts are not known with certainty and that the territories of the different tracts overlap one another considerably.

Dorsal Funiculi

The most important component of the dorsal funiculi is a large body of ascending axons derived from neurons located in the dorsal root ganglia. Other ascending fibers are axons of neurons in the dorsal horn. The ascending fibers are all ipsilateral. They are concerned especially with the discriminative qualities of sensation, including the ability to recognize readily changes in the positions of tactile stimuli applied to the skin. Conscious awareness of movement and of the positions of joints in the upper limb is also mediated by axons in the dorsal funiculi above the level of spinal segment T1. Fibers that carry the same proprioceptive modality from the lower limb travel in the dorsal funiculus only as far as the thoracic cord, where the axons end by synapsing in the nucleus dorsalis. The upward continuation of the pathway for position sense in the lower limb is located in the lateral funiculus. It was formerly thought that conscious appreciation of vibration required the integrity of the dorsal funiculi, but clinical observations indicate that this is not so. Both the dorsal and the lateral funiculi conduct impulses initiated by vibratory stimuli.

As the spinal cord is ascended, axons are added to the lateral side of each dorsal funiculus. Consequently, in the upper cervical cord, the lowest levels of segmental innervation are represented in the most medial part of the fasciculus gracilis and the uppermost levels in the most lateral part of the fasciculus cuneatus. These two fasciculi end, respectively, in the nucleus gracilis and nucleus cuneatus, which are located dorsally in the medulla. As a useful approximation, the gracile fasciculus and nucleus may be said to deal with sensations from the lower limb and the cuneate fasciculus and nucleus may be said to deal with sensations from the upper limb. The orderly arrangement of different levels of the body in the dorsal funiculi is an example of somatotopic lamination in a tract.

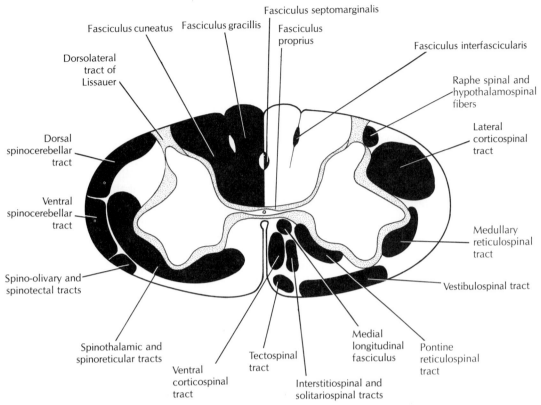

FIGURE 5-9.
Major tracts of the spinal white matter at midcervical level. Ascending tracts are on the left; descending tracts are on the right.

As will be seen, comparable lamination also exists in some other tracts of the spinal cord.

The ascending sensory fibers are not the only axons in the dorsal funiculi. Descending axons arise from three sources— the neurons in the nuclei gracilis and cuneatus, the spinal gray matter, and the dorsal root ganglia. The gracilo- and cuneatospinal pathways form part of a series of neural connections through which higher levels of the central nervous system are able to modify or edit the input of sensory messages from the cord. The spinospinal fibers, some of which run almost the full length of the cord in both directions, are probably involved in reflex coordination of the movements of the upper and lower limbs. The descending branches of incoming primary afferent axons provide a mechanism whereby the sensations arising in adjacent segmental levels of the body may be integrated so that meaningful patterns of impulses will ascend to the brain in the long ascending tracts.

Lateral Funiculus

The most conspicuous tract in the dorsal half of the lateral funiculus is the **lateral corticospinal tract,** which consists of axons of neurons in the cortex of the contralateral frontal and parietal lobes of the cerebral hemispheres. These fibers pass through the internal capsule, the basis pedunculi of the midbrain, the pons, and the medullary pyramid before decussating and entering the lateral funiculus of the cord. The corticospinal fibers from the frontal cortex terminate mainly in laminae IV through IX. Those from the parietal lobe end in laminae I through VII, but predominantly in laminae III and IV. The somatotopic lamination of the lateral corticospinal tract is such that fibers destined for the lowest levels of the spinal cord are the most laterally placed. In rodents and carnivores, the **rubrospinal tract,** arising from the contralateral red nucleus, is substantial and extends through most of the spinal cord immediately ventral to the lateral corticospinal tract. The rubrospinal tract is small in monkeys. In apes and man, it is rudimentary and ends in the second cervical segment.

The reticulospinal component of the dorsolateral funiculus arises in the nucleus raphe magnus in the reticular formation of the medulla and terminates in laminae I through III. These unmyelinated fibers, constituting the **raphe spinal tract** in the most dorsal part of the lateral funiculus, contain histochemically demonstrable quantities of serotonin, which they probably use as a neurotransmitter. The raphe spinal tract modifies the transmission from the dorsal horn of impulses initiated by noxious stimuli, which produce painful sensations. **Hypothalamospinal fibers,** similarly located, arise from the paraventricular nucleus of the hypothalamus and end among the preganglionic autonomic neurons in segments T1–L3 and S2–S4.

Ascending fibers in the dorsal part of the lateral funiculus arise from cells in the dorsal horn. They convey impulses initiated by most modalities of cutaneous and deep sensation, probably including vibration, to the nuclei gracilis and cuneatus of the medulla. The same region of the white matter also contains the fibers of the **spinocervical tract.** The axons of this tract arise ipsilaterally from cells in laminae IV through VI and terminate mainly in the lateral cervical nucleus, with a few ending in the nucleus cuneatus. The spinocervical tract is concerned with cutaneous sensation, but its importance relative to other ascending tracts is uncertain.

The ascending fibers just described are located deep in the white matter. Superficially located is the **dorsal spinocerebellar tract,** which is present only above level L2. The axons of this tract arise from the cells of the nucleus dorsalis (nucleus thoracicus) in lamina VII of the same side of the cord and terminate ipsilaterally in the cortex of the cerebellum, which they reach by traversing the inferior cerebellar peduncle. Collateral branches of some of the axons of the dorsal spinocerebellar tract are given off in the lower medulla, where they terminate in the nucleus Z of Brodal and Pompeiano. This nucleus is rostral to the nucleus gracilis and forms part of the pathway for conscious proprioception from the lower limb.

Several tracts are present in the ventral half of the lateral funiculus. The largest is the **spinothalamic tract,** which consists of the ascending axons of neurons located in the gray matter of the opposite half of the cord. The cells of origin are mostly in lamina V, although smaller numbers are present in laminae I, VII, and VIII. The axons cross the midline in the ventral white commissure close to the central canal and then traverse the ventral horn to enter the ventrolateral and ventral funiculi. The fibers of the spinothalamic tract end in thalamic nuclei. As they pass through the brain stem, these axons give off collateral branches to the reticular formation in the medulla and pons and to the periaqueductal gray matter in the midbrain. The spinothalamic tract conducts impulses concerned with tactile, thermal, and painful sensations. Its fibers are somatotopically arranged, with those for the lower limb lying most superficially and those for the upper limb lying closest to the gray matter. Distinct ventral and lateral spinothalamic tracts have been recognized by some, but there seems to be little justification for such a subdivision.

The **ventral spinocerebellar tract** is located superficially in the ventrolateral funiculus. It arises in the gray matter of the lower half of the spinal cord and consists largely of crossed fibers. The tract ascends as far as the midbrain and then makes a sharp turn caudally into the superior cerebellar peduncle. The fibers cross the midline for a second time within the cerebellum before ending in the cerebellar cortex. Thus, both spinocerebellar tracts convey sensory information (mainly proprioceptive) from one side of the body to the same side of the cerebellum. The other ascending components of the ventral half of the lateral funiculus are small. The **spinotectal tract** consists of fibers that cross the midline of the spinal cord and then project rostrally to the superior colliculus and the periaqueductal gray matter of the midbrain. The **spinoreticular tract**, originating in laminae V through VIII, includes crossed fibers that terminate in the pontine reticular formation and uncrossed fibers that end in the medullary reticular formation. These fibers form part of the ascending reticular activating system (Chapter 9), and may also be involved in the perception of pain and of various sensations originating in internal organs. The small **spino-olivary tract** projects to the accessory olivary nuclei of the medulla contralateral to the cells of origin; these nuclei, in turn, project across the midline to the cerebellar cortex.

A descending tract of the ventrolateral funiculus, the **medullary reticulospinal tract**, is derived from the gigantocellular reticular nucleus of the medulla. Most of its fibers are uncrossed, but a small proportion have crossed the midline in the medulla. This tract, together with the pontine reticulospinal tract (described below), is one of the descending pathways through which the brain directs and controls the

activity of motor neurons. Whereas the corticospinal tract is concerned mainly with skilled volitional movements, the reticulospinal tracts control ordinary activities that do not require constant conscious effort.

Ventral Funiculus

The long tracts in this part of the spinal white matter are all descending ones. The **ventral corticospinal tract** comprises a small proportion of the corticospinal fibers, those that did not cross the midline in the lower part of the medulla. The ventral corticospinal fibers decussate at segmental levels and terminate next to those of the larger lateral corticospinal tract. In a few people, most of the corticospinal fibers fail to decussate in the medulla and therefore descend ipsilaterally in the ventral funiculus. The **vestibulospinal tract** is an uncrossed pathway that arises from the lateral vestibular nucleus in the medulla. It is located in the lateral part of the ventral funiculus and its axons terminate in lamina VIII and in the medial part of lamina VII. A few vestibulospinal fibers synapse directly with motor neurons in the cell columns of lamina IX. This tract mediates equilibratory reflexes triggered mainly by the activity of the vestibular apparatus of the internal ear and which are put into effect by the axial musculature and the extensors of the limbs.

The **pontine reticulospinal tract** originates in the ipsilateral pontine reticular formation and terminates bilaterally in the spinal gray matter, with some of the axons decussating in the ventral white commissure. The remaining tracts of the ventral funiculus are small. The descending component of the **medial longitudinal fasciculus** (also called the medial vestibulospinal tract, in which case the vestibulospinal tract previously described is designated as lateral) arises in the medial vestibular nucleus in the medulla. It is involved in movements of the head required for maintaining equilibrium, and does not descend below the cervical levels of the spinal cord. Neither does the **tectospinal tract** from the contralateral superior colliculus, which functions in movements of the head required for fixation of gaze. The **interstitiospinal tract** is a small bundle originating in the interstitial nucleus of Cajal and in the Edinger–Westphal nucleus, both of which are located in the rostral part of the midbrain. This tract is probably involved in visuomotor coordination. A small **solitariospinal tract,** from the nucleus of the tractus solitarius in the medulla, is also present at all levels; it may mediate part of the higher control of autonomic functions.

The **fasciculus proprius** is a zone of myelinated fibers present in all the funiculi, immediately adjacent to the gray matter (see Fig. 5–9). It contains propriospinal (spinospinalis) fibers, which connect different segmental levels of the gray matter. The lengths of propriospinal fibers vary, from less than the length of one segment to almost the whole length of the cord. The axons run both rostrally and caudally; their most important functions relate to intersegmental spinal reflexes. Most of these fibers originate in laminae V through VIII

and terminate in the same laminae at other levels.

SPINAL REFLEXES

Certain neuronal connections in the spinal cord form the bases of spinal reflexes. The stretch reflex, gamma reflex loop, and flexor reflex are examples.

The **stretch reflex** is based on a two-neuron or monosynaptic reflex arc (Fig. 5–10). Slight stretching of a muscle stimulates the sensory endings in neuromuscular spindles, and the resultant excitation reaches the spinal cord by way of primary sensory neurons that have large group A processes. Axons of these cells in the dorsal funiculus give off collateral branches that excite alpha motor neurons, causing the stretched muscle to contract. This is an important postural reflex. The afferent impulses originate as an asynchronous discharge from the neuromuscular spindles, which are delicate monitors of change in the length of the muscle. The reflex alters tension in the muscle in such a way as to maintain a constant length. The stretch reflex forms the basis of the knee jerk test and other tendon reflex tests that are used in a neurological examination. A sharp tap on the patellar tendon causes synchronous

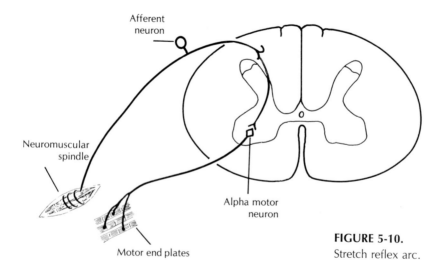

Afferent neuron

Neuromuscular spindle

Alpha motor neuron

Motor end plates

FIGURE 5-10.
Stretch reflex arc.

discharges from the spindles in the quadriceps femoris muscle, with prompt reflex contraction of the muscle and extension of the leg at the knee.

The reflex arc just described forms part of the **gamma reflex loop,** through which muscle tension comes under the control of descending motor pathways (Fig. 5–11). Fibers of these pathways (*e.g.,* reticulospinal, vestibulospinal) excite gamma motor neurons, causing contraction of intrafusal muscle fibers and an increase in the rate of firing from sensory endings in the neuromuscular spindles. The impulses are conveyed to alpha motor neurons that supply the main muscle mass through the monosynaptic reflex arc described for the stretch reflex.

The **flexor reflex,** which is protective as in withdrawal of the hand in response to a painful stimulus, is based on a series of at least three neurons and is therefore polysynaptic (Fig. 5–12). The cutaneous receptors are free nerve endings, and the afferent fibers synapse in the dorsal horn with interneurons. These end on alpha motor cells in several segments because a

withdrawal response requires the action of muscle groups.

The tension on a muscle is monitored by Golgi tendon spindles. When the tension reaches a certain level there is a distinct increase in the discharge from these spindles. The resulting nerve impulses reach interneurons in the spinal gray matter, these cells inhibit alpha motor neurons, and relaxation of the muscle follows. This reflex therefore tends to prevent excessive tension on the muscle and tendon.

ANATOMICAL AND CLINICAL CORRELATIONS

Lesions of the spinal cord result from trauma, degenerative and demyelinating disorders, tumors, infections, and impairment of blood supply. Testing for impairment or loss of cutaneous sensation is an important part of the neurological examination, and is particularly useful in detecting the site of a lesion that involves the spinal cord or nerve roots. The distribution of cutaneous areas (dermatomes) supplied by the spinal nerves is shown in Figure

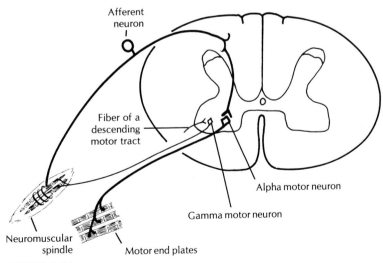

FIGURE 5-11.
Gamma reflex loop.

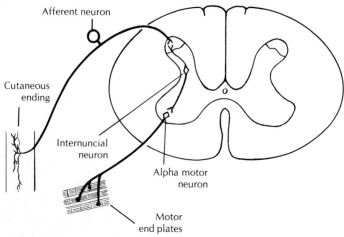

FIGURE 5-12.
Flexor reflex arc.

5–13. (Because different methods of investigation yield different results, a dermatomal map receiving general acceptance in all details has yet to be devised.) Cutaneous areas supplied by adjacent spinal nerves overlap. For example, the upper half of the area supplied by T6 is also supplied by T5, and the lower half by T7. There is therefore little sensory loss, if any, following interruption of a single dorsal root of a spinal nerve.

Reflex contraction of muscles is also used in testing for the integrity of segments of the cord and of the spinal nerves. The segments involved in the more commonly tested stretch or tendon reflexes are as follows: biceps reflex, C5 and C6; triceps reflex, C6 through C8; quadriceps reflex, L2 through L4; gastrocnemius reflex, S1 and S2.

Before specific pathological conditions are mentioned, it should be noted that a distinction is made between the effects of a lesion involving **lower motor neurons** as opposed to those involving **upper motor neurons.** Destruction or atrophy of lower motor neurons (in the present context, those of the ventral horn) results in flaccid paralysis of the affected muscles, diminished or absent tendon reflexes, and progressive atrophy of the muscles deprived of motor fibers. The term "upper motor neuron lesion," although regularly used clinically, leaves much to be desired. The lesion may be in the cerebral cortex or in another part of the cerebral hemisphere, in the brain stem, or in the spinal cord. Thus the "upper motor neuron" is a collective term, which includes all the descending pathways that control the activities of the principal neurons of lamina IX. In any event, the following signs are associated with an upper motor neuron lesion after the acute effects have worn off: varying degrees of voluntary paralysis, which is most severe in the upper limb; the sign of Babinski (upturning of the great toe and spreading of the toes upon stroking of the sole); and spasticity with exaggerated tendon reflexes.

The following elementary notes on selected lesions will show the necessity of understanding the intrinsic anatomy of the spinal cord in order to interpret signs and symptoms.

The cord may be damaged by spinal fracture or by dislocation, by penetrating wounds caused by projectile metal fragments, or by other traumatic events. Complete **transection** results in loss of all sen-

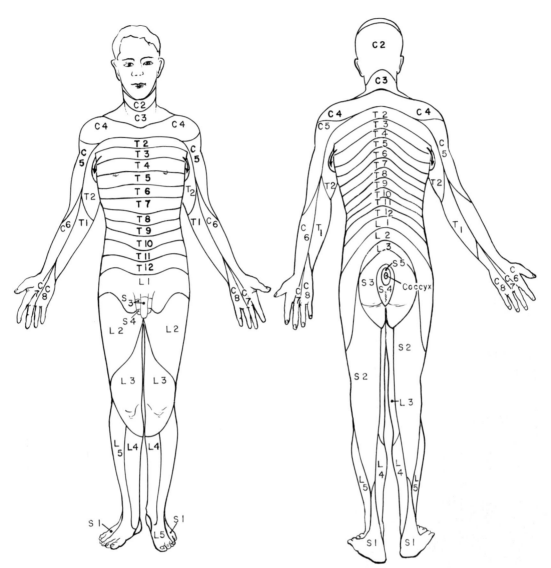

FIGURE 5-13.
Cutaneous distribution of spinal nerves (dermatomes).

sibility and voluntary movement below the lesion. The patient is tetraplegic (quadriplegic), with both arms and both legs paralyzed, if the upper cervical cord is transected, and paraplegic (both legs paralyzed) if the transection is between the cervical and lumbosacral enlargements. There is an initial period of spinal shock, lasting from a few days to several weeks, during which all somatic and vis-

ceral reflex activity is abolished. On return of reflex activity there is spasticity of muscles and exaggerated tendon reflexes. Bladder and bowel functions are no longer under voluntary control.

The events following partial transection of the spinal cord depend on the size and location of the lesion. **Hemisection**, although unusual in the literal sense, is an instructive lesion anatomically. The neurological signs caudal to the hemisected region of the cord constitute the Brown–Séquard syndrome. Position sense, tactile discrimination, and the feeling of vibration are lost *on the side of the lesion* because of interruption of the dorsal and dorsolateral funiculi. There is anesthesia for pain and temperature *on the opposite side* because of interruption of the spinothalamic tract. Light touch is not much affected because of essentially bilateral conduction in the dorsal and lateral funiculi. The patient is hemiplegic if the lesion is in the upper cervical cord, whereas hemisection of the thoracic cord results in paralysis of the leg (monoplegia). The paralysis is *ipsilateral* to the lesion and is of the upper motor neuron type, as has been described.

The following degenerative diseases also illustrate the anatomical basis of neurological signs. In **subacute combined degeneration** there is bilateral demyelination and loss of nerve fibers in the dorsal and dorsolateral funiculi. The principal etiological factor is vitamin B_{12} deficiency, and the disorder is typically encountered in association with pernicious anemia. The lesion results in loss of the senses of position, discriminative touch, and vibration. The gait is ataxic (without coordination) because the patient is unaware of the position of the legs.

Amyotrophic lateral sclerosis is a bilateral degenerative disease. The degenerative process is restricted to the motor system, affecting the corticobulbar and corticospinal tracts along with motor nuclei of cranial nerves and ventral horn motor cells. The signs are therefore a combination of upper and lower motor neuron lesions effects.

Syringomyelia is a disorder different from those already mentioned in that neuronal degeneration is not the primary pathological change. The condition is characterized by central cavitation of the spinal cord, usually beginning in the cervical region, with a glial reaction (gliosis) adjacent to the cavity. Decussating fibers for pain and temperature in the ventral white commissure are interrupted early in the disease. The cavitation and gliosis spread into the gray matter and white matter, and also longitudinally, leading to variable signs and symptoms depending on the regions involved. The classical clinical picture is that of "yokelike" anesthesia for pain and temperature over the shoulders and upper limbs, accompanied by lower motor neuron weakness and wasting of the muscles of the upper limbs. Spread of the cavitation and glial reaction into the lateral funiculi may result in voluntary paresis of the upper motor neuron type, affecting especially the lower limbs.

SUGGESTED READING

Abdel-Maguid TE, Bowsher D: The gray matter of the dorsal horn of the adult human spinal cord, including comparisons with general somatic and visceral afferent cranial nerve nuclei. J Anat 142:33–58, 1985

Barson AJ: The vertebral level of termination of the spinal cord during normal and abnormal development. J Anat 106:489–497, 1970

Brown AG: The dorsal horn of the spinal cord. Q J Exp Physiol 67:193–212, 1982

Brown AG: Organization in the Spinal Cord. Berlin, Springer-Verlag, 1984

Cervero F, Iggo A: The substantia gelatinosa of the spinal cord. A critical review. Brain 103:717–772, 1980

LaMotte C: Distribution of the tract of Lissauer and the dorsal root fibers in the primate spinal cord. J Comp Neurol 172:529–561, 1977

Nathan PN, Smith MC: The rubrospinal and central tegmental tracts in man. Brain 105:223–269, 1982

Noback CR, Demarest RJ: The Human Nervous System, 3rd ed. New York, McGraw-Hill, 1981

Ralston DD, Ralston HJ: The terminations of corticospinal tract axons in the macaque monkey. J Comp Neurol 242:325–337, 1985

Renshaw B: Central effects of centripetal impulses in axons of spinal nerve roots. J Neurophysiol 9:191–204, 1946

Rexed BA: Cytoarchitectonic atlas of the spinal cord in the cat. J Comp Neurol 100:297–379, 1954

Schoenen J: The dendritic organization of the

human spinal cord: The dorsal horn. Neuroscience 7:2057–2087, 1982

Smith MC, Deacon P: Topographical anatomy of the posterior columns of the spinal cord in man. The long ascending fibres. Brain 107:671–698, 1984

Truex RC, Taylor MJ, Smythe MQ, Gildenberg PL: The lateral cervical nucleus of the cat, dog and man. J Comp Neurol 139:93–104, 1965

SIX

Brain Stem: External Anatomy

The brain stem consists of the medulla oblongata, pons, and midbrain. Although each of the three regions has special features they have certain fiber tracts in common, and each region includes nuclei of cranial nerves. The fourth ventricle is partly in the medulla and partly in the pons. It is advantageous, therefore, to describe the medulla, pons, and midbrain together. (In names such as corticobulbar tract, also called the corticonuclear tract, "bulb" refers to the brain stem, in which motor nuclei of cranial nerves are located.)

MEDULLA OBLONGATA

The medulla oblongata (or medulla) is about 3 cm long and widens gradually in a rostral direction. It rests on the basilar portion of the occipital bone and is concealed from above by the cerebellum. The junction of the spinal cord and medulla is

at the upper rootlet of the first cervical nerve, which corresponds to the level of the foramen magnum. The spinal cord seems to pass imperceptibly into the medulla, insofar as surface markings are concerned, but internally there is an abrupt and extensive rearrangement of the gray matter and white matter. The rostral limit of the medulla is clearly marked on the ventral surface by the border of the pons (Fig. 6–1). In dorsal view (Fig. 6–3), the medulla is seen to consist of a **closed portion** containing a continuation of the central canal of the spinal cord, and an **open portion** in which part of the fourth ventricle is located. The ventricle results from a flexure of the embryonic brain with a dorsal concavity (the pontine flexure) and subsequent development of the large cerebellum with its thick peduncles. These events caused a divergence of the dorsal halves of the maturing brain stem, so that its lu-

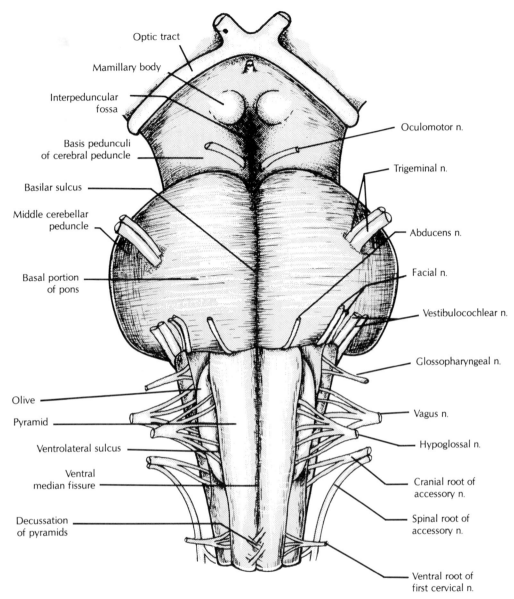

FIGURE 6-1.
Ventral aspect of the brain stem.

men widened out to form the fourth ventricle bounded by the medulla, pons, and cerebellum. The junction of the medulla and pons dorsally may be considered as a line passing along the inferior edges of the middle cerebellar peduncles.

The longitudinal grooves previously described for the spinal cord continue on

the medulla. The **ventral median fissure** is interrupted at the spinomedullary junction by bundles of decussating fibers. These are corticospinal fibers crossing from the pyramid of the medulla to the opposite side of the cord, where they constitute the lateral corticospinal tract. The **dorsal median sulcus** continues on the closed por-

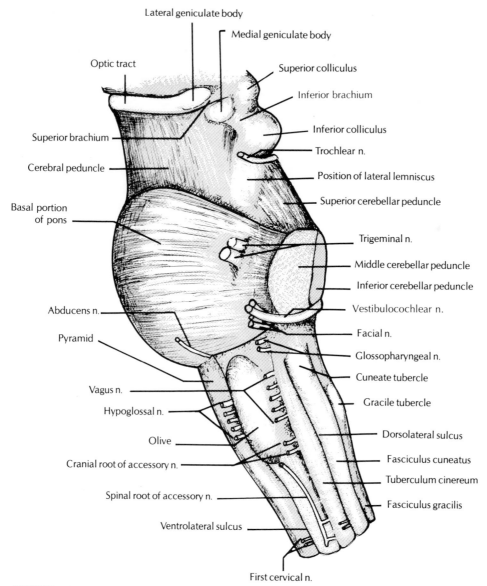

FIGURE 6-2.
Lateral aspect of the brain stem.

tion of the medulla, and the **ventrolateral** and **dorsolateral sulci** are in approximately the same position as they are in the spinal cord.

Three areas are thereby outlined on each side. The ventral area is occupied by the **pyramid,** which consists of cortico-spinal fibers (Fig. 6–1). This is the origin of the term pyramidal tract as a synonym for corticospinal tract. The lateral area (Fig. 6–2) includes a prominent oval swelling, the **olive,** which marks the position of the inferior olivary nucleus. Rootlets of the glossopharyngeal, vagus, and accessory nerves are attached to the lateral area just dorsal to the olive. The **tuberculum cine-**

reum is that part of the lateral area intervening between the attachment of the abovementioned nerves and the dorsolateral sulcus. The tuberculum cinereum marks the position of the spinal tract of the trigeminal nerve and the nucleus of the spinal tract, these being comparable to the dorsolateral tract (of Lissauer) and laminae I through IV of the dorsal gray horn in the spinal cord. The dorsal spinocerebellar tract is superficial to the trigeminal spinal tract in the rostral part of the tuberculum cinereum because the spinocerebellar fibers turn dorsally at this point to enter the inferior cerebellar peduncle. The **fasciculi gracilis** and **cuneatus** continue from the spinal cord into the dorsal area of the medulla (Fig. 6–3). The **gracile tubercle,** a slight elevation at the rostral end of the fasciculus gracilis, is produced by the nucleus gracilis, in which fibers of the fasciculus end. At a slightly more rostral level, the **cuneate tubercle** marks the position of the nucleus cuneatus or terminal nucleus of the fasciculus cuneatus. The apex of the V-shaped boundary of the inferior portion of the fourth ventricle is known as the **obex.**

Seven of the twelve cranial nerves are attached to the medulla or to the junction of the medulla and pons (Figs. 6–1, 6–2, and 6–3). The **abducens nerve** emerges from the ventral surface between the pons and the pyramid of the medulla. The nerve passes forward in the subarachnoid space beneath the pons, traverses the cavernous venous sinus just lateral to the body of the sphenoid bone, and enters the orbit through the superior orbital fissure. The **facial** and **vestibulocochlear nerves** are attached to the brain stem at the caudal border of the pons well out laterally, the facial nerve being the more medial. The facial nerve has two roots, motor and sensory. The sensory root, which includes some efferent parasympathetic fibers, lies between the larger motor root and the vestibulocochlear nerve; it is therefore known as the **nervus intermedius** (of Wrisberg).

The cochlear division of the vestibulocochlear nerve ends in the dorsal and ventral cochlear nuclei, which are situated on the base of the inferior cerebellar peduncle, whereas the vestibular division penetrates the brain stem deep to the root of the inferior cerebellar peduncle. The facial and vestibulocochlear nerves enter the internal acoustic meatus in the petrous temporal bone.

Roots of the **glossopharyngeal** and **vagus nerves,** as well as those of the cranial division of the **accessory nerve,** are attached to the medulla along a line between the olive and the tuberculum cinereum (the dorso-olivary sulcus). The accessory nerve is motor, whereas the glossopharyngeal and vagus nerves are mixed, having sensory and motor components. The cranial root of the accessory nerve is joined by the spinal root, and the glossopharyngeal, vagus, and accessory nerves leave the posterior cranial fossa through the jugular foramen. Roots of the **hypoglossal nerve,** a motor nerve, emerge along the ventrolateral sulcus between the pyramid and the olive, and the nerve leaves the posterior fossa through the hypoglossal canal.

PONS

This part of the brain stem owes its name to the appearance presented on its ventral surface (Fig. 6–1), which is that of a bridge connecting the right and left cerebellar hemispheres. However, the appearance is deceptive as far as the constituent nerve fibers are concerned, as noted below.

The pons consists of two quite different parts known as the basal (ventral) and dorsal portions of the pons, as is seen clearly in sections (see Figs. 7–9 and 7–10). The **basal portion** is distinctive of this part of the brain stem. Fibers from the cerebral cortex terminate ipsilaterally on nerve cells composing the pontine nuclei, and axons of the latter cells constitute the contralateral middle cerebellar peduncle. In

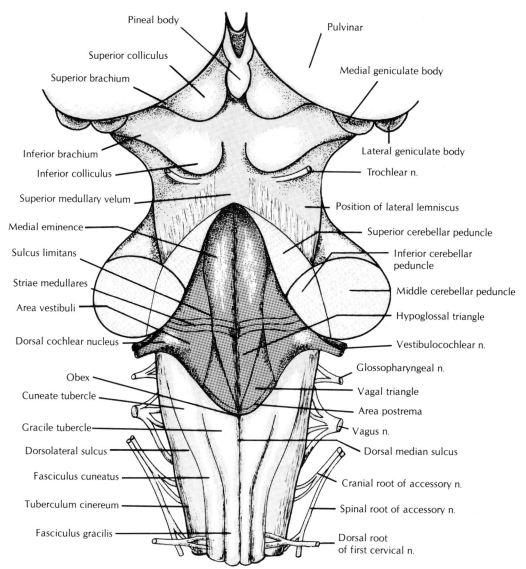

Pineal body

Pulvinar

Superior colliculus

Medial geniculate body

Superior brachium

Lateral geniculate body

Inferior brachium

Trochlear n.

Inferior colliculus

Superior medullary velum

Position of lateral lemniscus

Medial eminence

Superior cerebellar peduncle

Sulcus limitans

Inferior cerebellar peduncle

Striae medullares

Middle cerebellar peduncle

Area vestibuli

Hypoglossal triangle

Dorsal cochlear nucleus

Vestibulocochlear n.

Obex

Glossopharyngeal n.

Cuneate tubercle

Vagal triangle

Gracile tubercle

Area postrema

Dorsolateral sulcus

Vagus n.

Fasciculus cuneatus

Dorsal median sulcus

Tuberculum cinereum

Cranial root of accessory n.

Fasciculus gracilis

Spinal root of accessory n.

Dorsal root
of first cervical n.

FIGURE 6-3.
Dorsal aspect of the brain stem.

effect the basal pons is a large synaptic or relay station, providing a connection between the cortex of a cerebral hemisphere and that of the opposite cerebellar hemisphere as part of a circuit contributing to maximal efficiency of voluntary movements. The cerebral cortex, basal pons, and cerebellum all increased in size during mammalian evolution and are best developed in the human brain. The

corticospinal tracts traverse the basal portion of the pons before entering the pyramids.

The **dorsal portion** or **tegmentum** of the pons is similar to much of the medulla and midbrain in that it contains ascending and descending tracts and nuclei of cranial nerves. The dorsal surface of the pons contributes to the floor of the fourth ventricle.

The pons is about 2.5 cm in length. A

shallow groove, the **basilar sulcus,** runs along its ventral surface in the midline. The pons merges laterally into the middle cerebellar peduncles, with the attachment of the **trigeminal nerve** marking the transition between the pons and the peduncle (Fig. 6–1 and 6–2). The motor root of the trigeminal nerve is rostromedial to the larger sensory root. The trigeminal nerve enters the middle cranial fossa at the medial end of the petrous temporal bone, where the trigeminal ganglion is located. The three divisions of the nerve diverge from the ganglion, embedded in the dura mater. The ophthalmic division passes through the superior orbital fissure to reach the orbit. The maxillary division traverses the foramen rotundum, and the mandibular division traverses the foramen ovale, with both foramina being in the floor of the middle cranial fossa.

The rostral part of the pons is known as the **isthmus of the brain stem.** A slight bandlike elevation runs obliquely across the dorsolateral surface of the isthmus toward the inferior colliculus of the midbrain (Fig. 6–2). This elevation is produced by the lateral lemniscus, which is the main auditory tract of the brain stem.

FOURTH VENTRICLE

The **floor of the fourth ventricle (rhomboid fossa)** is broad in its midportion, narrowing toward the obex and the aqueduct of the midbrain (see Fig. 6–3). The floor is divided into symmetrical halves by a **median sulcus;** the **sulcus limitans** further divides each half into medial and lateral areas. The vestibular nuclear complex lies beneath most of the lateral area, which is therefore known as the **vestibular area** of the rhomboid fossa. Motor nuclei are located beneath the medial area, the caudal part of which is marked by two triangles or trigones. The rostral end of the dorsal nucleus of the vagus nerve lies beneath the **vagal triangle** (ala cinerea), and the rostral end of the hypoglossal nucleus lies beneath the **hypoglossal triangle.** The **area postrema** is a narrow strip between the vagal triangle and the margin of the ventricle. The appearance of this part of the rhomboid fossa suggested the tip of a pen to early anatomists, and the term calamus scriptorius (writing pen) was therefore applied to it.

The **facial colliculus,** a slight swelling at the lower end of the **medial eminence** (Fig. 6–3), is formed by fibers from the motor nucleus of the facial nerve looping over the abducens nucleus. There is a pigmented area, the **locus ceruleus,** at the rostral end of the sulcus limitans, indicating the site of a cluster of noradrenergic nerve cells containing melanin pigment. Delicate strands of nerve fibers emerge from the median sulcus, run laterally over the floor of the ventricle as the **striae medullares,** and enter the inferior cerebellar peduncle.

The tent-shaped roof of the fourth ventricle protrudes toward the cerebellum. The forepart of the roof is formed on each side by the superior cerebellar peduncles, which consist mainly of fibers proceeding from cerebellar nuclei into the midbrain. The V-shaped interval between the converging peduncles is bridged by the **superior medullary velum,** a thin sheet of tissue consisting of a layer of pia mater and one of ependyma, with some nerve fibers in between. The remainder of the roof consists of a thin pial-ependymal membrane, the **inferior medullary velum,** which often adheres to the undersurface of the cerebellum. A deficiency of variable size in the membrane constitutes the **median aperture of the fourth ventricle,** alternatively known as the **foramen of Magendie,** which provides the principal communication between the ventricular system and the subarachnoid space (Fig. 6–4).

The lateral walls of the fourth ventricle include the inferior cerebellar peduncles, which curve from the medulla into the cerebellum on the medial aspect of the middle peduncles (Fig. 6–3). Lateral recesses

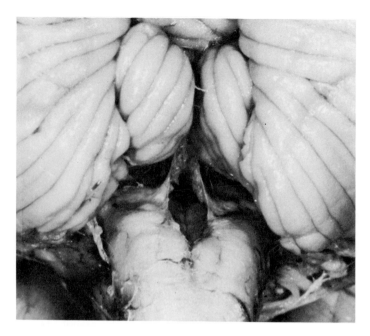

FIGURE 6-4.
Median aperture of the fourth ventricle (foramen of Magendie), opening from the fourth ventricle into the cerebellomedullary cistern of the subarachnoid space. (× 2½)

of the ventricle extend around the sides of the medulla and open ventrally as the **lateral apertures of the fourth ventricle** or the **foramina of Luschka,** through which cerebrospinal fluid enters the subarachnoid space (Fig. 6–5). These foramina are situated at the junction of the medulla, pons, and cerebellum (the cerebellopontine angles) near the attachment to the brain stem of the vestibulocochlear and glossopharyngeal nerves. The choroid plexus of the fourth ventricle is suspended from the inferior medullary velum; the plexus extends into the lateral recesses, and tufts even protrude into the foramina of Luschka.

MIDBRAIN

The ventral surface of the midbrain extends from the pons to the mamillary bodies of the diencephalon (Fig. 6–1). The prominent elevation on each side is formed by the **basis pedunculi** (crus cerebri), which consists of fibers of the pyramidal motor system and corticopontine fibers. Many small blood vessels penetrate

the midbrain in the floor of the **interpeduncular fossa,** and this region is therefore known as the **posterior perforated substance.** The **oculomotor nerve** emerges from the side of the interpeduncular fossa and passes forward through the cavernous venous sinus into the orbit.

The dorsal surface of the midbrain bears four rounded elevations, the paired **inferior** and **superior colliculi** (corpora quadrigemina) (Figs. 6–2 and 6–3). The colliculi make up the **roof** or **tectum** and indicate the extent of the midbrain on the dorsal surface (about 1.5 cm long). The major role of the inferior colliculus is that of a relay nucleus on the auditory pathway to the thalamus and thence to the cerebral cortex. Fibers connecting the inferior colliculus with the specific thalamic nucleus for hearing (medial geniculate nucleus) form an elevation known as the **inferior brachium** (Fig. 6–2 and 6–3). The superior colliculus is involved in the voluntary control of ocular movements and in movements of the eyes and head in response to visual and other stimuli. The **superior brachium** contains fibers proceeding from the

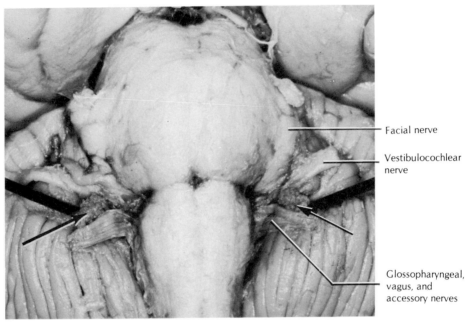

Facial nerve

Vestibulocochlear nerve

Glossopharyngeal, vagus, and accessory nerves

FIGURE 6-5.
Lateral apertures of the fourth ventricle (foramina of Luschka). Tufts of choroid plexus (*arrows*) occupy the foramina, into which marker sticks (*black*) have been inserted. (× 1⅕)

cerebral cortex and the retina to the superior colliculus. Other fibers in the superior brachium terminate in the **pretectal area** just in front of the superior colliculus; these fibers are part of a pathway from the retina for the pupillary light reflex. The **trochlear nerve** emerges from the brain stem immediately caudal to the inferior colliculus, curves around the midbrain, and enters the orbit after traversing the cavernous venous sinus.

The lateral surface of the midbrain (Fig. 6–2) is formed mainly by the **cerebral peduncle,** which constitutes the major portion of this region of the brain stem on each side.

The posterior part of the thalamus grows beyond the plane of transition between the diencephalon and the midbrain during maturation of the brain (Fig. 6–3). Consequently, transverse sections at the level of the superior colliculi include thalamic nuclei, in particular the medial and lateral geniculate nuclei, and a prominent nucleus of the thalamus known as the pulvinar (see Figs. 7–15 and 7–16).

SUGGESTED READING

Bertram EGM, Moore KL: An Atlas of the Human Brain and Spinal Cord. Baltimore, Williams & Wilkins, 1982

Montemurro DG, Bruni JE: The Human Brain in Dissection. Philadelphia, WB Saunders, 1981

Smith CG: Serial Dissections of the Human Brain. Baltimore, Urban & Schwarzenberg, 1981

SEVEN

Brain Stem: Nuclei and Tracts

The principal nuclei and fiber tracts of the brain stem are identified and discussed in this chapter. Long fiber tracts that traverse all or most of the brain stem are noted successively in the medulla, pons, and midbrain. A regional presentation of such tracts is not wholly desirable, and some pathways are reviewed as functional systems in Chapters 19 and 23. Nuclei of cranial nerves are included among the cell groups identified, although a description of the functional components of the cranial nerves is reserved for Chapter 8.

Sections stained by the Weigert method are used as illustrations; the levels of the sections are shown in Figure 7–1. Some tracts are difficult to identify in such sections, although their location has been established by experimental work using laboratory animals and clinicopathological correlations in humans. In the illustrations, therefore, the sites of these tracts are

indicated even though they cannot be distinguished from adjacent white matter.

The reticular formation is mentioned briefly here because the term is used in several contexts in the chapter. The reticular formation of the brain stem consists of neurons in areas not occupied by prominent nuclei or tracts. Most of the constituent cells defy organization into easily identifiable groups, and histological analysis therefore presents a formidable problem. The reticular formation has several functions of primary importance, including the following: an influence on levels of consciousness and degrees of alertness (ascending reticular activating system); a role in the control of movement through efferents to motor nuclei of cranial nerves and especially to the spinal cord; and a contribution to the autonomic nervous system through groups of neurons that function as cardiovascular and respiratory

92

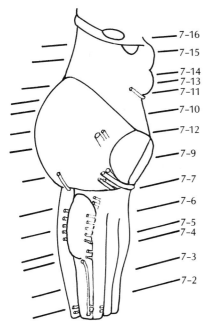

FIGURE 7-1.
Key to levels of the series of Weigert-stained sections of the brain stem that illustrate this chapter.

"centers." In view of its special histological characteristics and functional importance, the reticular formation is discussed separately in Chapter 9, as are several small nuclei of the brain stem.

MEDULLA

There is an extensive rearrangement of gray matter and white matter in the transitional zone between the spinal cord and the medulla, and this zone is coextensive with the pyramidal decussation. The ventral gray horns continue into the region of the decussation, where they include motor cells for the first cervical nerve and the spinal root of the accessory nerve. Here the gray matter is traversed obliquely by bundles of fibers that pass from the pyramids to the lateral corticospinal tracts (Figs. 7–2 and 7–3). Dorsal expansions of the gray matter at the level of the pyramidal decussation form the nuclei gracilis

and cuneatus. The dorsal gray horns of the spinal cord are replaced by the spinal trigeminal nuclei. The medulla has a complex internal structure above the decussation, a structure that is entirely different from that of the spinal cord (Figs. 7–4 through 7–7). The inferior olivary nucleus is the most prominent feature of the rostral half of the medulla. Near the pons, the base of the inferior cerebellar peduncle appears as a distinctive area of white matter in the dorsolateral part of the medulla (Fig. 7–7).

Ascending Pathways

Medial Lemniscus System

It will be recalled that long dorsal funiculus fibers reaching the medulla from the spinal cord transmit impulses for discriminative touch, proprioception, and vibration as an ipsilateral pathway. The **fasciculus gracilis** is concerned with tactile sensations for the leg and lower trunk, whereas impulses that mediate touch and proprioception from the upper trunk, arm, and neck are transmitted in the **fasciculus cuneatus.** Proprioceptive sensation from the lower limb is relayed to the medulla by collateral branches of some of the axons that constitute the dorsal spinocerebellar tract. These branches terminate in the nucleus Z of Brodal and Pompeiano, which is just rostral to the nucleus gracilis. Conduction for the vibratory sense was once thought to be confined to the dorsal funiculus. However, it is now known that a supplementary pathway exists in the lateral funiculus of the spinal cord.

The **nucleus gracilis,** in which fibers of the corresponding fasciculus terminate, is present throughout the closed portion of the medulla. The fibers of the fasciculus cuneatus end in the **nucleus cuneatus,** which first appears slightly rostral to the beginning of the nucleus gracilis and continues beyond the latter nucleus. There is a somatotopic representation in these nu-

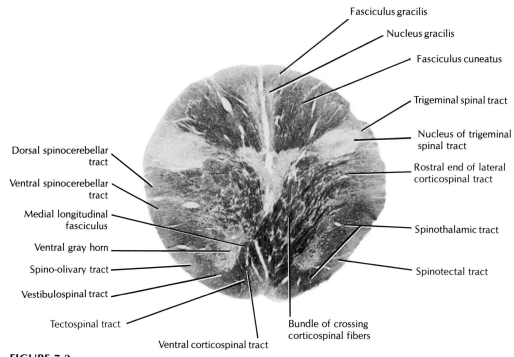

Fasciculus gracilis

Nucleus gracilis

Fasciculus cuneatus

Trigeminal spinal tract

Nucleus of trigeminal spinal tract

Rostral end of lateral corticospinal tract

Spinothalamic tract

Spinotectal tract

Dorsal spinocerebellar tract

Ventral spinocerebellar tract

Medial longitudinal fasciculus

Ventral gray horn

Spino-olivary tract

Vestibulospinal tract

Tectospinal tract

Ventral corticospinal tract

Bundle of crossing corticospinal fibers

FIGURE 7-2.

Junction of the medulla and spinal cord. (Weigert stain, × 5)

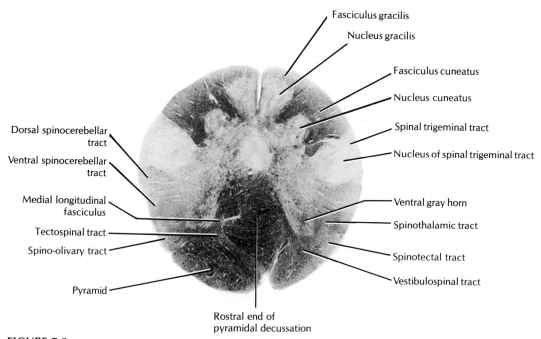

Fasciculus gracilis

Nucleus gracilis

Fasciculus cuneatus

Nucleus cuneatus

Spinal trigeminal tract

Nucleus of spinal trigeminal tract

Ventral gray horn

Spinothalamic tract

Spinotectal tract

Vestibulospinal tract

Dorsal spinocerebellar tract

Ventral spinocerebellar tract

Medial longitudinal fasciculus

Tectospinal tract

Spino-olivary tract

Pyramid

Rostral end of pyramidal decussation

FIGURE 7-3.

Medulla at the rostral end of the pyramidal decussation. (Weigert stain, × 4½)

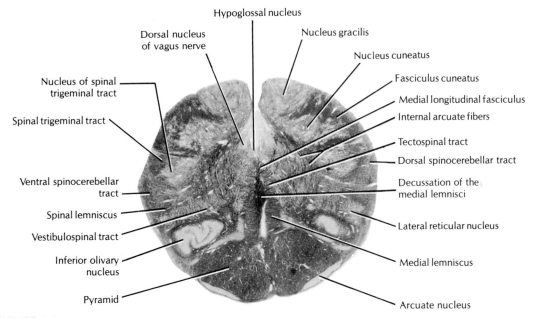

FIGURE 7-4.
Medulla at the caudal end of the inferior olivary nucleus. (Weigert stain, × 4)

clei—that is, fibers entering the spinal cord in a specific segment synapse with a specific group of cells in the nuclei. Such a point-to-point projection of fibers in sensory pathways forms an anatomical basis for recognition of the source of a stimulus.

The myelinated axons of the cells in the nucleus gracilis (and nearby nucleus Z) and the nucleus cuneatus pursue a curved course to the midline as **internal arcuate fibers,** which are shown clearly in Figure 7–4. After crossing the midline in the **decussation of the medial lemnisci,** the fibers turn rostrally in the **medial lemniscus.** This is one of the more substantial tracts of the brain stem, occupying the interval between the midline and the inferior olivary nucleus in the medulla (Figs. 7–4 through 7–7). Fibers conducting data from the contralateral foot are most ventral (*i.e.,* adjacent to the pyramid). The opposite side of the body is then represented sequentially, so that fibers for the neck are in the most dorsal part of the medial lemniscus. After traversing the pons and mid-

brain the tract ends in the thalamic nucleus for general sensation, which is the ventral posterior nucleus of the thalamus. Cervicothalamic fibers from the opposite lateral cervical nucleus (when present) reach the same thalamic nucleus by joining the medial lemniscus.

Spinothalamic and Spinotectal Tracts

The spinothalamic tract for pain, temperature, and touch on the opposite side of the body continues into the medulla without appreciable change in position. This is also true of the spinotectal tract, which conveys somesthetic data to the superior colliculus of the midbrain. However, the two tracts soon merge to form the **spinal lemniscus,** which traverses the lateral area of the medulla dorsal to the inferior olivary nucleus (Figs. 7–4 through 7–7). The spinotectal fibers leave the spinal lemniscus in the rostral midbrain, and the spinothalamic fibers continue to the ventral posterior nucleus of the thalamus. Collateral branches of the same fibers go to the intra-laminar and posterior groups of nuclei of the thalamus. (The thalamic nuclei are de-scribed in Chapter 11.)

Spinoreticular Fibers

Spinoreticular fibers in the ventrolateral white matter of the cord continue into the brain stem, where they synapse with cells of the reticular formation. They transmit somesthetic data, especially that of cuta-neous origin, and data from the viscera. Axons of cells in the reticular formation project caudally to the spinal cord and ros-trally to the thalamus, and impulses trans-mitted by the ascending fibers influence neuronal activity throughout much of the cerebral cortex through a thalamic relay.

There are, therefore, alternative con-duction routes from the spinal cord to the thalamus and cerebral cortex. The direct lemniscal route (medial and spinal lem nisci) proceeds without interruption, mainly to the ventral posterior thalamic nucleus, which in turn projects to the pri-mary sensory area of the cerebral cortex. This is the more recent pathway, which became increasingly important as the thal-amus and cerebral cortex increased in size and functional significance during mam-malian evolution. Alternatively, sensory data reach the intralaminar group of tha-lamic nuclei through an extralemniscal route that involves the reticular formation. The intralaminar nuclei project to the ce-rebral cortex generally. The latter pathway influences levels of consciousness and de-grees of alertness, and is also involved in the awareness (but not the localization) of pain.

The **lateral reticular nucleus,** whose af-ferents include spinoreticular fibers and which is related functionally to the cere-bellum, is an exceptionally distinct group of cells of the reticular formation situated dorsal to the inferior olivary nucleus and near the surface of the medulla (Figs. 7–4, 7–5, and 7–6).

Spinocerebellar Tracts

The **dorsal** and **ventral spinocerebellar tracts** traverse the medulla in the periph-ery of the lateral area (Figs. 7–2 through 7–6). The dorsal tract, which is uncrossed, originates in the nucleus dorsalis (nucleus thoracicus or Clarke's column) of the tho-racic and upper lumbar segments of the spinal cord. The ventral tract, on the other hand, is crossed, and many of the cells of origin are in the lumbosacral enlargement of the cord. The dorsal spinocerebellar fi-bers enter the inferior cerebellar peduncle (Figs. 7–7 and 7–9), whereas the ventral spinocerebellar tract continues through the pons and enters the cerebellum by way of the superior cerebellar peduncle.

Medullary Nuclei Connected with the Cerebellum

Inferior Olivary Complex

Several nuclei in the medulla receive af-ferents from various sources and project to the cerebellum. These nuclei include the components of the inferior olivary com-plex. The largest component is the **inferior olivary nucleus,** which is shaped like a crumpled bag or purse with the hilus fac-ing medially (Figs. 7–5, 7–6, and 7–7). The **medial accessory olivary nucleus** lies be-tween the medial lemniscus and the infe-rior olivary nucleus, and the **dorsal acces-sory olivary nucleus** is immediately dorsal to the inferior olivary nucleus (Fig. 7–6). The relatively small accessory nuclei are phylogenetically older than the principal inferior olivary nucleus. The connections of the inferior olivary complex are sum-marized in Figure 7–8.

The **central tegmental tract** is in part a pathway from the midbrain to the inferior olivary complex. These descending fibers originate in the red nucleus and the peri-aqueductal gray matter, and from neurons elsewhere in the tegmentum of the mid-brain; these sources relay data from the

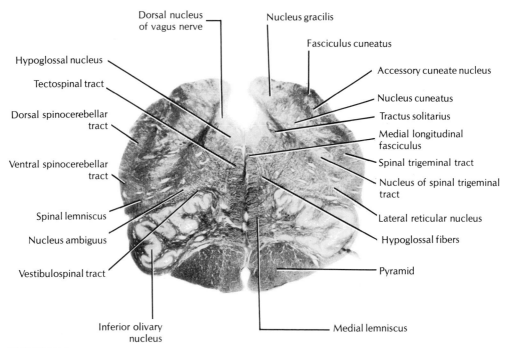

FIGURE 7-5.
Medulla at the level of transition between its closed and open portions. (Weigert stain, × 3)

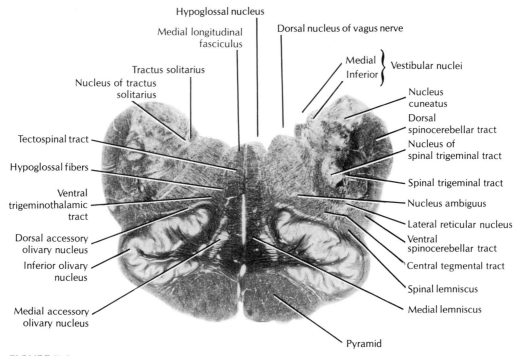

FIGURE 7-6.
Medulla at the midolivary level. (Weigert stain, × 3¼)

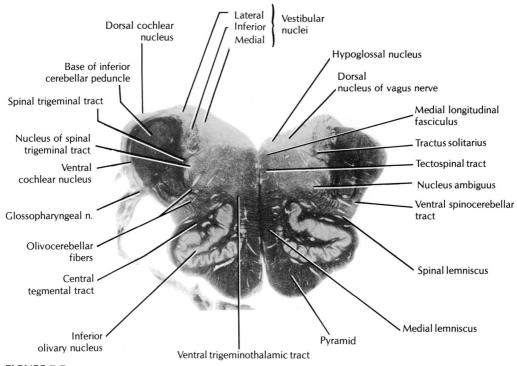

FIGURE 7-7.
Rostral end of the medulla. (Weigert stain, × 2½)

cerebral cortex, the cerebellum, and other sites that have yet to be identified clearly. The terminal portion of the central tegmental tract forms a dense layer on the dorsal surface of the inferior olivary nucleus, best seen in Figure 7–7. The tract also contains numerous ascending fibers that proceed to the diencephalon, many of which originate in the reticular formation of the brain stem.

Other afferents to the inferior olivary complex come from the cerebral cortex, spinal cord, and cerebellum. **Cortico-olivary fibers** originate in the sensorimotor strip of cerebral cortex, lying on each side of the boundary between the frontal and parietal lobes. These fibers, which terminate mainly in the principal nucleus, accompany the corticospinal tract through the midbrain and pons. The inferior oli-

vary nucleus receives impulses originating in proprioceptors by way of afferent fibers from the nucleus Z rostral to the nucleus gracilis and from the nucleus cuneatus. The **spino-olivary tract** continues from the cord into the ventrolateral area of the medulla (Figs. 7–2 and 7–3), and its fibers end in the accessory olivary nuclei. A modest number of **cerebello-olivary fibers,** which are collateral branches of fibers entering the midbrain from the cerebellum through the superior cerebellar peduncle, convey impulses from the central nuclei of the cerebellum.

Olivocerebellar fibers constitute the projection from the inferior olivary complex. Fibers from the principal nucleus occupy its interior and leave through the hilus. After decussating in the midline, the strands of myelinated olivocerebellar fi-

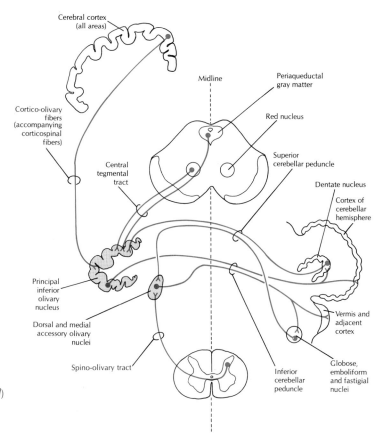

FIGURE 7-8.
Afferent (*blue*) and efferent (*red*)
connections of the inferior
olivary complex of nuclei.

bers curve in a dorsolateral direction and
enter the inferior cerebellar peduncle, of
which they are the largest single component (Fig. 7–7). The accessory olivary nuclei project to regions of the cerebellum
that are concerned with the maintenance
of equilibrium and the generally stereotyped movements of postural changes and
locomotion. The inferior olivary nucleus
projects to the part of the cerebellum that
ensures efficiency of voluntary movements, especially those requiring precision. The inferior olivary complex is the
main source of a type of afferent to the
cerebellar cortex called climbing fibers,
which terminate on, and excite, the Purkinje cells. Physiological studies indicate
that the inferior olivary complex of nuclei
channels programs of instructions into the
cerebellum for subsequent use in the co-

ordination of learned patterns of movement.

Arcuate Nucleus

The arcuate nucleus, on the surface of the
pyramid (Fig. 7–4), receives collateral
branches of corticospinal fibers. Fibers
from the nucleus enter the cerebellum by
way of the inferior cerebellar peduncle,
which they reach by two routes. Some
travel over the lateral surface of the medulla as the external arcuate fibers; the remainder run dorsally in the midline of the
medulla and then laterally in the striae
medullares in the floor of the fourth ventricle. The connections of the arcuate nucleus are similar to those of the cell groups
in the basal portion of the pons—both re-

ceive afferents from the cerebral cortex and project to the cerebellum.

Accessory Cuneate Nucleus

The accessory (lateral) cuneate nucleus is embedded in the fasciculus cuneatus external to the cuneate nucleus (Fig. 7–5). The afferents to the accessory cuneate nucleus are fibers that entered the spinal cord in cervical dorsal roots; many such afferents are in fact collateral branches of fibers that end in the cuneate nucleus. Efferents from the accessory cuneate nucleus, accompanied by a few fibers from the cuneate nucleus, enter the cerebellum by way of the inferior peduncle. These **cuneocerebellar fibers** supplement the dorsal spinocerebellar tract by providing a pathway from proprioceptive and other sensory endings in the neck and upper limb.

Descending Tracts

Corticospinal Tract

The corticospinal (pyramidal) tract is among the larger and more important tracts of the human brain and spinal cord. The parent cell bodies are situated in a substantial area of cerebral cortex that occupies adjoining regions of the frontal and parietal lobes. The corticospinal fibers traverse the medullary center of the cerebral hemisphere and the internal capsule to reach the brain stem. The fibers continue as a compact fasciculus in the basis pedunculi of the midbrain, but the tract is broken up into bundles on entering the basal portion of the pons. These coalesce in the caudal pons, and the corticospinal tract is again a compact fasciculus in the pyramid of the medulla (Figs. 7–4 through 7–7).

Each pyramid contains approximately one million fibers of varying size. The thickest and most rapidly conducting fibers are thought to come from the giant pyramidal cells of Betz in the primary motor area.

The proportion of fibers that cross over in the **decussation of the pyramids** varies among people, but on the average about 85% enter the decussation. The rostral limit of the pyramidal decussation appears in Figure 7–3, and a bundle of fibers passing through the gray matter from a pyramid to the opposite lateral corticospinal tract is shown in Figure 7–2. The 15% of nondecussating fibers continue into the ventral funiculus of the cord as the ventral corticospinal tract. The corticospinal fibers terminate in laminae IV through IX of the spinal gray matter, and a few of them synapse directly with motor neurons. The corticospinal tract is often thought of as being exclusively motor, and this is indeed its major functional aspect. However, it includes axons of cortical origin that terminate on neurons involved in sensory pathways and modulate the transmission of general sensory information to the brain.

Tracts Originating in the Midbrain

The **central tegmental tract** has already been mentioned as arising from the ipsilateral red nucleus and other gray areas of the midbrain. It runs caudally in the lateral area, dorsal to the inferior olivary nucleus, throughout most of the medulla (Fig. 7–7), and terminates in the inferior olivary complex. A bundle of axons from the contralateral red nucleus continues caudally as the **rubrospinal tract,** which comes to occupy a position just ventral to the lateral corticospinal tract in the spinal cord. Rubrospinal fibers are numerous in most mammals, but in humans the tract consists of only a few fibers that end in the upper two cervical segments of the spinal cord.

The **tectospinal tract** originates in the superior colliculus of the midbrain, and the fibers cross at that level to the opposite side of the brain stem. The tract lies next to the midline and dorsal to the medial lemniscus throughout most of the medulla (Figs. 7–4 through 7–7). The tectospinal tract is deflected ventrally at the level of the pyramidal decussation (Figs. 7–2 and 7–3), and continues into the ventral funiculus of the spinal cord.

Nuclei of Cranial Nerves and Associated Tracts

Hypoglossal, Accessory, Vagus, and Glossopharyngeal Nerves

The **hypoglossal nucleus** for innervation of the tongue muscles consists of a column of motor cells near the midline throughout most of the medulla. The nucleus is situated in the central gray matter in the closed part of the medulla (Fig. 7–4) and beneath the hypoglossal triangle of the rhomboid fossa (Figs. 7–5, 7–6, and 7–7). The myelinated axons leaving the nucleus are directed ventrally between the medial lemniscus and the inferior olivary nucleus (Figs. 7–5 and 7–6); they continue lateral to the pyramid and emerge as the hypoglossal nerve roots along the ventrolateral sulcus. The **nucleus ambiguus** is situated dorsal to the inferior olivary nucleus in the position shown in Figures 7–5, 7–6, and 7–7. This important cell column supplies muscles of the soft palate, pharynx, larynx, and upper esophagus through the cranial root of the accessory nerve and the vagus and glossopharyngeal nerves. It also contains parasympathetic neurons whose axons end in the cardiac ganglia and control the heart rate. The **dorsal nucleus of the vagus nerve** is the largest of the parasympathetic nuclei in the brain stem; it contains the cell bodies of preganglionic neurons for smooth muscle and for glandular elements of the thoracic and abdominal viscera. The nucleus lies lateral to the hypoglossal nucleus in the gray matter surrounding the central canal (Fig. 7–4), and extends rostrally beneath the vagal triangle of the rhomboid fossa (Figs. 7–5, 7–6, and 7–7).

There is a bundle of visceral afferent fibers known as the **tractus solitarius,** which lies along the lateral side of the dorsal nucleus of the vagus nerve (Figs. 7–5, 7–6, and 7–7). This tract consists of caudally directed fibers whose cell bodies are in the inferior ganglia of the vagus and glossopharyngeal nerves and in the geniculate ganglion of the facial nerve. The fibers terminate in the **nucleus of the tractus solitarius,** a column of cells that lies adjacent to, and partly surrounds the tract. The vagal and glossopharyngeal afferents have an important role in visceral reflexes, and transmit impulses for taste from the epiglottis and posterior one third of the tongue. The fibers contributed by the facial nerve are for taste in the anterior two thirds of the tongue and in the palate.

Vestibulocochlear Nerve

Nuclei in which the cochlear and vestibular divisions of the eighth cranial nerve terminate are situated in the rostral part of the medulla. The **dorsal cochlear nucleus,** lying on the base of the inferior cerebellar peduncle, is shown in Figure 7–7, and a portion of the **ventral cochlear nucleus** appears lateral to the peduncle in the same figure. Fibers leaving the cochlear nuclei are noted later in the description of the pons.

The **vestibular nuclear complex,** situated beneath the vestibular area of the rhomboid fossa, is divided into **superior, lateral, medial,** and **inferior vestibular nuclei** according to their cytoarchitecture and connections. The superior nucleus is in the pons, in the position shown in Figure 7–9, whereas the remaining nuclei are in the medulla (Figs. 7–6 and 7–7). The vestibular nerve penetrates the brain stem deep to the fibers of the inferior cerebellar peduncle. This occurs slightly rostral to the attachment of the cochlear nerve, so the vestibular nerve is not included in Figure 7–7. Most vestibular nerve fibers terminate in the vestibular nuclear complex, and the remainder enter the cerebellum through the inferior peduncle. Descending branches of vestibular nerve fibers that terminate in the inferior vestibular nucleus, together with vestibulospinal fibers from the lateral vestibular nucleus, give the inferior nucleus a stippled appearance in sections (Fig. 7–7). In addition to the primary vestibulocerebellar fibers, numerous secondary fibers proceed from the vestibular nuclei into the cerebellum through the inferior peduncle.

Vestibular nuclei project to the spinal cord by way of two tracts. The larger of these is the **vestibulospinal tract,** for which the cells of origin are in the lateral vestibular (Deiters') nucleus. Vestibulospinal fibers run caudally, dorsal to the inferior olivary nucleus, in the position indicated in Figures 7–4 and 7–5. The tract is deflected ventrally at the level of the pyramidal decussation (Figs. 7–2 and 7–3), and continues into the ipsilateral ventral funiculus of the spinal cord.

Fibers from the vestibular nuclei account for most of those in the **medial longitudinal fasciculus,** which extends rostrally and caudally adjacent to the midline. (The ascending fibers will be identified later for the pons and midbrain.) The parent cell bodies of the descending fibers are in the medial vestibular nucleus, and are mainly ipsilateral. The fasciculus is dorsal to the tectospinal tract until the level of the pyramidal decussation is reached (Figs. 7–4 through 7–7). It is then deflected ventrally (Figs. 7–2 and 7–3) and continues into the ventral white matter of the spinal cord. The tectospinal tract is deflected ventrally in a similar manner. The fibers of the medial longitudinal fasciculus and the tectospinal tract are joined by the ventral corticospinal tract below the pyramidal decussation, and there is considerable intermingling of the three categories of fibers in the ventral funiculus of the cervical cord.

Trigeminal Nerve

The trigeminal nerve contributes a tract and associated nucleus to the internal structure of the medulla. Many fibers of the trigeminal sensory root turn caudally on entering the pons. They constitute the **spinal trigeminal tract,** so named because some of the fibers extend as far as the third cervical segment of the spinal cord. The spinal tract transmits data for pain, temperature, and touch from the extensive area of distribution of the trigeminal nerve. The fibers terminate in the subjacent **nucleus of the spinal trigeminal tract.** The tract and nucleus lie deep to the root of the inferior cerebullar peduncle and the dorsal spinocerebellar tract in the rostral part of the medulla (Figs. 7–4 through 7–7). More caudally, they lie under the surface area of the medulla known as the tuberculum cinereum (Figs. 7–2 and 7–3). Many of the descending fibers are unmyelinated or thinly myelinated, and the nucleus consists principally of small neurons. The spinal trigeminal tract and its nucleus share, therefore, some structural and functional characteristics with the dorsolateral tract of Lissauer and laminae I through IV of the spinal gray matter. The **ventral trigeminothalamic tract** (Fig. 7–6) is a crossed fasciculus that arises from neurons in the nucleus of the spinal tract (and the pontine trigeminal nucleus) and in the adjacent part of the reticular formation, and ends in the ventral posterior nucleus of the thalamus. Conducting sensory data from the head, the ventral trigeminothalamic tract is comparable functionally to the spinothalamic tract for the body generally.

PONS

The main features in Weigert-stained sections through the pons are its division into basal (ventral) and dorsal regions, and the prominent cerebellar peduncles (Figs.

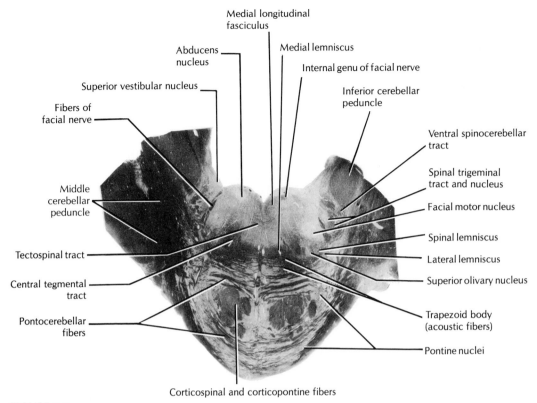

FIGURE 7-9.
Caudal region of the pons. (Weigert stain, × 2⅖)

7–9 and 7–10). The basal portion consists of longitudinal fiber bundles, transverse fibers, and collections of nerve cells in the intervals between longitudinal and transverse fasciculi. The longitudinal bundles are numerous and small at rostral levels (Figs. 7–10 and 7–11), although many of them coalesce as they approach the medulla (Fig. 7–9). The inferior and middle cerebellar peduncles appear in Figure 7–9, and the superior peduncles in Figure 7–10.

Dorsal Portion (Tegmentum)

The pontine tegmentum is structurally similar to the medulla and midbrain. There are therefore tracts that were en-

countered in the medulla, together with components of several cranial nerves.

Ascending and Descending Tracts; Inferior and Superior Cerebellar Peduncles

The **medial lemniscus** "rotates" in passing from the medulla into the pons, where it takes up a position in the most ventral part of the tegmentum. The lemniscus has a roughly oval outline at the level shown in Figure 7–9; it moves laterally farther forward and becomes straplike in shape (Figs. 7–10 and 7–11). The medial lemniscus rotates in such a way that fibers from the nucleus cuneatus are medial to those from the nucleus gracilis. The somatotopic representation is therefore neck, arm, trunk, and leg, in a medial to lateral se-

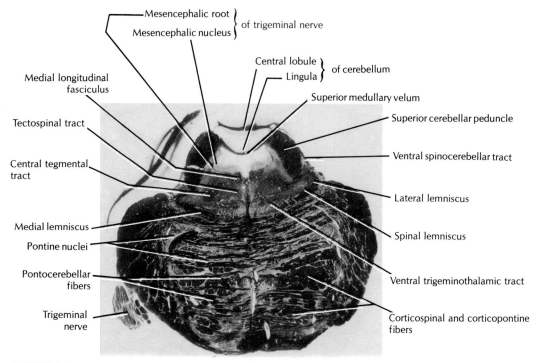

FIGURE 7-10.
Pons at approximately midlevel. (Weigert stain, × 2⅓)

quence. The **spinal lemniscus** is situated near the lateral edge of the medial lemniscus throughout the pons (Figs. 7–9, 7–10, and 7–11). The **ventral spinocerebellar tract** traverses the most lateral part of the tegmentum (Fig. 7–9) and then curves dorsally and enters the cerebellum through the superior peduncle (Figs. 7–10 and 7–12).

With respect to descending tracts, the **central tegmental tract** is medial to the fibers of the superior cerebellar peduncle at the level of the pontine isthmus (Fig. 7–11), in the central area of the tegmentum at midpons levels (Fig. 7–10), and just dorsal to the medial lemniscus in the caudal region of the pons (Fig. 7–9). The **tectospinal tract** is near the midline in the pontine tegmentum (Figs. 7–9, 7–10, and 7–11), a position that is maintained throughout the course of this tract in the medulla and spinal cord.

The **inferior cerebellar peduncles** enter the cerebellum from the caudal part of the pons. In this location, they are on the medial aspects of the middle cerebellar peduncles, forming the lateral walls of the fourth ventricle (Fig. 7–9). Olivocerebellar fibers are the most numerous in the inferior peduncle, followed by fibers of the dorsal spinocerebellar tract. Smaller components are contributed by cuneocerebellar fibers from the accessory cuneate nucleus, by fibers from the arcuate nucleus and the reticular formation of the medulla, and by others from the pontine trigeminal nucleus and nucleus of the spinal tract of the trigeminal nerve. The region of the inferior cerebellar peduncle immediately adjoining the fourth ventricle consists of fibers entering the cerebellum from the vestibular nerve and vestibular nuclei, together with cerebellar efferents from portions of the cerebellum that are concerned

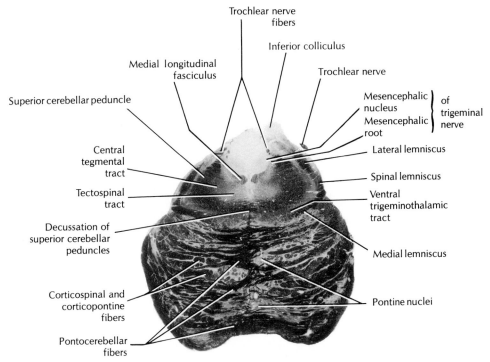

FIGURE 7-11.
Rostral portion of the pons, including the isthmus region of the pontine tegmentum. (Weigert stain, × 2⅕)

with maintaining equilibrium. The latter fibers terminate in vestibular nuclei and in the reticular formation of the medulla and pontine tegmentum.

The **superior cerebellar peduncles** (Fig. 7–10) consist mainly of cerebellar efferent fibers that originate in cerebellar nuclei and enter the brain stem immediately caudal to the inferior colliculi of the midbrain. The fibers cross the midline at the level of the inferior colliculi in the **decussation of the superior cerebellar peduncles** (Fig. 7–11, 7–13, and 7–14). Most of them continue rostrally to a thalamic nucleus (ventral lateral nucleus) from which fibers project to the motor cortex in the frontal lobe, and the remainder end in the red nucleus and in the reticular formation. The superior cerebellar peduncles also contain fibers that enter the cer-

ebellum. These consist of the ventral spinocerebellar tract and of some fibers from the red nucleus and from the mesencephalic nucleus of the trigeminal nerve.

Nuclei of Cranial Nerves and Associated Tracts

Vestibulocochlear Nerve

Fibers from the cochlear nuclei cross the pons to ascend in the lateral lemniscus of the opposite side. These slender bundles of auditory (acoustic) fibers are directed across the brain stem in the deepest part of the tegmentum, and it is difficult to distinguish them from nearby fascicles of pontocerebellar fibers. The transverse strands of acoustic fibers, some of which intersect the medial lemniscus, compose the **trapezoid body** (Fig. 7–9). Some fibers from the cochlear nuclei end in the **superior olivary nucleus** (Fig. 7–9) of either side, from which efferent fibers are added to the auditory pathway. Fibers originating in the cochlear and superior olivary nuclei turn rostrally in the lateral part of the tegmentum to form the **lateral lemniscus** (Fig. 7–9). This tract is situated at the lateral edge of the medial lemniscus in the first part of its course (Fig. 7–10), and then moves dorsally to end in the inferior colliculus of the midbrain (Fig. 7–11). The auditory pathway continues through the inferior brachium to the medial geniculate nucleus of the thalamus, and then to the auditory area of cortex in the temporal lobe.

Of the four vestibular nuclei, only the **superior vestibular nucleus** is as far rostral as the level shown in Figure 7–9. Fibers from all the vestibular nuclei, some crossed and some uncrossed, ascend in the **medial longitudinal fasciculus,** which runs near the midline and close to the floor of the fourth ventricle throughout the pons (Figs. 7–9, 7–10, and 7–11). The fibers terminate mainly in the abducens, trochlear, and oculomotor nuclei; the connections thereby established coordinate movements of the eyes with movements of the head. The medial longitudinal fasciculus also contains other groups of fibers concerned with movement of the eyes. These are discussed in Chapter 8.

Facial and Abducens Nerves

The **motor nucleus of the facial nerve** for the muscles of expression consists of a prominent group of typical motor neurons in the ventrolateral part of the tegmentum (Fig. 7–9). Fibers from the nucleus course in a dorsomedial direction and then form a compact bundle, the **internal genu,** which loops over the caudal end of the abducens nucleus beneath the facial colliculus of the rhomboid fossa. The bundle of fibers that forms the genu then runs for-

ward along the medial side of the abducens nucleus and curves again over its rostral end (right side of Fig. 7–9). After leaving the genu, the fibers pass between the nucleus of origin and the nucleus of the spinal trigeminal tract, emerging as the motor root of the facial nerve at the junction of the pons and medulla.

The **abducens nucleus,** for innervation of the lateral rectus muscle of the eye, is located beneath the facial colliculus, as noted above (see Fig. 7–9). The efferent fibers of the nucleus proceed in a ventral direction, with a caudal inclination, and leave the brain stem as the abducens nerve between the pons and the pyramid of the medulla.

Trigeminal Nerve

The **spinal trigeminal tract** and **nucleus** are situated in the lateral part of the tegmentum of the caudal portion of the pons (Fig. 7–9). The pontine tegmentum also contains two additional trigeminal nuclei, the pontine trigeminal and motor nuclei (Fig. 7–12). The **pontine trigeminal nucleus** (also known as the chief, or principal, nucleus) is situated at the rostral end of the spinal trigeminal nucleus and receives fibers for touch, especially discriminative touch. Fibers from the pontine trigeminal nucleus project to the thalamus, along with fibers from the nucleus of the spinal tract, in the **ventral trigeminothalamic tract** (Figs. 7–10 and 7–11). A **dorsal trigeminothalamic tract,** consisting of crossed and uncrossed fibers, originates in the pontine trigeminal nuclei exclusively. (Alternatively, all the trigeminothalamic fibers are said to compose the **trigeminal lemniscus.**) The **motor nucleus,** which is medial to the pontine trigeminal nucleus (Fig. 7–12), consists of typical motor neurons for the muscles of mastication and a few other muscles.

The **mesenecephalic nucleus of the trigeminal nerve** is a slender strand of cells beneath the lateral edge of the rostral part

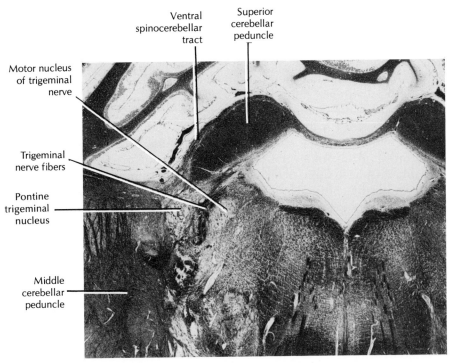

Motor nucleus of trigeminal nerve

Ventral spinocerebellar tract

Superior cerebellar peduncle

Trigeminal nerve fibers

Pontine trigeminal nucleus

Middle cerebellar peduncle

FIGURE 7-12.
Portion of a section through the middle of the pons, at the level of the pontine and motor nuclei of the trigeminal nerve. (This particular level was missing from the series of Weigert-stained sections that illustrate this chapter. This figure is from another brain specimen. × 5½)

of the fourth ventricle (Figs. 7–10 and 7–11), extending into the midbrain. These unipolar cells are unusual because they are cell bodies of primary sensory neurons and the only such cells that are not in cerebrospinal ganglia. Fibers from the nucleus form the **mesencephalic root of the trigeminal nerve** (Figs. 7–10 and 7–11); most of them are distributed through the mandibular division of the nerve to proprioceptive endings in the muscles of mastication.

Basal Portion

The basal or ventral portion of the pons (Figs. 7–9, 7–10, and 7–11) is especially large in humans because of its relationship to those parts of the cortex of the cerebral and cerebellar hemispheres that increased in size and functional importance during mammalian evolution.

The longitudinal fasciculi consist of fibers that entered the pons from the basis pedunculi of the midbrain. Many of them are **corticospinal fibers** that pass through the pons to reassemble as the pyramids of the medulla. The fasciculi also contain numerous **corticopontine fibers,** which originate in widespread areas of cerebral cortex and establish synaptic contact with cells of the **pontine nuclei** of the same side. Except in the caudal one third of the pons, in which there are large regions of pontine gray matter (Fig. 7–9), the pontine nuclei are small groups of cells scattered among the longitudinal and transverse fasciculi (Figs. 7–10 and 7–11). The nuclei consist of small and medium-sized polygonal cells. Their axons cross the midline, forming the conspicuous transverse bundles of **pontocerebellar fibers,** and enter the cerebellum through the **middle cerebellar peduncle.** Data from the cerebral cortex, in which most of the neural events underlying volitional movements occur, are made available to the cerebellar cortex through the relay in the pontine nuclei. Activity in the cerebellar cortex influences motor area in the frontal lobe of the cerebral hemisphere through a pathway that includes the dentate nucleus of the cerebellum and the ventral lateral nucleus of the thalamus. The well-developed circuit linking the cerebral and cerebellar cortices contributes to precision and efficiency of voluntary movements.

MIDBRAIN

The internal structure of the midbrain is illustrated in Figures 7–13 through 7–16. The sections shown in Figures 7–13 and 7–14 are through the inferior colliculi. The planes of the sections are such that Figure 7–13 includes the basal pons and Figure 7–14 shows the extreme rostral lip of the basal pons (see Fig. 7–1). Figures 7–15 and 7–16 illustrate more rostral levels that include the superior colliculi. These also include certain thalamic nuclei that are in the transverse plane of the rostral midbrain.

For descriptive purposes the midbrain is divided into the following regions (refer to Fig. 7–15 for their identification): the **tectum** or **roof,** which is special to this part of the brain stem, consists of the paired inferior and superior colliculi (corpora quadrigemina); the **basis pedunculi** is a dense mass of descending fibers; the **substantia nigra** appears as a prominent zone of gray matter, immediately dorsal to the basis pedunculi; and the remainder of the midbrain comprises the **tegmentum,** which contains fiber tracts, the prominent red nuclei, and the periaqueductal gray matter surrounding the cerebral aqueduct (aqueduct of Sylvius). The term **cerebral**

peduncle refers to all of the midbrain, on each side, exclusive of the tectum.

Tectum and Associated Tracts

Inferior Colliculus

The inferior colliculus, which consists of a large nucleus made up of small and medium-sized cells, is incorporated into the auditory pathway to the cerebral cortex. Fibers of the lateral lemniscus envelop the nucleus and enter it from superficial and deep aspects (Fig. 7–13). Fibers from the nucleus of the inferior colliculus traverse the inferior brachium to reach the medial geniculate nucleus of the thalamus (Figs. 7–14, 7–15, and 7–16), which in turn projects to the auditory area of cortex in the temporal lobe. There are commissural fibers between the inferior colliculi, accounting in part for the bilateral cortical projection from each ear. The inferior colliculi evolved as increasingly significant structures in mammals concurrent with the development of the cortical area for hearing.

Some fibers from the inferior colliculus pass forward into the superior colliculus. From the latter site, through a polysynaptic pathway described in Chapter 8, nerve impulses reach cranial nerve nuclei that supply the extraocular muscles, and tectospinal fibers influence spinal motor neurons in the cervical region. A pathway is thereby established for reflex turning of the eyes and head toward the source of an unexpected sound.

Superior Colliculus

The superior colliculi (Figs. 7–15 and 7–16) differ from the inferior colliculi both in phylogenetic background and in function. The optic tectum of the midbrain in lower vertebrates is the homologue of the superior colliculi. The optic tectum constitutes an important integrating center for visual and somesthetic data, especially in

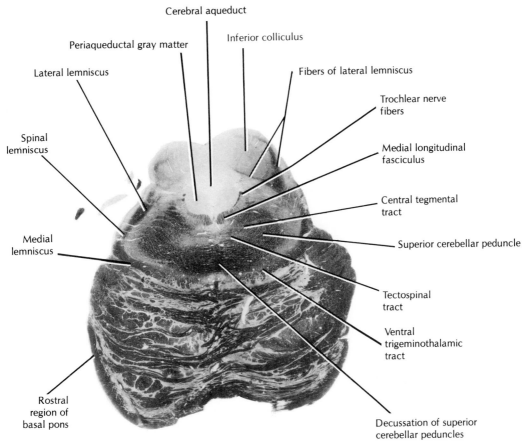

Cerebral aqueduct

Periaqueductal gray matter

Inferior colliculus

Lateral lemniscus

Fibers of lateral lemniscus

Trochlear nerve fibers

Spinal lemniscus

Medial longitudinal fasciculus

Central tegmental tract

Medial lemniscus

Superior cerebellar peduncle

Tectospinal tract

Ventral trigeminothalamic tract

Rostral region of basal pons

Decussation of superior cerebellar peduncles

FIGURE 7-13.
Section through the basal pons and inferior colliculi of the midbrain. (Weigert stain, × 3)

fishes and amphibia, in which it is larger than the telencephalon. In some of the lower mammals, such as rodents, most of the axons of the optic tract terminate in the superior colliculus. In higher mammals, including humans, most of the fibers constituting the visual pathway from the retina go to the lateral geniculate nucleus of the thalamus instead. The importance of the optic tectum in lower vertebrates has left an imprint in the human superior colliculus in the form of a complex histological structure consisting of seven alternating layers of white matter and gray matter.

The cortex of the occipital lobe is an important source of afferent fibers to the superior colliculus in humans. Corticotec-tal fibers come from the primary visual area and from the visual association cortex in the occipital lobe; this cortex surrounds the primary visual area on which the retina projects after a synaptic relay in the lateral geniculate nucleus of the thalamus. Other corticotectal afferents are derived from an area of the frontal lobe called the frontal eye field. Corticotectal fibers (which are ipsilateral) make up most of the **superior brachium,** which reaches the superior colliculus by passing between two thalamic nuclei, the pulvinar and the medial geniculate nucleus (Figs. 7–15 and 7–16). Through collicular efferents (to be described), this connection between the cortex and the superior colliculus is re-

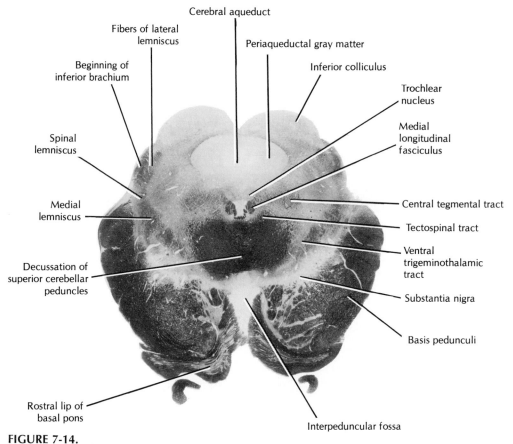

FIGURE 7-14.

Midbrain at the level of the rostral portions of the inferior colliculi. (Weigert stain, × 3)

sponsible for both voluntary and involuntary movements of the eyes and head, as when rapidly shifting the direction of gaze (saccadic movements) or when following objects passing across the visual field (smooth pursuit movements). Corticotectal fibers originating in the occipital cortex also appear to function in the ocular response of accommodation (*i.e.*, thickening of the lens and constriction of the pupil), which accompanies convergence of the eyes when viewing a near object.

Some fibers of the optic tract, originating in the retina, reach the superior colliculus by way of the superior brachium. These fibers constitute the afferent limb of a reflex pathway that assists in turning of the eyes and head in order to follow an object moving across the field of vision. In addition, spinotectal fibers terminate in the superior colliculus and transmit data from general sensory endings, of which those in the skin are the most important. The connections thereby established presumably function in directing the eyes and head toward the source of cutaneous stimuli.

Efferents from the superior colliculus are distributed to the spinal cord and nuclei of the brain stem. Fibers destined for the spinal cord curve around the periaqueductal gray matter, cross to the opposite side in the **dorsal tegmental decussation** (of Meynert), and continue caudally near the midline as the **tectospinal tract** (Figs. 7–13 and 7–14). Efferents to the

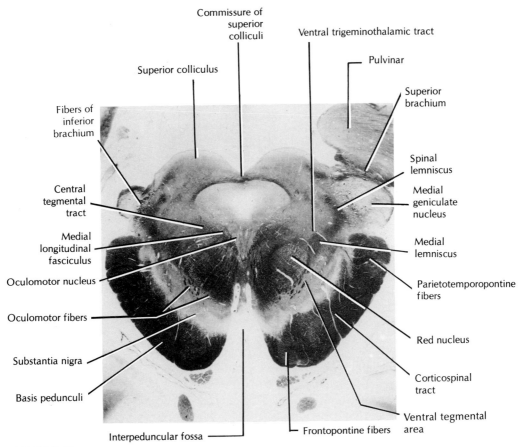

FIGURE 7-15.
Midbrain at the level of the superior colliculi. (Weigert stain, × 3)

brain stem (tectobulbar fibers) are for the most part directed bilaterally. They go to the pretectal area, to the accessory oculomotor nuclei, and to the paramedian pontine reticular formation. These regions project to the nuclei of the oculomotor, trochlear, and abducens nerves, which supply the eye muscles. (Neural control of these muscles is discussed in Chapter 8.) Other efferent fibers from the superior colliculus terminate in the reticular formation near the motor nucleus of the facial nerve, providing a reflex pathway for protective closure of the eyelids when there is a sudden visual stimulus. Still other efferents terminate in the red nucleus. An indirect projection to the cerebellum consists of

tectopontine fibers to the dorsolateral region of the nuclei pontis in the basal pons and pontocerebellar fibers in the contralateral middle cerebellar peduncle.

The superior colliculi are interconnected by the **commissure of the superior colliculi** (Figs. 7–15 and 7–16). The **posterior commissure** is a robust bundle running transversely, just dorsal to the transition between the cerebral aqueduct and the third ventricle. A small piece of the commissure in the midline is included in the section illustrated in Figure 7–16. In spite of the substantial size of the posterior commissure, the source and termination of its fibers are not all known. Some have been identified as coming from the supe-

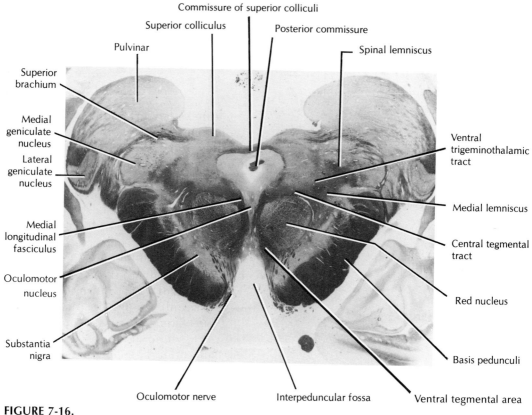

FIGURE 7-16.

Midbrain at the level of the rostral portions of the superior colliculi. (Weigert stain, × 2)

rior colliculus and the following smaller nuclei nearby: pretectal area, habenular nuclei (in the epithalamus of the diencephalon), and the accessory oculomotor nuclei.

Pretectal Area

The pretectal area consists of four small nuclei that are situated immediately in front of the lateral edge of the superior colliculus. The pretectal area receives fibers from the retina by way of the optic tract and the superior brachium. These fibers are probably all collateral branches of axons destined for the lateral geniculate nucleus of the thalamus. Efferent fibers travel to the Edinger–Westphal nucleus

(origin of preganglionic parasympathetic fibers in the oculomotor nerve) of each side. The pretectal area is thereby included in a reflex pathway for the pupillary response to light, with the pupils becoming smaller as the intensity of light increases. Other afferents to the pretectal area come from the superior colliculus, the visual cortex, and the frontal eye fields, and other efferent fibers go from the pretectal area to the accessory oculomotor nuclei. Through these connections, the pretectal area is included in the pathways for the cortical control of eye movement (Chap. 8).

Both the pretectal area and the superior colliculus send some fibers to the nuclei comprising the pulvinar of the thalamus.

In some laboratory animals, neurons in the pretectal area have axons that enter the optic tract and terminate in the retina.

Tegmentum

Fasciculi Proceeding to the Thalamus

The **medial lemniscus** continues to be a readily identifiable fasciculus as it traverses the midbrain in the lateral area of the tegmentum to its termination in the ventral posterior nucleus of the thalamus (Figs. 7–14, 7–15, and 7–16). The **spinal lemniscus** is dorsolateral to the medial lemniscus, this spatial relationship being continued from the pontine tegmentum. Spinotectal fibers leave the spinal lemniscus to enter the superior colliculus, and some end in the periaqueductal gray matter. The spinothalamic fibers continue into the diencephalon, where they end in the ventral posterior nucleus of the thalamus and, in smaller numbers, in other thalamic nuclei.

Red Nucleus and Associated Tracts

The red nucleus is a prominent motor component of the tegmentum. The nucleus is egg-shaped (round in transverse section), extending from the caudal limit of the superior colliculus into the subthalamic region of the diencephalon. The nucleus has a pinkish hue in a fresh specimen because it is more vascular than the surrounding tissue. Myelinated nerve fibers passing through the nucleus give it a punctate appearance in Weigert-stained sections (Figs. 7–15 and 7–16).

The red nucleus is differentiated into two regions, the **pars magnocellularis**, consisting of large cells in the midst of small neurons, and the **pars parvicellularis**, which contains small cells only. The former, which occupies the caudal region of the nucleus, is strongly developed in lower mammals but is rudimentary in hu-

mans. The converse is true for the small-celled portion, which accounts for nearly all of the human red nucleus.

Although some of the connections of the red nucleus are well known, the evidence for others is equivocal and they are still under investigation. Those afferents that come from the cerebellum and the cerebral cortex are best documented. Fibers originating in the cerebellar nuclei constitute the superior cerebellar peduncles and enter the midbrain. Some of these fibers terminate in the red nucleus, whereas the majority pass through or around it en route to a thalamic nucleus (the ventral lateral nucleus), which in turn projects to the motor cortex of the frontal lobe. This same cortex gives rise to numerous corticorubral fibers, and there are afferents to the red nucleus from the superior colliculus.

In regard to efferent connections of the red nucleus, fibers of the rubrospinal tract cross the midline in the **ventral tegmental decussation** (of Forel) and continue through the brain stem into the lateral funiculus of the spinal cord. Since the tract originates in the pars magnocellularis, it is a minor pathway in the human brain, and its few fibers terminate in the first two segments of the cervical spinal gray matter. Some descending fibers accompany the rubrospinal fibers initially and then end in the motor nucleus of the facial nerve as well as in those nuclei of the reticular formation that project to the cerebellum. In addition to these crossed projections, rubro-olivary fibers travel in the ipsilateral central tegmental tract to terminate in the inferior olivary complex, which projects across the midline to the cerebellum. These fibers originate in the pars parvicellularis, and are therefore abundant in the human brain. A few direct rubrocerebellar fibers traverse the superior cerebellar peduncles and end in certain central nuclei of the cerebellum (globose and emboliform nuclei).

Nuclei of Cranial Nerves and Associated Tracts

Vestibulocochlear Nerve

Certain tracts that originate in the sensory nuclei of cranial nerves continue into the midbrain, and two of them are associated with the vestibulocochlear nerve. The **lateral lemniscus** for auditory conduction was identified in the discussion of the inferior colliculus. The **medial longitudinal fasciculus** is situated adjacent to the midline (Figs. 7–13 through 7–16), in the same general position as at lower brain stem levels. Most of its fibers originate in vestibular nuclei, and those reaching the midbrain terminate in the trochlear, oculomotor, and accessory oculomotor nuclei. The fasciculus also contains association fibers connecting the abducens, trochlear, and oculomotor nuclei.

Trigeminal Nerve

The **ventral trigeminothalamic tract,** which arises from the nucleus of the spinal tract and the pontine trigeminal nucleus, continues through the midbrain near the medial lemniscus (Figs. 7–13 through 7–16). **Dorsal trigeminothalamic fibers** from the pontine trigeminal nuclei of both sides traverse the midbrain tegmentum some distance dorsal to the ventral tract. The **mesencephalic nucleus** of the trigeminal nerve continues from the pons into the lateral region of the periaqueductal gray matter throughout most of the midbrain.

Trochlear and Oculomotor Nerves

The **trochlear nucleus** is in the periaqueductal gray matter at the level of the inferior colliculus, where it lies just dorsal to the medial longitudinal fasciculus (Fig. 7–14). Fibers from the nucleus curve dorsally around the periaqueductal gray matter, with a caudal slope (Figs. 7–11 and 7–13). On reaching the dorsal surface of the brain stem, the fibers decussate in the superior medullary velum and emerge as the trochlear nerves just behind the inferior colliculi. The trochlear nerve supplies the superior oblique muscle of the eye.

The **oculomotor nucleus** is in the ventral part of the periaqueductal gray matter at the level of the superior colliculus; the paired nuclei have a V-shaped outline in sections (Figs. 7–15 and 7–16). Bundles of fibers from the nucleus pursue a curved course through the tegmentum, with many of them passing through the red nucleus (Fig. 7–15), and then emerge along the side of the interpeduncular fossa to form the oculomotor nerve (Fig. 7–16). The oculomotor nerve supplies the extraocular muscles, with the exception of the lateral rectus and superior oblique. It also supplies the striated fibers of the levator palpebrae superioris muscle. The oculomotor nucleus includes a parasympathetic component, the **Edinger–Westphal nucleus,** for the ciliary and sphincter pupillae muscles of the eye.

Substantia Nigra; Ventral Tegmental Area

The substantia nigra is a large nucleus, situated between the tegmentum and the basis pedunculi throughout the midbrain (Figs. 7–14, 7–15, and 7–16), and extending into the subthalamic region of the diencephalon. The nucleus is rudimentary in lower vertebrates, makes its first definitive appearance in mammals, and is largest in the human brain. The neurons are multipolar and of medium size. The dopaminergic cells composing the **pars compacta** adjacent to the tegmentum contain cytoplasmic inclusion granules of melanin pigment. These pigment-containing cells are most numerous in primates, especially in humans. The number of melanin granules is few at birth, increases rapidly during childhood, and then more slowly throughout life. The pigment is present in albinos.

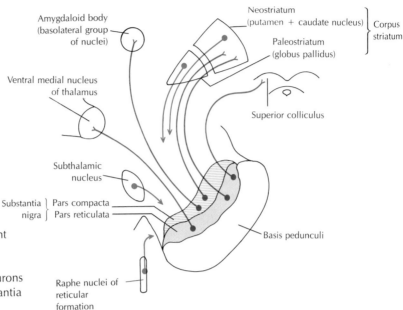

FIGURE 7-17.
Afferent (*blue*) and efferent
(*red*) connections of the
substantia nigra. Afferent
fibers terminate upon neurons
of both parts of the substantia
nigra.

The region of the nucleus bordering the basis pedunculi consists of cells lacking pigment and is called the **pars reticulata.** It is extensively penetrated by the dendrites of the cells of the pars compacta, so that afferent fibers are likely to synapse with neurons of both parts of the substantia nigra. These afferents arise from the corpus striatum (caudate and lentiform nuclei) and, in smaller numbers, from the subthalamic nucleus and from the raphe nuclei of the midbrain and pontine reticular formation. Efferent fibers arising from the cells of the pars compacta go mainly to the neostriatum (caudate nucleus plus the outer part, known as the putamen, of the lentiform nucleus). Some also end in the amygdaloid body in the temporal lobe. Cells of the pars reticulata project to the neostriatum, to the ventral medial nucleus of the thalamus, and to the superior colliculus. The major connections of the substantia nigra just noted are shown in Figure 7–17.

The importance of the substantia nigra is manifest when the disturbances of motor function in paralysis agitans (Parkinson's disease) are considered. In this crippling disorder there is muscular rigidity, a fine tremor, a slow and shuffling gait, masklike facies, and other abnormalities. The most consistent pathological finding in Parkinson's disease is degeneration of the melanin-containing cells in the pars compacta of the substantia nigra. Results of biochemical and histochemical studies provided data for therapy. Under normal circumstances dopamine is present in the pigmented cells of the substantia nigra and in the neostriatum of the corpus striatum, whereas it is virtually absent at these sites in Parkinson's disease. These observations have led to the suggestion that the substantia nigra, as part of an undoubtedly complex role, has a regulatory effect on the neostriatum through the action of dopamine as a neurotransmitter substance. Administration of dopamine has been an obvious form of biochemical therapy to be explored. However, dopamine does not cross the blood–brain barrier, so a metabolic precursor that does gain access to brain tissue has been used instead. This precursor is dihydroxyphenylalanine (dopa), and its conversion to dopamine probably occurs in the surviving neurons of the pars compacta. The administration of L-dopa ameliorates some of the motor abnormalities in Parkinson's disease.

The significance of melanin in the substantia nigra is not known, except that it is related chemically to the metabolic sequence that includes dopamine. The pigment may be an inert byproduct of the essential biochemical reactions in the substantia nigra, which would be consistent with the increase in the amount of pigment with age.

The ventral tegmental area (of Tsai) (Figs. 7–15 and 7–16), between the substantia nigra and the red nucleus, is a population of dopaminergic neurons. The axons of these cells end in the hypothalamus, the hippocampal formation, and other parts of the limbic system. These projections, sometimes called the "mesolimbic dopaminergic system," have been intensively studied in animals because their actions are blocked by drugs that are useful in the clinical management of schizophrenia and other mental disorders. The drugs antagonize dopamine at its postsynaptic receptors.

Basis Pedunculi

The basis pedunculi (crus cerebri) consists of fibers of the pyramidal and corticopontine systems (see Figs. 7–14, 7–15, and 7–16). **Corticospinal fibers** constitute the middle three fifths of the basis pedunculi; the somatotopic arrangement is that of fibers for the neck, arm, trunk, and leg in a medial to lateral direction. Many **corticobulbar (corticonuclear) fibers** leave the basis pedunculi and continue to their destinations through the tegmentum of the midbrain and pons. Those corticobulbar fibers that remain continue caudally in the basis pedunculi, where they are situated between the corticospinal and frontopontine tracts. The great majority of the corticobulbar fibers end in the reticular formation near the motor trigeminal nucleus, the motor facial nucleus, the nucleus ambiguus, and the hypoglossal nucleus. A few make direct synaptic contacts with the motor neurons in these nuclei. In addition to these pathways, which have obvious motor functions, there are corticobulbar fibers to the pontine and spinal trigeminal nuclei and to the nucleus of the tractus solitarius. Axons of cortical origin that end in the nuclei gracilis and cuneatus are also classified as corticobulbar. Some of these are collaterals of fibers of the corticospinal tract. Thus, corticobulbar connections are involved in modulating the transmission of sensory information rostrally from the brain stem as well as in the control of movement.

Corticopontine fibers are divided into two large fasciculi. The **frontopontine tract** occupies the medial one fifth of the basis pedunculi. The lateral one fifth consists of the **parietotemporopontine tract**, most of whose fibers originate in the parietal lobe. Corticopontine fibers terminate in the nuclei pontis of the basal pons.

VISCERAL PATHWAYS IN THE BRAIN STEM

Primary visceral afferent neurons at spinal cord levels accompany the parasympathetic division of the autonomic system in the sacral region and the sympathetic division in the thoracic and upper lumbar regions. In addition to their involvement in spinal visceral reflexes, the sacral afferents convey information related to the feeling of fullness in the bladder and rectum and to pain in pelvic viscera. The thoracic and upper lumbar afferents are concerned with pain originating in all other viscera, as well as spinal visceral reflexes. The **ascending visceral pathways** in the spinal cord are in the ventral and ventrolateral funiculi. They may be considered to be parts of the spinothalamic and spinoreticular tracts. Data of visceral origin reach the reticular formation, the thalamus, and the hypothalamus.

The more important physiological visceral afferents reach the nucleus of the tractus solitarius in the medulla by way of the vagus and glossopharyngeal nerves. These nerves include general visceral afferents for visceral reflexes, in which the dorsal nucleus of the vagus nerve and the nucleus ambiguus are the principal efferent components. The nucleus of the tractus solitarius also receives afferents for taste through the vagus, glossopharyngeal, and facial nerves. Ascending fibers from the nucleus of the tractus solitarius travel ipsilaterally in the central tegmental tract and terminate in the hypothalamus and, with a relay in the pontine reticular formation, in the ventral medial basal nucleus of the thalamus. From the latter site information with respect to taste is relayed to a cortical taste area in the parietal lobe. A small **solitariospinal tract** originating in the nucleus of the tractus solitarius terminates on preganglionic autonomic neurons in the spinal cord.

There are two descending pathways whose cells of origin are located in the hypothalamus. **Mamillotegmental fibers** originate in the mamillary body of the hypothalamus; they terminate in the reticular formation of the midbrain, from which impulses reach autonomic nuclei in the brain stem and spinal cord. Fibers from other hypothalamic nuclei, notably the paraventricular nucleus, run caudally in the **dorsal longitudinal fasciculus** (of Schütz), a bundle of unmyelinated fibers in the periaqueductal gray matter of the midbrain. Some terminate in the reticular formation of the brain stem and the dorsal nucleus of the vagus nerve, while the hypothalamospinal fibers proceed to autonomic nuclei in the spinal cord. Thus, impulses of hypothalamic origin reach the preganglionic sympathetic and sacral parasympathetic neurons both directly and through relays in the reticular formation. Clinical evidence indicates that fibers influencing the sympathetic nervous system descend ipslaterally through the lateral part of the medulla.

ANATOMICAL AND CLINICAL CORRELATIONS

Vascular lesions are among the more important of the various pathological conditions affecting the brain stem. Hemorrhage into the brain stem usually has serious consequences because of the presence of nuclei that control the vital functions of respiration and circulation. The neurological signs resulting from vascular occlusion depend on the location and size of the affected region. The following examples are presented to show the correlation between neurological signs and the location of the lesion.

The **medial medullary syndrome** results from occlusion of a medullary branch of the vertebral artery; the size of the infarction depends on the distribution of the particular artery involved. In the example shown in Figure 7–18 the affected area includes the pyramid and most of the medial lemniscus on one side. The lesion extends far enough laterally to include fibers of the hypoglossal nerve as they pass between the medial lemniscus and the inferior olivary nucleus. A patient with this particular lesion has contralateral hemiparesis, as well as impairment of the sensations of position and movement, and of discriminative touch, on the opposite side of the body. Paralysis of the tongue muscles is ipsilateral, however, and the tongue deviates to the affected side on protrusion because the action of the healthy genioglossus muscle is unopposed. This is an example of crossed or alternating paralysis, in which the body is affected on the side opposite the lesion, whereas muscles supplied by a cranial nerve are affected on the same side as the lesion.

Occlusion of a vessel supplying the lateral area of the medulla results in the **lateral medullary**, or **Wallenberg's, syndrome.** The occluded vessel may be the posterior inferior cerebellar artery, or it may be a medullary branch of this artery or of the vertebral artery. The extent of the

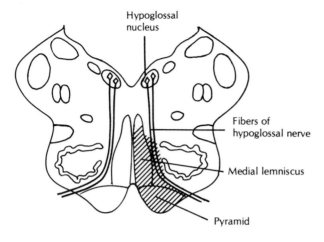

FIGURE 7-18.
Site of a lesion producing the medial medullary syndrome.

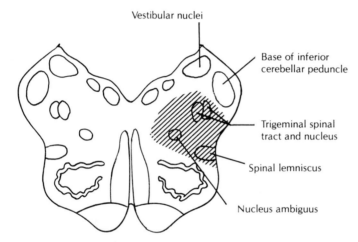

FIGURE 7-19.
Site of a lesion producing the lateral medullary syndrome.

infarcted area is typically as shown in Figure 7–19. Inclusion of the spinal trigeminal tract and its nucleus is responsible for ipsilateral loss of pain and temperature sensibility in the area of distribution of the trigeminal nerve. There is sensory loss, especially for pain and temperature, on the opposite side of the body because of interruption of fibers of the spinothalamic tract in the spinal lemniscus. Because the medial lemniscus is intact, touch sensation is diminished rather than abolished. Destruction of the nucleus ambiguus causes paralysis of muscles of the soft palate, pharynx, and larynx on the side of the lesion, with difficulty in swallowing and phonation. The descending pathway to the intermediolateral cell column of the spinal cord may be included in the area of degeneration. The signs of a lateral medullary lesion may therefore include Horner's syndrome, which consists of a small pupil, slight drooping of the upper eyelid (ptosis), slight enophthalmos, and sometimes warm, dry skin of the face, all on the side of the lesion. The infarcted region may extend dorsally to include the base of the inferior cerebellar peduncle and vestibular nuclei, causing dizziness, cerebellar ataxia, and nystagmus. Cerebellar signs are more pronounced, of course, if infarction of part of the cerebellum is added to that of the medulla (posterior inferior cerebellar artery thrombosis).

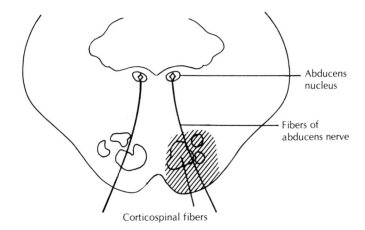

FIGURE 7-20.
Site of a basal pontine lesion involving the pyramidal tract and abducens nerve.

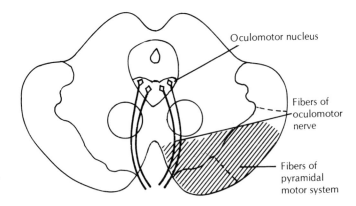

FIGURE 7-21.
Site of a lesion in the midbrain involving the pyramidal and corticopontine tracts and oculomotor nerve.

Lesions in the basal region of the pons or the midbrain may produce alternating paralysis, similar to that described for the medial medullary syndrome. Figure 7–20 illustrates an area of infarction in one side of the caudal region of the pons, resulting from occlusion of a pontine branch of the basilar artery. Interruption of corticospinal fibers causes contralateral hemiparesis, and inclusion of abducens nerve fibers in the lesion causes paralysis of the lateral rectus muscle on the ipsilateral side and a medial strabismus or squint.

The position of a vascular lesion in the basal region of a cerebral peduncle, such as might follow occlusion of a branch of the posterior cerebral artery, is shown in Figure 7–21. A lesion at this site causes **Weber's syndrome,** in which there is contralateral hemiparesis because of interrup-

tion of corticospinal fibers and ipsilateral paralysis of ocular muscles because of inclusion of oculomotor nerve fibers in the infarcted area. There is paralysis of all the extraocular muscles except the lateral rectus and superior oblique muscles. The most obvious signs are loss of ability to raise the upper eyelid and lateral strabismus, together with dilation of the pupil because of interruption of parasympathetic fibers supplying the sphincter pupillae muscle.

SUGGESTED READING

Armstrong DM: Functional significance of connections of the inferior olive. Physiol Rev 54:358–417, 1974
Carpenter MB, Sutin J: Human Neuroanatomy, 8th ed. Baltimore, Williams & Wilkins, 1983
Crosby EC, Humphrey T, Lauer EW: Correla-

tive Anatomy of the Nervous System. New York, Macmillan, 1962

Kuypers HGJM, Lawrence DG: Cortical projections to the red nucleus and the brain stem in the rhesus monkey. Brain Res 4:151–188, 1967

Miller RA, Burack E: Atlas of the Central Nervous System in Man. Baltimore, Williams & Wilkins, 1968

Nieuwenhuys R, Voogd J, van Huijzen C: The Human Central Nervous System. A Synopsis and Atlas. Berlin, Springer-Verlag, 1981

Nathan PW, Smith MC: The rubrospinal and central tegmental tracts in man. Brain 105:223–269, 1982

Nathan PW, Smith MC: The location of descending fibres to sympathetic neurons supplying the head and neck. J Neurol Neurosurg Psychiat 49:187–194, 1986

Oades RD, Halliday GM: Ventral tegmental (AIO) system: Neurobiology. I. Anatomy and connectivity. Brain Res 12:117–165, 1987

Olszewski J, Baxter D: Cytoarchitecture of the Human Brain Stem. Basel, S Karger, 1954

Riley HA: An Atlas of the Basal Ganglia, Brain Stem and Spinal Cord. New York, Hafner, 1960

Saper CB: Anatomical substrates for the hypothalamic control of the autonomic nervous system. In Brooks C McC, Koizumi K, Sato A (eds): Integrative Actions of the Autonomic Nervous System, Chap. 24. Amsterdam, Elsevier-North Holland, 1979

Szabo J: Strionigral and nigrostriatal connections. Appl Neurophysiol 42:9–12, 1979

EIGHT

Cranial Nerves

The cranial nerves, listed in the order in which numbers are assigned to them, are as follows:

1. Olfactory
2. Optic
3. Oculomotor
4. Trochlear
5. Trigeminal
6. Abducens
7. Facial
8. Vestibulocochlear
9. Glossopharyngeal
10. Vagus
11. Accessory
12. Hypoglossal

In addition to motor and general sensory functions, five systems for the special senses are served by various cranial nerves. In these the receptors are localized and highly specialized, in contrast to general sensory endings, which are scattered throughout the tissues of the body and are relatively simple in structure. Of the special senses, the olfactory system is an integral part of the forebrain (Chap. 17). The optic and vestibulocochlear nerves will be discussed in the section on systemic neuroanatomy, in which the visual, auditory, and vestibular systems are described (Chaps. 20, 21, and 22). The special sense of taste (gustatory system) is dealt with in this chapter because the primary sensory neurons for taste are included with sensory neurons that have other functions in the facial, glossopharyngeal, and vagus nerves.

OCULOMOTOR, TROCHLEAR, AND ABDUCENS NERVES

The third, fourth, and sixth cranial nerves supply the extraocular muscles with motor fibers; their nuclei therefore consist of multipolar motor neurons and receive afferents from the same sources. The oculomotor nucleus includes a parasympathetic component, the Edinger–Westphal nucleus, for the sphincter pupillae and ciliary muscles of the eye.

Oculomotor Nerve

The **oculomotor nucleus** is situated in the periaqueductal gray matter of the midbrain, ventral to the aqueduct at the level of the superior colliculus (Fig. 8–1). The paired nuclei have a triangular outline in transverse section and are bounded laterally by the medial longitudinal fasciculi. The cells for individual extraocular muscles (including the levator palpebrae superioris muscle) are localized in longitudinal groups; these subnuclei are represented bilaterally, except for one, which is situated dorsocaudally in the midline. According to Warwick's schema for the oculomotor nucleus of the monkey there are three laterally disposed cell groups, which supply the inferior rectus, inferior oblique, and medial rectus muscles. On the medial side of these there is a subnucleus for the superior rectus muscle. The unpaired cell group, which is called the caudal central nucleus, supplies the levator palpebrae superioris muscle on each side. Myelinated axons from the oculomotor nucleus curve ventrally through the tegmentum, with many of them passing through the red nucleus. The fibers emerge as a series of roots along the side of the interpeduncular fossa, and these roots converge immediately to form the oculomotor nerve.

Oculomotor fibers are partly crossed and partly uncrossed. Although full details are lacking for humans, it appears that only uncrossed fibers supply the inferior rectus, inferior oblique, and medial rectus muscles. The superior rectus muscle receives crossed fibers only, and the levator palpebrae superioris muscle is supplied by the unpaired caudal central nucleus. (Smooth

muscle fibers of the levator are innervated by sympathetic nerves.) The small size of the motor unit, in which about six muscle fibers are supplied by a nerve fiber, attests to the delicate neuromuscular mechanisms required for coordinated movement of the eyes in binocular vision.

Mixed with the motor neurons of the oculomotor nucleus are neurons whose axons pass in the medial longitudinal fasciculus to the trochlear and especially the abducens nuclei of the same and the opposite side. These **internuclear neurons** mediate inhibition of antagonistic muscles whenever the eyes are moved.

The **Edinger–Westphal nucleus** is dorsal to the rostral two thirds of the main oculomotor nucleus, and its small spindle-shaped cells are similar to other preganglionic parasympathetic neurons. Fibers from the Edinger–Westphal nucleus accompany other oculomotor fibers into the orbit, where they terminate in the ciliary ganglion. Postganglionic fibers then pass through short ciliary nerves to the eyeball, in which they supply the sphincter pupillae muscle of the iris and the ciliary muscle. The Edinger–Westphal nucleus also contributes fibers to the small interstitiospinal tract, which is probably concerned with visuomotor coordination.

A lesion that interrupts fibers of the oculomotor nerve causes paralysis of all extraocular muscles except the superior oblique and lateral rectus muscles. The sphincter pupillae muscle in the iris and the ciliary muscle in the ciliary body are functionally paralyzed, although they are not denervated. The consequences of such a lesion are lateral strabismus caused by unopposed action of the lateral rectus muscle, inability to direct the eye medially or vertically, and drooping of the upper eyelid (ptosis). Interruption of the parasympathetic fibers causes dilation of the pupil, enhanced by unopposed action of the dilator pupillae muscle in the iris, which has a sympathetic innervation. There is no

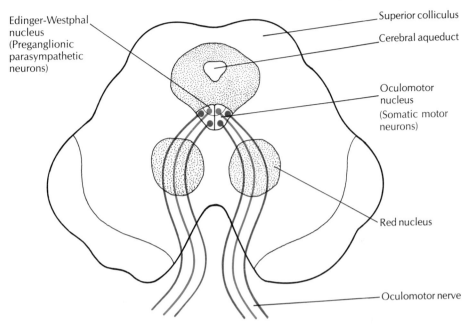

FIGURE 8-1.
Origin of the oculomotor nerve in the midbrain.

longer pupillary constriction in response to an increase of light intensity or in accommodation for near objects, nor does the ciliary muscle contract to allow the lens to increase in thickness for focusing on a near object. The preganglionic parasympathetic fibers run superficially in the nerve and are therefore the first axons to suffer when the nerve is affected by external pressure. Consequently, the first sign of compression of the oculomotor nerve is ipsilateral slowness of the pupillary response to light.

Trochlear Nerve

The **trochlear nucleus** for the superior oblique muscle is immediately caudal to the oculomotor nucleus, at the level of the inferior colliculus (Fig. 8–2). Trochlear nerve fibers have an unusual course, and this is the only nerve to emerge from the dorsum of the brain stem. Small bundles of fibers curve around the periaqueductal gray matter with a caudal slope and de-

cussate in the superior medullary velum with fibers from the companion nucleus; the slender nerve emerges immediately caudal to the inferior colliculus. The superior oblique muscle, as with the superior rectus, is therefore supplied by crossed fibers. The function of the superior oblique muscle is to rotate and depress the eyeball. Paralysis of the muscle, as in the rare occurrence of an isolated lesion of the trochlear nerve, causes vertical diplopia (double vision). The diplopia is maximal when the eye is directed downward and inward, and a person so affected may experience difficulty in walking downstairs.

Abducens Nerve

The **abducens nucleus** for the lateral rectus muscle is situated beneath the facial colliculus in the floor of the fourth ventricle (Fig. 8–3). A bundle of facial nerve fibers curves over the nucleus, contributing to the facial colliculus. The motor neu-

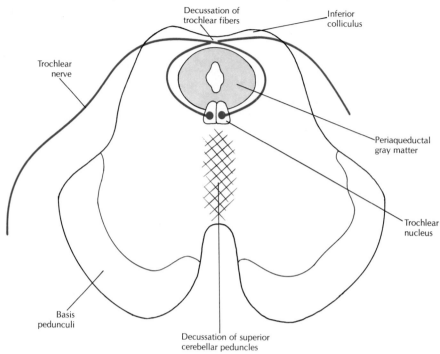

FIGURE 8-2.
Origin of the trochlear nerve in the midbrain.

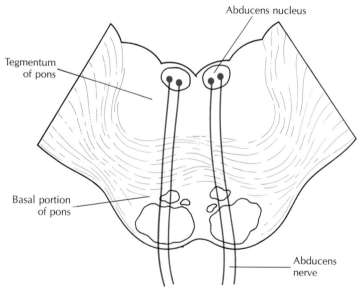

FIGURE 8-3.
Origin of the abducens nerve in the pons.

rons in the abducens nucleus give rise to axons that pass through the pons in a ventrocaudal direction, emerging from the brain stem at the junction of the pons and the pyramid. The abducens nucleus also contains internuclear neurons whose axons travel to the part of the oculomotor nucleus concerned with supplying the medial rectus muscle.

Interruption of the abducens nerve causes medial strabismus and inability to direct the affected eye laterally. Functional impairment of any of the extraocular muscles causes diplopia. The separation between the two images is greatest when the patient attempts to look in the direction of action of the weak or paralyzed muscle.

An understanding of the neuroanatomical basis of ocular movements, which will now be discussed, is essential for the clinical analysis of impairment of these movements.

Afferents to Nuclei Supplying Extraocular Muscles

The main part of the oculomotor nucleus (*i.e.*, all but the parasympathetic component) and the trochlear and abducens nuclei receive fibers from the same sources, as is to be expected. These afferents are concerned with the control of both voluntary and involuntary eye movements. Voluntarily initiated conjugate movements of the eyes include those that occur when scanning a landscape or reading a printed page. These movements, known as **saccadic eye movements,** are very rapid, with each being completed in 20 to 50 msec. Slower movements of the eyes are possible only when tracking a moving object in the visual field. These largely involuntary **smooth pursuit movements** are mentioned later in connection with visual fixation.

Voluntary Eye Movements

The area of the cerebral cortex that controls voluntary eye movements is the **fron-tal eye field,** located anterior to the motor cortex. Electrical stimulation of the frontal eye field results in conjugate deviation of the eyes to the opposite side. A destructive lesion there causes the eyes to deviate to the same side—looking away from the paralyzed side of the body if the motor cortex has been damaged by the same lesion. However, there are no direct corticobulbar fibers from any part of the cerebral cortex to the nuclei of cranial nerves 3, 4, and 6. Instead, the voluntary control of eye movements is mediated by a polysynaptic pathway that involves the frontal cortex, the superior colliculus, the pretectal area, the accessory oculomotor nuclei, and finally the oculomotor, trochlear, and abducens nuclei (Fig. 8–4). (The accessory oculomotor nuclei consist of four pairs of nuclei, which are shown in Fig. 9–8.) The internuclear neurons, whose axons travel in the medial longitudinal fasciculus to interconnect the three motor nuclei, inhibit all motor neurons supplying muscles that are passively lengthened as the eyes move. For example, the coordinated contraction of the left lateral rectus and the right medial rectus is associated with inhibition of the left medial rectus and the right lateral rectus.

The medial longitudinal fasciculus also transmits impulses from the vestibular nuclei and provides for coordinated movements of the eyes and head. With respect to conjugate movements of the eyes, cells in the reticular formation near the abducens nucleus constitute the **paramedian pontine reticular formation (PPRF),** which functions as a "center for lateral gaze" (Fig. 8–5). The PPRF receives fibers from the superior colliculus and the vestibular nuclei, and from other parts of the reticular formation. It sends fibers to the ipsilateral abducens nucleus and, through the medial longitudinal fasciculus, to those cells of the contralateral oculomotor nucleus that supply the medial rectus muscle. The actions of the medial and lateral recti are thereby coordinated in horizontal move-

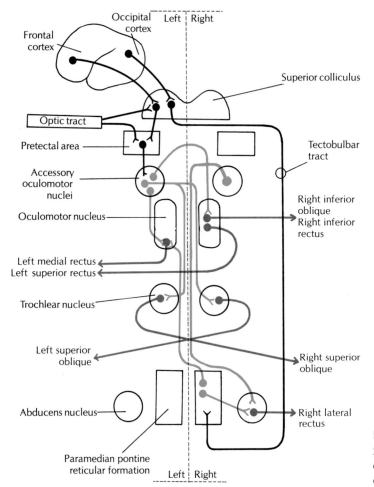

FIGURE 8-4.
Some pathways for the control of eye movements by the cerebral cortex and superior colliculus.

ments of the eyes.* A lesion in the PPRF causes paralysis of conjugate gaze to the ipsilateral side.

A small lesion in the medial longitudinal fasciculus in the upper part of the pons causes **internuclear ophthalmoplegia,** in which the ipsilateral eye cannot adduct when the contralateral eye abducts and also exhibits nystagmus. These abnormalities are evident only when the patient is

asked to gaze to the side opposite that of the lesion; contraction of the medial rectus occurs normally with convergence of the eyes for looking at a near object. The paralysis of adduction of the ipsilateral eye is attributed to transection of fibers from the contralateral PPRF and the ipsilateral abducens nucleus to the ipsilateral oculomotor nucleus. The associated nystagmus in the abducting (contralateral) eye is a useful diagnostic sign, but a neuroanatomical explanation for it has not yet been found.

Comparable "centers" for conjugate movement of the eyes in the vertical plane are present in the upper midbrain bilaterally. A lesion involving the rostral inter-

---

* This coordination is a function of both the PPRF and the internuclear neurons contained in the abducens nucleus. Formerly both populations of cells were thought to reside in a region named the parabducens nucleus, but this term is now obsolete since it does not refer to any real anatomical entity.

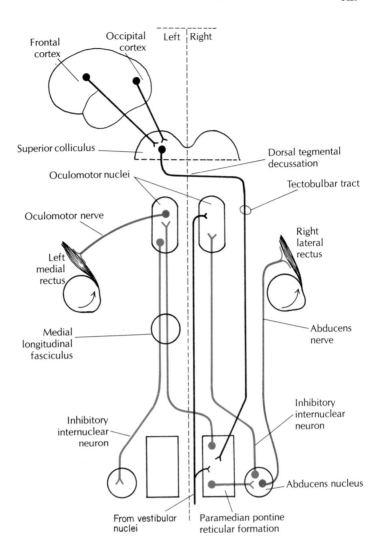

FIGURE 8-5.
Pathways involved in conjugate movements of the eyes.

stitial nucleus of the medial longitudinal fasciculus (one of the accessory oculomotor nuclei) causes paralysis of downward gaze. A lesion located a little further caudally, or alternatively one that transects the posterior commissure, causes paralysis of upward gaze. These disorders of vertical eye movements can result from pressure by a tumor of the pineal gland.

Fixation and Convergence

Normally the eyes are directed toward some object in the center of the field of vision. If the object moves both eyes will execute smooth pursuit movements in or-

der to maintain visual fixation, which contributes importantly to awareness of the position of the head and, integrated with other sensory information, helps in the maintenance of the body's equilibrium. These slow eye movements are largely involuntary. They are controlled by the cortex of the occipital lobe, including both the primary visual area and the surrounding visual association cortex. Electrical stimulation of these areas results in conjugate movement of the eyes to the opposite side. The descending connections of the occipital cortex are essentially the same as those of the frontal eye field (Fig. 8–4). The direct visual input from the retina to the superior colliculus may also be involved in reflex eye movements for visual fixation.

Convergence of the eyes occurs when both eyes are focused on a near object. The neuroanatomical substrates of convergence are poorly understood but are presumed to be similar to those just described for visual fixation. Convergence requires the integrity of the occipital cortex but not that of the frontal eye field or of the PPRF. The descending pathway probably includes synaptic relays in the superior colliculus and in the accessory oculomotor nuclei.

Light and Accommodation Reflexes

The Edinger–Westphal nucleus is a parasympathetic autonomic nucleus concerned mainly with reflex responses to light and accommodation. An increase in the intensity of light falling on the retina causes constriction of the pupil. The afferent limb of the reflex arc involves fibers in the optic nerve and optic tract reaching the pretectal area by way of the superior brachium (Fig. 8–6). The pretectal area projects to the Edinger–Westphal nucleus, from which fibers traverse the oculomotor nerve to the ciliary ganglion in the orbital cavity. Postganglionic fibers travel through the short ciliary nerves to the sphincter pupillae muscle of the iris. Some neurons in the pretectal area send their axons across the midline in the posterior commissure to the contralateral Edinger–Westphal nucleus. Consequently, both pupils constrict when a light is shone into only one eye. This

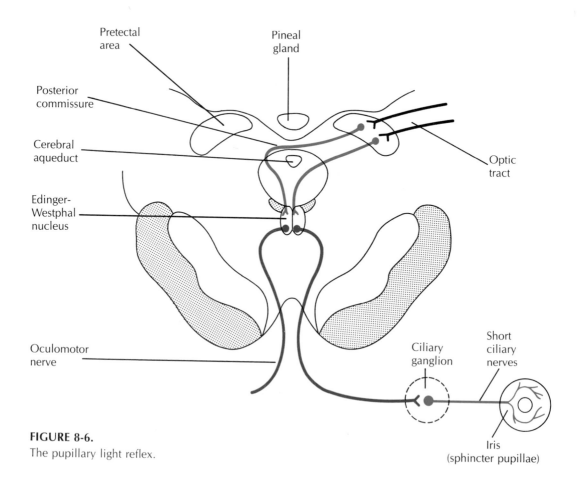

FIGURE 8-6.
The pupillary light reflex.

response of the contralateral iris is known as the consensual light reflex.

The response of accommodation of the lens accompanies ocular convergence produced by visual fixation on a near object. Impulses originating in the occipital cortex and relayed to the Edinger–Westphal nucleus through the superior colliculus appear to initiate the accommodation response. The efferent part of the pathway consists of pre- and postganglionic fibers from the Edinger–Westphal nucleus and the ciliary ganglion, respectively. The postganglionic fibers supply the ciliary muscle, which on contraction allows the lens to increase in thickness and thereby increases refractive power for focusing on a near object. The sphincter pupillae muscle contracts at the same time, sharpening the image by decreasing the diameter of the pupil and reducing spherical aberration in the refractive media.

The difference in the pathways for pupillary responses to light and accommodation is reflected in how these responses are affected by disease. For example, in the Argyll Robertson pupil there is constriction of the pupil when attention is directed to a near object, although pupillary constriction in response to light is absent. The Argyll Robertson pupil is characteristically seen in patients with tabes dorsalis, a syphilitic disease of the central nervous system. Loss of the pupillary light reflex alone could be the result of a small lesion in the pretectal or periaqueductal region, but the site of pathological change has not yet been discovered. The Argyll Robertson pupil is irregular and smaller than normal, probably because of disease of the iris itself. Normal people occasionally have one pupil that responds more slowly than the other to both light and accommodation.

TRIGEMINAL NERVE

The trigeminal nerve is the principal sensory nerve for the head and is the motor nerve for the muscles of mastication and several small muscles.

Sensory Components

The cell bodies of most of the primary sensory neurons are in the **trigeminal** (semilunar or gasserian) **ganglion,** with the remainder being in the mesencephalic nucleus. The peripheral processes of trigeminal ganglion cells constitute the ophthalmic and maxillary nerves and the sensory component of the mandibular nerve. The cell bodies of sensory neurons for the three divisions of the nerve occupy anatomically discrete regions within the ganglion. The mandibular nerve also includes proprioceptive fibers from the mesencephalic nucleus. The trigeminal nerve is responsible for sensation from the skin of the face and forehead, the scalp as far back as the vertex of the head, the mucosa of the oral and nasal cavities and the paranasal sinuses, and the teeth (Fig. 8–7). The trigeminal nerve also contributes sensory fibers to most of the dura mater. The scalp of the back of the head and an area of skin at the angle of the jaw are supplied by the second and third cervical nerves. The external ear has a complicated and overlapping innervation. The anterior border of the auricle, the anterior wall of the external acoustic meatus, and the anterior part of the tympanic membrane receive trigeminal fibers. The concha of the auricle, much of the acoustic meatus and tympanic membrane, and a cutaneous area behind the ear are supplied by the facial and vagus nerves. The helix and the posterior surface are supplied by the second and third cervical nerves.

Pontine Trigeminal Nucleus

The central processes of trigeminal ganglion cells make up the large sensory root of the trigeminal nerve; these fibers enter the pons and terminate in the pontine tri-

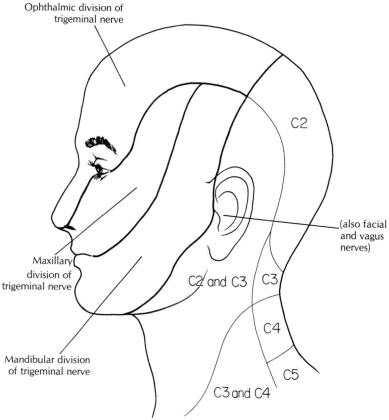

Ophthalmic division of
trigeminal nerve

C2

(also facial
and vagus
nerves)

Maxillary
division of
trigeminal nerve

C2 and C3   C3

C4

Mandibular division
of trigeminal nerve

C5

C3 and C4

FIGURE 8-7.
Cutaneous innervation of the head and neck. The boundaries between the
territories supplied by the three divisions of the trigeminal nerve do not
overlap appreciably, as do the boundaries between spinal dermatomes.

geminal nucleus and in the nucleus of the
spinal trigeminal tract. The pontine trigeminal nucleus, also called the chief or
superior sensory nucleus, is in the dorsolateral area of the pontine tegmentum at
the level of entry of the sensory fibers (Fig.
8–8). Large diameter fibers for discriminative touch terminate in the pontine trigeminal nucleus. Other fibers divide on
nearing the nucleus; one branch enters it
and the other branch turns caudally in the
spinal tract and ends in the nucleus of the
spinal tract. These afferents are mainly for
light touch, and both nuclei must therefore
participate in this sensory modality.

Spinal Trigeminal Tract and Nucleus of the
Spinal Tract

Large numbers of sensory root fibers of
intermediate size and many fine, unmyelinated fibers turn caudally on entering
the pons. These fibers for pain, temperature, and light touch combine with descending branches of the afferents mentioned above to form the spinal trigeminal
tract (Fig. 8–8). The tract includes a small
complement of fibers from the facial, glossopharyngeal, and vagus nerves. The latter
fibers conduct general sensory data from
part of the external ear and from the mu-

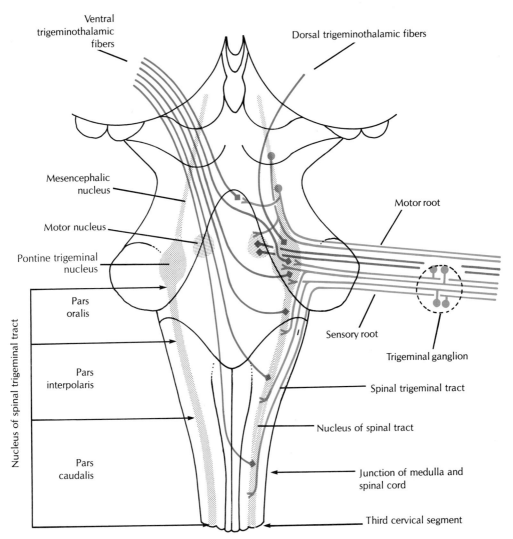

FIGURE 8-8.
Nuclei of the trigeminal nerve and their connections.

cosa of the posterior part of the tongue, the pharynx, and the larynx. Some fibers of the spinal tract descend as far as the upper three segments of the cord, where they intermingle with fibers of the dorsolateral tract of Lissauer. There is a spatial arrangement of fibers in the sensory root and spinal tract, corresponding to the three divisions of the trigeminal nerve. In the sensory root, ophthalmic fibers are dorsal, mandibular fibers are ventral, and maxil-

lary fibers are in between. There is a rotation of the fibers as they enter the brain stem, with the result that the mandibular fibers are dorsal and the ophthalmic fibers ventral in the trigeminal spinal tract. Fibers from the facial, glossopharyngeal, and vagus nerves are dorsal to the mandibular fibers.

Fibers of the spinal tract terminate in the subjacent nucleus of the spinal tract (Fig. 8–8), and also in the reticular formation medial to the nucleus. This nucleus extends from the pontine trigeminal nucleus to the caudal limit of the medulla; the nucleus of the spinal tract and the dorsal portion (laminae I through IV) of the dorsal gray horn are indistinguishable from one another in the upper three cervical segments of the spinal cord. The nearby reticular formation corresponds to lamina V of the spinal gray matter. Trigeminothalamic fibers arise from cells in this region as well as from those of the spinal and pontine trigeminal nuclei.

Based on cytoarchitecture, the nucleus of the spinal tract is divided into three subnuclei. The **pars caudalis,** which extends from the level of the pyramidal decussation to spinal segment C3, receives fibers for pain and temperature. The integrity of the pars caudalis and of the caudal end of the spinal trigeminal tract are essential for the perception of pain originating in the same side of the head. In the first three cervical segments, laminae I through IV of the dorsal gray horn are concerned with pain and temperature in both the trigeminal area of distribution and in that of the most rostral cervical nerves (neck and back of the head).

Of the remaining two regions of the nucleus of the spinal tract (see Fig. 8–8), the **pars interpolaris** extends from the level of the rostral third of the inferior olivary nucleus to that of the pyramidal decussation. It contains rather large cells scattered among diffusely arranged small and medium-sized neurons. In the **pars oralis,** which extends from the pars interpolaris rostrally to the pontine trigeminal nucleus, there is a more dense arrangement of small and medium-sized cells. This subnucleus closely resembles the pontine trigeminal nucleus. Fibers of the spinal tract terminating in these regions appear to be mainly concerned with touch, including some discriminative touch in the case of the pars oralis, although there is evidence that the pars interpolaris receives some

pain afferents from the teeth. Some of the fibers are descending branches of afferents that also send a branch to the pontine trigeminal nucleus.

Some efferent fibers from the sensory trigeminal nuclei terminate in motor nuclei of the trigeminal and facial nerves, the nucleus ambiguus, and the hypoglossal nucleus for reflex responses to stimuli arising in the area of distribution of the trigeminal nerve. For example, touching the cornea causes the eyelids to close reflexly; the afferent fibers are in the ophthalmic nerve and the efferent fibers of the reflex arc are in the facial nerve. As a further example, irritation of the nasal mucosa causes sneezing. For this reflex, afferent impulses in the maxillary nerve are relayed to motor nuclei of the trigeminal and facial nerves, the nucleus ambiguus, the hypoglossal nucleus, and (through a reticulospinal relay) to the phrenic nucleus and motor cells in the spinal cord that supply the intercostal and other respiratory muscles.

Projections from the spinal trigeminal nuclei to the reticular formation provide an important source of cutaneous stimuli for the parts of the reticular formation concerned with consciousness and arousal. Other fibers enter the cerebellum through the inferior peduncle. The principal pathway from the pontine and spinal trigeminal nuclei to the thalamus is the crossed **ventral trigeminothalamic tract** (see Fig. 8–8), which ascends close to the medial lemniscus. Smaller numbers of fibers, crossed and uncrossed, proceed from the pontine trigeminal nucleus to the thalamus in the **dorsal trigeminothalamic tract.** The combined tracts are commonly referred to as the **trigeminal lemniscus.**

Mesencephalic Nucleus

The mesencephalic nucleus consists of a slender strand of cells that extends from the pontine trigeminal nucleus through the midbrain (see Fig. 8–8). The nucleus is located beneath the lateral edge of the floor of the fourth ventricle in the pons and in the lateral region of the periaqueductal gray matter in the midbrain. The unipolar cells are primary sensory neurons in an unusual location; they are the only such cells that are incorporated into the central nervous system, rather than being in cerebrospinal ganglia. Fibers from the nucleus constitute the slender **mesencephalic root** of the trigeminal nerve that runs alongside the mesencephalic nucleus. The single process of each cell divides into a peripheral and a central branch. Most of the peripheral branches enter the motor root of the trigeminal nerve and are distributed within the mandibular division (Fig. 8–8). These fibers end in deep proprioceptive-type receptors adjacent to the teeth of the lower jaw and in neuromuscular spindles in the muscles of mastication. Some fibers from the mesencephalic nucleus traverse the sensory root and the trigeminal ganglion for distribution by way of the maxillary division to endings in the hard palate, adjacent to the teeth of the upper jaw. Central branches of the single processes of some cells of the mesencephalic nucleus terminate in the motor nuclei of the trigeminal nerve. This connection establishes the stretch reflex that originates in neuromuscular spindles in the masticatory muscles, together with a reflex for control of the force of the bite. Other central branches synapse with cells of the reticular formation, from which fibers proceed to the thalamus along with other trigeminothalamic fibers. In addition, a few fibers from the mesencephalic nucleus enter the cerebellum through the superior peduncle.

Motor Component

The **motor nucleus** of the trigeminal nerve, consisting of typical multipolar neurons, is situated medial to the chief sensory nucleus (see Fig. 8–8). Fibers from the motor nucleus constitute the bulk of the motor root, which joins sensory fibers of the mandibular nerve just distal to the trigeminal ganglion. This nerve supplies the muscles of mastication (masseter, temporalis, and lateral and medial pterygoid muscles) and several smaller muscles—the tensor tympani, tensor veli palatini, digastric (anterior belly), and mylohyoid muscles. The motor nucleus receives afferents from the corticobulbar tract; most of these are crossed, but there is a significant proportion of uncrossed fibers. Some of the corticobulbar neurons contact the motor neurons directly but the majority end in the nearby reticular formation and influence the motor trigeminal nucleus through interneurons.

Afferents for reflexes come mainly from the sensory trigeminal nuclei, including the mesencephalic nucleus. In addition to the stretch reflex there is also a jaw-opening reflex in which the contractions of the masseter, temporalis, and medial pterygoid muscles are inhibited as a result of painful pressure applied to the teeth. Cells supplying the tensor tympani muscle receive acoustic fibers from the superior olivary nucleus. The tensor tympani muscle, by reflex contraction, checks excessive movement of the tympanic membrane caused by loud sounds.

Clinical Considerations

Of the pathological conditions that affect the trigeminal complex, major trigeminal neuralgia, or **tic douloureux,** is of special importance because of the excruciating pain. Tic douloureux is characterized by paroxysms of pain in the area of distribution of one of the trigeminal divisions, usually with periods of remission and exacerbation. The maxillary nerve is most frequently involved, then the mandibular nerve, and least frequently the ophthalmic nerve. The paroxysm, which is of sudden onset, may be set off by mild stimulation of the face, such as touching the skin; there is often an especially sensitive "trigger zone." The cause of tic douloureux is unknown, although in many cases the symptoms are relieved if a small aberrant artery is moved away from the sensory root of the nerve. Other surgical procedures aim to interrupt the pain pathway from the affected cutaneous area to the nucleus of the spinal tract of the trigeminal nerve. It is important to preserve corneal sensitivity, which affords protection from damage that might lead to corneal ulceration. Transection of the spinal trigeminal tract in the lower medulla abolishes the ability to feel pain in the face. The somatotopic lamination of the tract permits placement of a small lesion that restricts the analgesic area to the territory of a single division of the trigeminal nerve.

The sensory and motor nuclei of the trigeminal nerve may be included in areas of degeneration in the brain stem, or the intracranial portion of the nerve may be affected by trauma, by tumor growth, or by another lesion. Interruption of the motor fibers causes paralysis and eventual atrophy of the muscles of mastication. The mandible deviates to the affected side because of the unopposed action of the contralateral lateral pterygoid muscle, with the function of this muscle being to protrude the jaw. Interruption of corticobulbar fibers does not cause complete paralysis of the masticatory muscles on the side opposite the lesion because the motor nucleus also receives some uncrossed fibers from the motor cortex.

FACIAL NERVE

The facial nerve has two sensory components; one supplies taste buds and the other contributes cutaneous fibers to part of the external ear. There are also two efferent components, one for the facial muscles of expression and one for the submandibular and sublingual salivary glands and the lacrimal gland.

Sensory Components

The cell bodies of primary sensory neurons are in the **geniculate ganglion,** situated at the bend of the nerve as it traverses the facial canal in the petrous temporal bone.

Gustatory Fibers

The peripheral processes of cells for taste, with these cells composing most of the ganglion, enter the chorda tympani branch of the facial nerve, which joins the lingual branch of the mandibular nerve (see Fig. 8–10). The fibers are distributed to taste buds in the anterior two thirds of the tongue, most of which are along its lateral border. Fibers for palatal taste buds follow a complicated route and, as is true also of parasympathetic fibers in the facial and glossopharyngeal nerves, an understanding of the gross anatomy of the head is necessary to visualize their course. In brief, these sensory fibers leave the facial nerve in the greater petrosal branch at the level of the geniculate ganglion; this branch proceeds into the pterygopalatine fossa above the palate, where the fibers join palatine branches of the maxillary division of the trigeminal nerve. The trigeminal fibers of the palatine nerves provide for general sensation in the palate and on the inner surface of the gums, whereas the fibers from the facial nerve terminate in taste buds in the hard and soft palates.

The central processes of geniculate ganglion cells that subserve taste enter the brain stem in the sensory root of the facial nerve (nervus intermedius) and turn caudally in the tractus solitarius (Fig. 8–9). The facial nerve fibers in this fasciculus are joined more caudally by gustatory fibers from the glossopharyngeal and vagus nerves. Fibers from these three sources terminate in the **nucleus of the tractus so-**

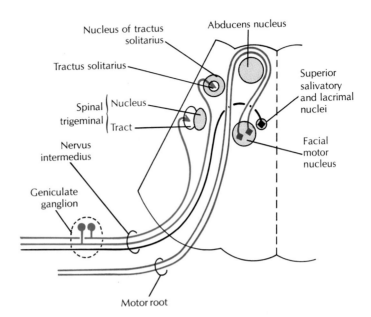

FIGURE 8-9.
Components of the facial nerve in the pons.

litarius, a column of cells adjacent to and partly surrounding the tract. Only the large-celled rostral part of the nucleus receives taste fibers; it is often called the **gustatory nucleus.** The caudal part, whose cells are small, receives general visceral afferents. Fibers from the gustatory nucleus run rostrally, perhaps in the central tegmental tract. Some terminate in the ipsilateral **parabrachial nucleus,** in the lateral part of the midbrain reticular formation; others continue rostrally to the hypothalamus. Gustatory fibers from the parabrachial nucleus project to the **ventral medial basal nucleus** of the thalamus. This thalamic nucleus projects to the cortical area for taste, which is posterior to the general sensory area for the mouth. Physiological evidence has shown that gustatory sensations are transmitted to the thalamus and cortex bilaterally.

Cutaneous Fibers

The cutaneous sensory fibers leave the facial nerve just after it leaves the facial canal at the stylomastoid foramen (Fig. 8–10). These fibers are distributed to the skin of the concha of the auricle, a small area behind the ear, the wall of the external acoustic meatus, and the external surface of the tympanic membrane. The central processes of the geniculate ganglion cells for cutaneous sensation enter the brain stem in the nervus intermedius. They continue into the spinal tract of the trigeminal nerve (Fig. 8–9) and terminate in the subadjacent nucleus of the spinal tract.

Efferent Components

For Supply of Striated Muscles

The motor component of the facial nerve for the muscles of expression and certain additional muscles is the most important part of the nerve from the clinical viewpoint. The **facial motor nucleus** is situated in the caudal one third of the ventrolateral part of the pontine tegmentum (see Fig. 8–9). Efferent fibers of the nucleus pursue an unexpected course. Directed initially toward the floor of the fourth ventricle, the fibers form a compact bundle that loops over the caudal end of the abducens nucleus, runs forward along its medial side, and loops again over the rostral end of the

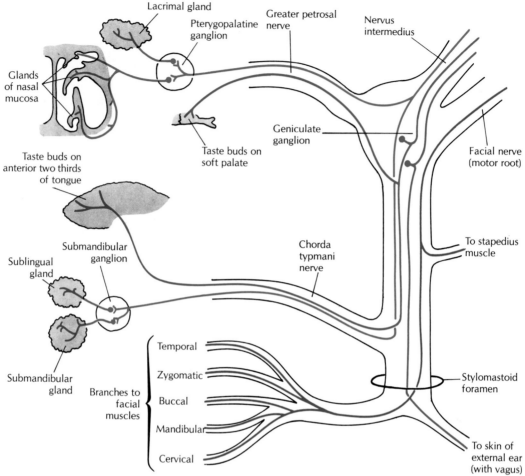

FIGURE 8-10.
Components of the peripheral parts of the facial nerve.

nucleus. The fibers then proceed to the point of emergence of the motor root of the facial nerve by passing between the nucleus of origin and the nucleus of the spinal trigeminal tract. The configuraton of the fiber bundle around the abducens nucleus is called the **internal genu,** with the external genu of the facial nerve being in the facial canal at the level of the geniculate ganglion.

The explanation for the course of facial motor fibers in the pons is based on a migration of cells in the embryo. It has been suggested that neurons destined to form the abducens and facial nuclei are inter-

mingled at an early embryonic stage. The facial neurons subsequently move in a ventrolateral direction under the influence of the spinal trigeminal tract and its nucleus. Concurrently the abducens neurons move dorsomedially toward the medial longitudinal fasciculus. The fibers extending from the facial nucleus to the region of the abducens nucleus indicate the direction and extent of the change in position of the nuclei during embryonic development. Such shifts in position of groups of nerve cells during development are said to be the result of **neurobiotaxis,** a term introduced by Ariëns Kappers in

1914 to indicate the tendency of neurons to migrate toward major sources of stimuli.

The motor root of the facial nerve consists entirely of fibers from the motor nucleus. They supply the muscles of expression (mimetic muscles), the platysma and stylohyoid muscles, and the posterior belly of the digastric muscle. The facial nerve also supplies the stapedius muscle of the middle ear; this small muscle is inserted on the stapes and, by reflex contraction in response to loud sounds, prevents excessive movement of the stapes.

The motor nucleus receives afferents from several sources, including important connections for reflexes. Tectobulbar fibers from the superior colliculus complete a reflex pathway that provides for closure of the eyelids in response to intense light or a rapidly approaching object. Fibers from trigeminal sensory nuclei function in the corneal reflex and in chewing or sucking responses on placing food in the mouth. Fibers from the superior olivary nucleus on the auditory pathway permit reflex contraction of the stapedius muscle.

Corticobulbar afferents are crossed, except for those terminating on cells that supply the frontalis and orbicularis oculi muscles, which receive both crossed and uncrossed fibers. Contralateral voluntary paralysis of the *lower facial muscles* is therefore a feature of upper motor neuron lesions. However, under such circumstances, the facial muscles continue to respond involuntarily to changing moods and emotions. Emotional changes of facial expression are typically lost in Parkinson's disease (masklike facies), although voluntary use of the facial muscles is retained. The neuroanatomical basis for the two types of control of facial movement is not known.

Parasympathetic Nuclei

The **superior salivatory** and **lacrimal nuclei** consist of indefinite clusters of small cells, partly intermingled, that are medial to the motor nucleus (see Fig. 8–9). The exact positions of these nuclei in the human brain are not known with certainty. They contain the cell bodies of preganglionic neurons for the submandibular and sublingual salivary glands and for the lacrimal gland. Fibers from the nuclei leave the brain stem in the nervus intermedius and continue in the facial nerve until branches are given off in the facial canal in the petrous temporal bone. The fibers follow devious routes to their destinations, running part of the way in branches of the trigeminal nerve (Fig. 8–10). Briefly stated, fibers from the superior salivatory nucleus leave the facial nerve in the chorda tympani branch and join the lingual branch of the mandibular nerve to reach the floor of the oral cavity. There they terminate in the submandibular ganglion and on scattered nerve cells in the submandibular gland. Short postganglionic fibers are distributed to the parenchyma of the submandibular and sublingual glands, where the impulses stimulate secretion and cause vasodilation.

Fibers from the lacrimal nucleus leave the facial nerve in the greater petrosal branch and terminate in the pterygopalatine ganglion located in the pterygopalatine fossa. Postganglionic fibers for the stimulation of secretion and vasodilation reach the lacrimal gland through the zygomatic branch of the maxillary nerve. Other postganglionic fibers are distributed to mucous glands in the mucosa that lines the nasal cavity and the paranasal sinuses.

The superior salivatory nucleus comes under the influence of the hypothalamus, perhaps through the dorsal longitudinal fasciculus, and of the olfactory system through relays in the reticular formation. Data from taste buds and from the mucosa of the oral cavity are received by way of the nucleus of the tractus solitarius and sensory trigeminal nuclei, respectively. The chief sources of impulses to the lacrimal nucleus are presumed to be the hypothalamus for emotional responses and the nucleus of the spinal trigeminal tract for lacrimation caused by irritation of the cornea and conjuctiva.

Clinical Considerations

A facial paralysis commonly accompanies hemiplegia caused by occulsion of a blood vessel supplying the internal capsule or the motor cortex. For reasons already stated, only the lower half of the face is affected. When a unilateral facial paralysis involves the musculature around the eyes and in the forehead in addition to that around the mouth, the lesion must involve the cell bodies in the facial nucleus or their axons. In the most common condition, known as **Bell's palsy,** the facial nerve is affected as it traverses the facial canal in the petrous temporal bone, with rapid onset of weakness (paresis) or paralysis of the facial muscles on the affected side. The etiology is thought to be an infection of the facial nerve and adjacent tissue in the facial canal. The signs of Bell's palsy depend not only on the severity of the infection, but also on where the facial nerve is affected in its passage through the facial canal. All functions of the nerve are lost if the damage is proximal to the geniculate ganglion. In addition to the paralysis of facial muscles, there is a loss of taste sensation in the anterior two thirds of the tongue and in the palate of the affected side, together with impairment of secretion by the submandibular, sublingual, and lacrimal glands. Also, sounds seem abnormally loud (hyperacusis) because of paralysis of the stapedius muscle.

In mild cases most of the nerve fibers are not so severely damaged as to result in wallerian degeneration, and the prognosis is favorable. Recovery is slow and frequently incomplete when it must rely on nerve fiber regeneration. There is no regeneration into the brain stem of sensory fibers that have been interrupted on the central side of the geniculate ganglion. In the case of such a lesion in the proximal part of the nerve, some regenerating sali-

vary fibers may find their way into the greater petrosal nerve and reach the pterygopalatine ganglion. This results in lacrimation (crocodile tears) when aromas and taste sensations cause stimulation of cells in the superior salivatory nucleus. When the nerve is affected in the distal part of the facial canal after the greater petrosal and chorda tympani branches are given off, the condition is limited to paresis or paralysis involving both the upper and lower facial muscles on the side of the lesion.

GLOSSOPHARYNGEAL, VAGUS, AND ACCESSORY NERVES

The ninth, tenth, and eleventh cranial nerves have much in common functionally, and share certain nuclei in the medulla. Although it is customary to discuss these nerves individually, repetition is avoided by considering them together.

Afferent Components

The glossopharyngeal and vagus nerves include sensory fibers for the special visceral sense of taste from the posterior one third of the tongue, pharynx, and epiglottis, together with general visceral afferents from the carotid sinus, carotid body, and viscera of the thorax and abdomen. There are also general sensory fibers for pain, temperature, and touch from the mucosa of the back of the tongue, from the pharynx and nearby regions, and from the skin of part of the ear. The cell bodies of primary sensory neurons are in the superior and inferior ganglia of each of the nerves.

Visceral Afferents

The cell bodies for the **gustatory fibers** are in the inferior ganglia of the glossopharyngeal and vagus nerves. The fibers are distributed through the glossopharyngeal nerve to taste buds on the back of the tongue and also to the few that occur in the pharyngeal mucosa. Vagal fibers supply taste buds on the epiglottis; these are unimportant because few persist into adult life. Central processes of the ganglion cells join the tractus solitarius and terminate in the rostral portion of the nucleus of the tractus solitarius—the gustatory nucleus (Figs. 8–11 and 8–12).

The cell bodies of afferent neurons for **general visceral reflexes** are also in the inferior ganglia of the glossopharyngeal and vagus nerves. These fibers in the glossopharyngeal nerve supply the carotid sinus at the bifurcation of the common carotid artery and the adjacent carotid body. Nerve endings in the wall of the carotid sinus function as baroreceptors, which monitor arterial blood pressure, whereas the carotid body contains chemoreceptors that monitor oxygen tension in the circulating blood. Vagal fibers similarly supply baroreceptors in the aortic arch and chemoreceptors in the small aortic bodies adjacent to the arch. The vagus nerve contains many afferent fibers that are distributed to the viscera of the thorax and abdomen; impulses conveyed centrally are important in

reflex control of cardiovascular, respiratory, and alimentary functions. The central processes of the primary sensory neurons for these reflexes descend in the tractus solitarius and end in the more caudal part of its nucleus (Figs. 8–11 and 8–12). Connections from the latter site are established bilaterally with several regions of the reticular formation. Reticulobulbar and reticulospinal connections provide pathways for reflex responses mediated by parasympathetic and sympathetic efferents.

Some axons from the nucleus of the tractus solitarius proceed rostrally to the hypothalamus. Still others constitute the small solitariospinal tract, which terminates on preganglionic autonomic neurons in the spinal cord.

Other Afferent Fibers

The glossopharyngeal nerve includes fibers for the general sensations of pain, temperature, and touch in the mucosa of the posterior one third of the tongue, up-

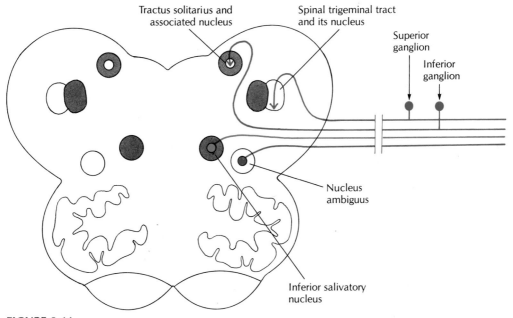

FIGURE 8-11.
Components of the glossopharyngeal nerve in the medulla.

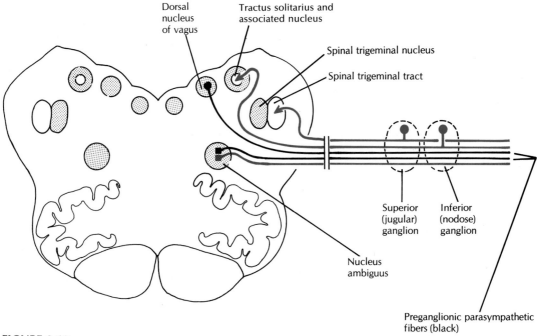

FIGURE 8-12.
Components of the vagus nerve in the medulla.

per part of the pharynx (including the tonsillar area), auditory or eustachian tube, and middle ear. The vagus nerve carries fibers having the same functions to the lower part of the pharynx, the larynx, and the esophagus. The cell bodies of these sensory neurons are thought to be in the superior ganglia of the glossopharyngeal and vagus nerves. Their central processes descend in the spinal tract of the trigeminal nerve and terminate in the corresponding nucleus (Figs. 8–11 and 8–12). The afferents for touch from the pharynx are important in the "gag reflex" through a reflex pathway that includes the nucleus ambiguus and the hypoglossal nucleus.

Finally, the vagus nerve, through its auricular branch, contributes sensory fibers to the concha of the external ear, a small area behind the ear, the wall of the external acoustic meatus, and the tympanic membrane. The cell bodies are in the superior ganglion of the nerve and the cen-

tral processes join the spinal tract of the trigeminal nerve. The area of skin and tympanic membrane supplied by the auricular branch of the vagus nerve is coextensive with that supplied by the facial nerve.

Efferent Components

The ninth, tenth, and eleventh cranial nerves include motor fibers for striated muscles, and the ninth and tenth nerves contain parasympathetic efferents.

For Supply of Striated Muscles

The **nucleus ambiguus** is a column of typical motor neurons situated dorsal to the inferior olivary nucleus (Figs. 8–11 and 8–12; see also Fig. 8–14). Fibers from the nucleus are directed dorsally at first. They then turn sharply to mingle with other fibers in the glossopharyngeal and vagus nerves, and some of them constitute the entire cranial root of the accessory nerve. The nucleus ambiguus supplies muscles of the soft palate, pharynx, and larynx, together with striated muscle fibers in the upper part of the esophagus. The only muscle in these regions not supplied by this nucleus is the tensor veli palatini muscle, which is innervated by the trigeminal nerve.

A small group of cells in the rostral end of the nucleus ambiguus supplies the stylopharyngeus muscle through the glossopharyngeal nerve (see Fig. 8–11). A large region of the nucleus supplies the remaining pharyngeal muscles, the cricothyroid muscle (an external muscle of the larynx), and the striated muscle of the esophagus

through the vagus nerve (Fig. 8–12). Fibers from the caudal part of the nucleus leave the brain stem in the cranial root of the accessory nerve (Fig. 8–14). They join the spinal root of the accessory nerve temporarily and then constitute the internal ramus of the nerve, which passes over to the vagus nerve in the region of the jugular foramen (Fig. 8–13). These fibers supply muscles of the soft palate and the intrinsic muscles of the larynx. It would be simpler, although contrary to convention, to consider the cranial root of the accessory nerve as part of the vagus nerve, leaving the spinal root as the definitive accessory nerve.

The nucleus ambiguus is not composed solely of motor neurons. As described further on, some of its cells are preganglionic

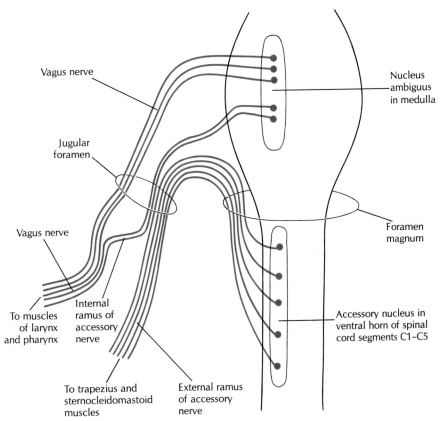

FIGURE 8-13.
Spinal and cranial roots of the accessory nerve.

parasympathetic neurons for control of the heart rate.

The nucleus ambiguus receives afferents from sensory nuclei of the brain stem, most importantly from the nucleus of the spinal tract of the trigeminal nerve and from the nucleus of the tractus solitarius. These connections establish reflexes for coughing, gagging, and vomiting, with the stimuli arising in the mucosa of the respiratory and alimentary passages. Corticobulbar afferents are both crossed and uncrossed; muscles supplied by the nucleus ambiguus are therefore not paralyzed in the event of a unilateral lesion of the upper motor neuron type.

Motor neurons for the sternocleidomastoid and trapezius muscles differentiate in the embryo near cells that are destined to form the nucleus ambiguus. The former cells migrate into the spinal cord (segments C1 through C5) and take up a position in the lateral part of the ventral gray horn. Arising as a series of rootlets along the side of the cord just dorsal to the denticulate ligament, the spinal root of the accessory nerve ascends next to the spinal cord, thus retracing the migration of cells of origin (see Fig. 8–13). On reaching the side of the medulla by passing through the foramen magnum, the spinal and cranial roots unite and continue as the accessory nerve as far as the jugular foramen. Fibers from the nucleus ambiguus then join the vagus nerve, as already noted, and those of spinal origin proceed to the sternocleidomastoid and trapezius muscles as the external ramus of the accessory nerve. Corticospinal fibers that control the spinal accessory neurons are almost all crossed. There is therefore contralateral weakness (paresis) of the sternocleidomastoid and trapezius muscles if an upper motor neuron lesion is present.

Parasympathetic Nuclei

There are parasympathetic fibers in the glossopharyngeal nerve, and these are es-

pecially numerous in the vagus nerve. The **inferior salivatory nucleus** for the parotid gland is a small collection of cells caudal to the superior salivatory nucleus and near the rostral tip of the nucleus ambiguus (see Fig. 8–11). (Its exact location in the human brain is uncertain.) Fibers from the inferior salivatory nucleus are included in the glossopharyngeal nerve, enter its tympanic branch, and reach the otic ganglion by way of the tympanic plexus and the lesser petrosal nerve. Postganglionic fibers join the auriculotemporal branch of the mandibular nerve and thus reach the parotid gland. The parasympathetic supply to the parotid gland is secretomotor and vasodilatory. The inferior salivatory nucleus is influenced by stimuli from the hypothalamus, olfactory system, nucleus of the tractus solitarius, and sensory trigeminal nuclei.

The largest parasympathetic nucleus is the **dorsal nucleus of the vagus nerve.** This column of cells extends throughout most of the medulla in the gray matter around the central canal and beneath the vagal triangle in the floor of the fourth ventricle (see Fig. 8–12). The axons of the cells in the dorsal nucleus constitute the majority of the preganglionic parasympathetic fibers of the vagus nerve. They end in the pulmonary plexus and in abdominal viscera, mostly in the myenteric and submucous plexuses of the alimentary canal. Other vagal parasympathetic neurons have their cell bodies in the nucleus ambiguus. The axons of these neurons terminate in small ganglia associated with the heart. It has been demonstrated in several animal species that the cardiac ganglia receive all their afferent fibers from the nucleus ambiguus and none from the dorsal nucleus of the vagus nerve. There is no reason to believe that these anatomical arrangements are any different in humans.

The dorsal nucleus of the vagus nerve and the visceral efferent neurons of the nucleus ambiguus are influenced, directly or indirectly, by the hypothalamus, the olfactory system, autonomic "centers" in the reticular formation, and the nucleus of the tractus solitarius.

Isolated lesions involving the ninth, tenth, or eleventh cranial nerves separately are uncommon. However, several pathological events, most frequently of vascular origin, cause destructon of the central nuclei. A unilateral lesion of the nucleus ambiguus, for example, results in ipsilateral paralysis of the soft palate, pharynx, and larynx, with the expected signs of hoarseness and difficulty in breathing and swallowing. Extensive lesions, especially if bilateral, carry a poor prognosis. Complete laryngeal paralysis leads to asphyxia unless immediate precautions are taken to restore the airway.

HYPOGLOSSAL NERVE

The **hypoglossal nucleus** lies between the dorsal nucleus of the vagus nerve and the midline of the medulla (Fig. 8–14). The hypoglossal triangle in the floor of the fourth ventricle marks the position of the rostral part of the nucleus. Fibers from the hypoglossal nucleus course ventrally on the lateral side of the medial lemniscus and emerge along the sulcus between the

pyramid and the olive. The hypoglossal nerve supplies the intrinsic muscles of the tongue and the three extrinsic muscles (genioglossus, styloglossus, and hyoglossus). The nucleus receives afferents from the nucleus of the tractus solitarius and the sensory trigeminal nuclei for reflex movements of the tongue in swallowing, chewing, and sucking in response to gustatory and other stimuli from the oral and pharyngeal mucosae. Corticobulbar afferents are predominantly crossed; a unilateral upper motor neuron lesion therefore causes paresis of the opposite side of the tongue.* Paralysis and eventual atrophy of the affected muscles follow destruction of the hypoglossal nucleus or interruption of the nerve. The tongue *deviates to the weak side* on protrusion because of the unopposed protrusor action of the contralateral genioglossus muscle.

---

* Only corticobulbar fibers are usually mentioned when discussing upper motor neuron lesions and their effects on muscles supplied by cranial nerves. In fact, voluntary control of the musculature generally is also mediated through pathways from the cortex that include the reticular formation. Corticoreticular as well as corticobulbar fibers are typically interrupted in an upper motor neuron lesion.

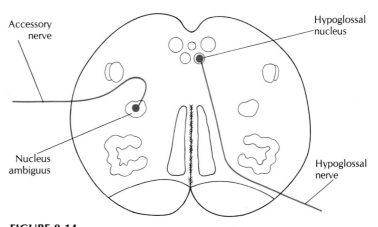

FIGURE 8-14.
Hypoglossal nerve and origin of the cranial root of the accessory nerve in the medulla.

SENSORY NERVE SUPPLY OF NEUROMUSCULAR SPINDLES

The striated skeletal muscles supplied by cranial nerves all execute movements that are delicately controlled. Proprioceptive input is therefore physiologically important. The following account is based on the results of animal experimentation; there is as yet no reliable information relating to humans. The information so obtained indicates that the mesencephalic nucleus of the trigeminal nerve is concerned primarily with the supply of neuromuscular spindles in the muscles of mastication.

The extraocular muscles contain spindles of a special type. Their sensory fibers in the ophthalmic nerve come from cells in the trigeminal ganglion whose central processes terminate in the pars oralis of the nucleus of the spinal tract of the trigeminal nerve.

Sensory fibers originating in the mesencephalic nucleus of the trigeminal nerve supply neuromuscular spindles in muscles innervated by the mandibular division, together with other proprioceptors associated with the muscles of mastication and proprioceptorlike endings adjacent to the teeth and in the hard palate. However, cell bodies for afferents from the temporomandibular joint have been located in the trigeminal ganglion.

The presence of spindles in the facial muscles has not been conclusively established. Sensory fibers for spindles in laryngeal muscles have been identified in the vagus nerve; the cell bodies must be in a ganglion of the vagus nerve because the fibers persist after section of the nerve proximal to the ganglia. Proprioceptors in the sternocleidomastoid and trapezius muscles receive sensory fibers through the second, third, and fourth cervical nerves, which provide the muscles with innervation additional to that from the accessory nerve.

Some of the cell bodies of sensory neurons supplying spindles in the tongue are in the inferior ganglion of the vagus nerve, with the fibers passing over to the hypoglossal nerve through an anastomotic connection. The muscles of the tongue also receive proprioceptive fibers from cells in dorsal root ganglia of the second and third cervical nerves. They enter the hypoglossal nerve through the ansa hypoglossi in the anterior triangle of the neck.

CLASSIFICATION OF CRANIAL AND SPINAL NERVE COMPONENTS

The components, including associated sensory nuclei, of the cranial and spinal nerves can be classified under seven headings. Four of these are present in both cranial and spinal nerves; three more are added in the former to include the special senses and to recognize the different embryonic origins of the muscles of the head. Cranial nerve nuclei in the brain stem are shown in Figure 8–15 according to the following classification, which is based on the classical embryological and comparative anatomical studies of C. J. Herrick.

Afferent Components

The **special somatic afferent** group consists of those special senses that relate the body to the external environment. This group consists of the optic nerve (included by convention) and the cochlear and vestibular nuclei.

General somatic afferent nuclei receive impulses from general sensory endings and are therefore concerned with pain, temperature, touch, and proprioception. The cells are in the nuclei gracilis and cuneatus, the sensory trigeminal nuclei, and the dorsal gray horn of the spinal cord.

Special visceral afferents are for taste, with second-order neurons located in the rostral part of the nucleus of the tractus solitarius (gustatory nucleus). The olfactory nerves are conventionally considered as special visceral afferent because of the influence of smell on visceral functions.

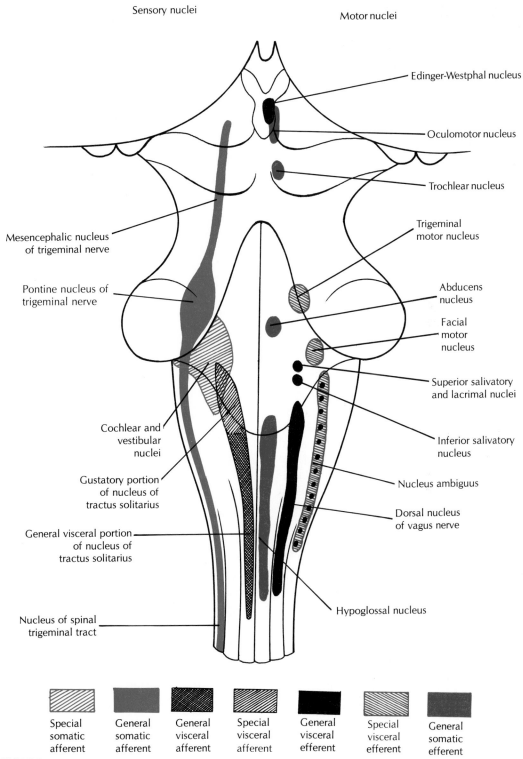

FIGURE 8-15.
Classification of the nuclei of cranial nerves.

General visceral afferent components are for visceral reflexes and for sensations such as fullness of hollow organs and pain of visceral origin. The second-order neurons are in the caudal portion of the nucleus of the tractus solitarius and the dorsal gray horn of the spinal cord.

Efferent Components

Groups of motor neurons included under the heading of **general somatic efferents** supply muscles derived from myotomes of the embryonic somites. They are the oculomotor, trochlear, abducens, and hypoglossal nuclei and the ventral horn cells of the spinal cord.

Special visceral efferents supply muscles derived from the branchial or gill arches of the embryo. They are classified as "visceral" because of the respiratory function of the gill arches in aquatic forms. There are three special visceral efferent nuclei: the trigeminal motor nucleus for the muscles of mastication, which develop from the first branchial arch, the facial motor nucleus for the muscles of expression, of second branchial arch derivation, and the nucleus ambiguus for muscles of the palate, pharynx, larynx, and upper esophagus, with these muscles being derived from the third, fourth, and fifth branchial arches. The spinal accessory nucleus is also usually included in the special visceral efferent category.

General visceral efferents are the preganglionic neurons of the autonomic nervous system. In the brain stem they include the Edinger–Westphal nucleus, lacrimal nucleus, superior and inferior salivatory nuclei, dorsal nucleus of the vagus nerve, and some of the cells in the nucleus ambiguus. In the spinal cord, this category consists of the intermediolateral cell column in the thoracic and upper lumbar segments and the parasympathetic cells in the sacral cord.

Centrifugal fibers in the optic nerve and especially the vestibulocochlear nerve are not included in the classical list of components because they were not known at the time the classification was devised. The name **special somatic efferent** is appropriate for efferent axons that modify the activities of the special sensory receptors.

SUGGESTED READING

Beckstead RM, Morse JR, Norgren R: The nucleus of the solitary tract in the monkey: Projections to the thalamus and brain stem nuclei. J Comp Neurol 190:259–282, 1980

Bender MB: Brain control of conjugate horizontal and vertical eye movements. A survey of the structural and functional correlates. Brain 103:23–69, 1980

Brodal A: Neurological Anatomy in Relation to Clinical Medicine, 3rd ed. New York, Oxford University Press, 1981

Büttner-Ennever JA, Büttner U, Cohen B, Baumgartner G: Vertical gaze paralysis and the rostral interstitial nucleus of the medial longitudinal fasciculus. Brain 105:125–149, 1982

Calaresu FR, Faiers AA, Mogenson, GJ: Central neural regulation of heart and blood vessels in mammals. Progr Neurobiol 5:1–35, 1975

Ferguson GG, Brett DC, Peerless SJ, Barr HWK, Girvin JP: Trigeminal neuralgia: A comparison of the results of percutaneous rhizotomy and microvascular decompression. Can J Neurol Sci 8:207–214, 1981

FitzGerald MJT, Comerford PT, Tuffery AR: Sources of innervation of the neuromuscular spindles in sternomastoid and trapezius. J Anat 134:471–490, 1982

FitzGerald MJT, Sachithanandan SR: The structure and source of lingual proprioceptors in the monkey. J Anat 128:523–552, 1979

Karim MA, Leong SK: Neurons of origin of cervical vagus nerves in the rat and monkey. Brain Res 186:208–210, 1980

Loewy AD: Neural regulation of the pupil. In Brooks C McC, Koizumi K, Sato A (eds): Integrative Functions of the Autonomic Nervous System, pp 131–141. Amsterdam, Elsevier–North Holland, 1979

May M (ed): The Facial Nerve. New York, Thieme, 1986

Norgren R, Leonard CM: Ascending central gustatory pathways. J Comp Neurol 150:217–237, 1973

Porter JD, Guthrie BL, Sparks DL: Innervation of monkey extraocular muscles: Localization of sensory and motor neurons by retrograde transport of horseradish peroxidase. J Comp Neurol 218:208–219, 1983

Ruskell GL: Spiral nerve endings in human extraocular muscles terminate in motor end plates. J Anat 139:33–43, 1984

Sparks DL: Translation of sensory signals into commands for control of saccadic eye movements: Role of primate superior colliculus. Physiol Rev 68:118–171, 1986

Travers JB, Travers SP, Norgren R: Gustatory neural processing on the hindbrain. Ann Rev Neurosci 10:595–632, 1987

Walberg F: On the morphology of the mesencephalic trigeminal cells. New data based on tracer studies. Brain Res 322:119–123, 1984

Wurtz RH, Albano JE: Visual-motor function of the primate superior colliculus. Annu Rev Neurosci 3:189–226, 1980

Zahm DS, Munger BL: The innervation of the primate fungiform papilla—Development, distribution and changes following selective ablation. Brain Res Rev 9:147–186, 1985

NINE

Reticular Formation

This chapter contains an account of the essentials of the reticular formation of the brain stem, followed by descriptions of a few nuclei that are not discussed in Chapters 7 and 8.

Broadly defined, the reticular formation consists of a substantial portion of the brain stem in which the groups of neurons and bundles of fibers present a netlike ("reticular") appearance. It excludes nuclei of cranial nerves, long tracts that pass through the brain stem, and the more conspicuous masses of gray matter. The neurons of the reticular nuclei all have unusually long dendrites that extend into parts of the brain stem remote from the cell bodies. Their architecture enables them to receive and integrate synaptic inputs from most or all of the systems of neurons projecting to or through the brain stem. Caudally the reticular formation blends imperceptibly into lamina VII of the spinal gray matter. It is important to appreciate that the "ascending reticular activating system," to be considered presently, is not identical with the reticular formation. The system includes large parts of the reticular formation, together with parts of the diencephalon and telencephalon.

The reticular formation receives data from most of the sensory systems and has efferent connections, direct or indirect, with all levels of the central nervous system. It contributes to several functions, including the sleep–arousal cycle, the motor system of the brain and spinal cord, and the regulation of visceral activity. Although such adjectives as "primitive" and "diffuse" have been applied to the reticular formation, it is not a mass of randomly interconnected neurons. The parts of the reticular formation differ from one another in their cytoarchitecture, connections, and physiological functions. Aggregations of neurons are thereby recognized, and they are called nuclei even though they are not as clearly circumscribed as most nuclei elsewhere. In fact, information obtained through research has revealed higher and higher degrees of orderly structural organization than were previously thought to exist.

NUCLEI AND CYTOARCHITECTURE

The nuclei of the reticular formation can be classified as follows: the precerebellar nuclei, the raphe nuclei, the central and lateral groups of nuclei, and the catecholamine nuclei.

Precerebellar Reticular Nuclei

Three nuclei—the lateral reticular nucleus, the paramedian reticular nucleus, and the pontine reticulotegmental nucleus (Fig. 9–1)—project to the cerebellum. These, the precerebellar reticular nuclei, are functionally quite separate from the rest of the reticular formation; they are therefore considered in Chapter 10, which deals with the cerebellum.

Raphe Nuclei

The raphe nuclei are in the midline of the brain stem. The cells are interspersed among bundles of decussating myelinated axons, which are the most conspicuous feature of the raphe in sections stained for myelin. The raphe nuclei form a contiguous column, but individual nuclei with different cytoarchitecture and efferent projections are recognized at different levels. Some of these are named in Figure 9–1. The nucleus raphe magnus, in the medulla, is the best understood member of the group, and certain aspects of the nucleus are discussed later in the chapter. The neurons of the raphe produce serotonin, and are believed to use this amine as a transmitter.

Central and Lateral Groups of Nuclei

On each side of the midline is the central group of nuclei—the ventral reticular and the gigantocellular reticular nuclei in the medulla, and the caudal and oral pontine reticular nuclei. The lateral group of reticular nuclei includes the parvicellular reticular nucleus in the medulla and pons, and the cuneiform, pedunculopontine, and parabrachial nuclei in the midbrain (see Fig. 9–1). The approximate positions of the precerebellar, central, and lateral nuclei are shown in Figures 9–1 through 9–5, but it should be remembered that the formally designated territories of the populations of cells overlap, both in the rostrocaudal and in the medial to lateral directions.

The dendrites of neurons of the central group of reticular nuclei spread out in a plane at right angles to the long axis of the brain stem. The long axons run rostrally and caudally, with many collateral branches that synapse with the dendrites of other reticular neurons (Fig. 9–6A). Terminal branches of the axons end in other nuclei of the reticular formation or in more remote regions, such as the thalamus and spinal cord. Some of the neurons in the central group of nuclei have axons that branch close to the cell body in such a way that a single cell may give rise to a reticulothalamic and a reticulospinal fiber (Fig. 9–6B). Because groups of rostrally projecting neurons are mostly situated caudal to caudally projecting groups, there is considerable interaction between the ascending and descending outputs of the central group of nuclei. The reticular formation contains no interneurons with short axons, but synapses are very numerous because of the abundant collateral axonal branches. The laterally placed parvicellular reticular nucleus consists of neurons whose axons generally project medially into the central group of nuclei.

The major afferent connections of the central and some of the lateral nuclei of the reticular formation are summarized in

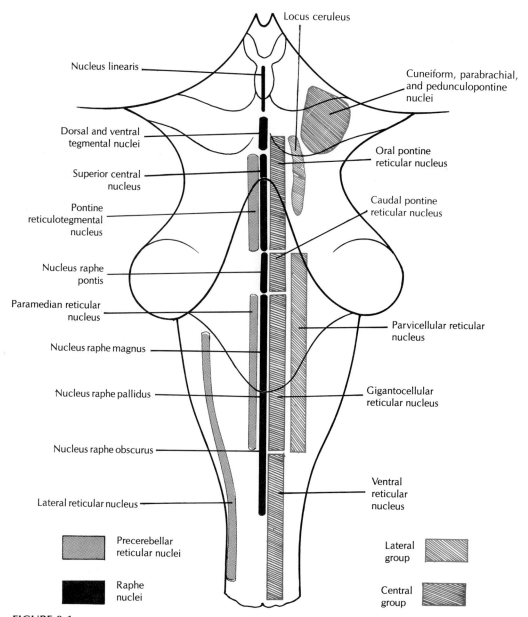

FIGURE 9-1.

Nuclei of the reticular formation of the brain stem.

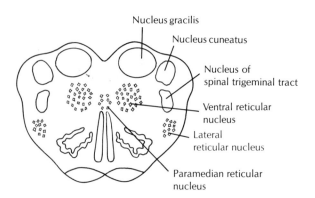

FIGURE 9-2.

Reticular nuclei at the level of the caudal portion of the inferior olivary nucleus.

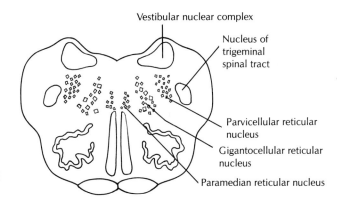

FIGURE 9-3.
Reticular nuclei at the level of the rostral portion of the inferior olivary nucleus.

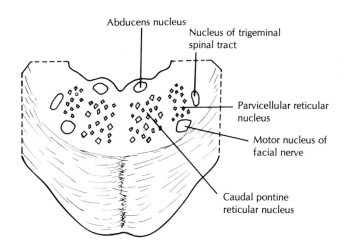

FIGURE 9-4.
Reticular nuclei in the caudal region of the pontine tegmentum.

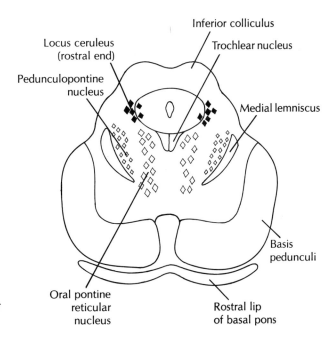

FIGURE 9-5.
Reticular nuclei at the level of the inferior colliculus.

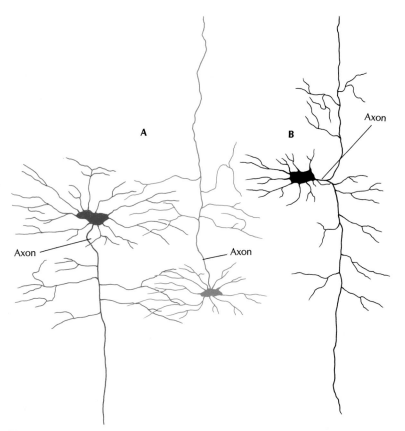

FIGURE 9-6.
Neurons of the reticular formation. **(A)** Interaction between dendrites and collateral axonal branches of neurons with ascending (*blue*) and descending (*red*) projections. **(B)** A neuron whose axon divides into long ascending and descending branches.

Figure 9–7. The largest contingents of afferent fibers come from the spinal cord, from the primary motor cortex of the frontal lobe, and from much of the cortex of the parietal lobe, including the somesthetic area. Other afferents include those that originate in the vestibular nuclei, in the cerebellar nuclei, and in the superior colliculus. The main efferent projections arise in the central group of nuclei and proceed rostrally to the thalamus and caudally to the spinal cord. All connections except those of the pontine reticulospinal tract (which is ipsilateral) include both crossed and uncrossed fibers.

Lateral nuclei other than the parvi-cellular reticular nucleus have various connections and functions. Thus, the cuneiform and pedunculopontine nuclei are involved in the control of movement. The parabrachial nucleus is connected with the limbic system, and also forms part of the ascending pathway for taste sensation.

Catecholamine Nuclei

The **locus ceruleus** at the rostral end of the floor of the fourth ventricle on each side marks the position of a nucleus with a rich vascular supply and consisting of neurons containing melanin pigment. The nucleus (also known as the nucleus pigmentosus)

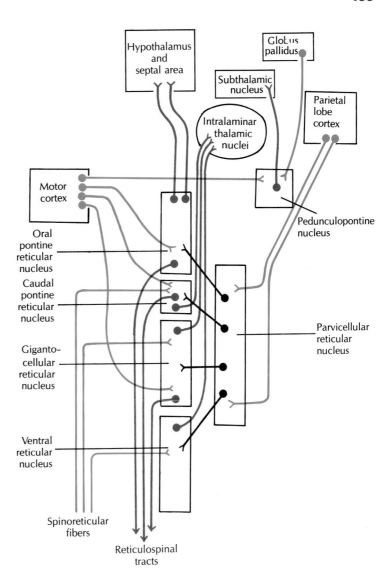

FIGURE 9-7.
Connectons of the central and lateral groups of reticular nuclei.

is partly in the pons and partly in the mid-brain, lying dorsolateral to the oral pontine reticular nucleus (Figs. 9–1 and 9–5). The neurons of the locus ceruleus contain large quantities of norepinephrine (noradrena-line), which they use as a transmitter sub-stance. The axons are greatly branched and very long, extending into all parts of the central nervous system, including the cerebral cortex, diencephalon, brain stem, cerebellum, and spinal cord. Individual axons branch close to the cell body, and the branches commonly proceed to widely

separated places. The dendrites of the neurons are also extensive, spreading well outside the anatomical confines of the nu-cleus.

Little is known of the afferent connec-tions of the locus ceruleus. In experimen-tal animals, fibers have been found to come from some of the raphe nuclei, from the hypothalamus, and from two telence-phalic regions, the amygdaloid body and the cingulate gyrus. The functions of the nucleus are unknown. The widespread dissemination of its efferent axons indicates that the noradrenergic neurons probably exert some rather general effect on the brain as a whole. A neuromodulatory action at synapses has been suggested. Another proposal is that the efferent fibers contact supposedly contractile cells (pericytes) associated with capillary blood vessels in the central nervous system, thereby providing an intrinsic central vasomotor regulatory system.

The locus ceruleus is the largest of about a dozen nuclei in the brain stem that produce catecholamines. Most produce norepinephrine, but some of those in the medulla produce epinephrine (adrenaline). A third catecholamine is dopamine, the transmitter used by the large neurons of the substantia nigra and ventral tegmental area, and by certain nuclei of the hypothalamus.

FUNCTIONAL ORGANIZATION

Despite the close anatomical association between the rostrally and caudally projecting neurons, it is convenient to consider the functional organization as consisting of three systems with overlapping functions. The ascending reticular activating system is concerned with arousal and consciousness. The reticulospinal and reticulobulbar system is concerned with motor and visceral functions. A system involving the serotonergic raphe nuclei modulates the transmission of signals in ascending pathways and may also influence the level of consciousness.

Ascending Reticular Activating System

The ascending reticular activating system consists of the sensory input to the reticular formation and rostral transmission to certain thalamic nuclei, from which activity spreads to the cerebral cortex. The reticular nuclei included in the system are the four constituting the central group, the parvicellular reticular nucleus, and possibly some of the catecholamine nuclei. The

name "ascending reticular activating system" is the one most widely used. Synonyms include "nonspecific afferent system" and "ascending activating system."

Sensory Input

The sensory input to the ascending reticular activating system is as follows. Neurons giving rise to spinoreticular fibers are located in laminae V through VIII of the spinal gray matter. These cells are stimulated as a result of activity in primary afferent fibers that mediate all modalities of external and visceral sensation. The spinoreticular tract ascends through the ventrolateral funiculus of the cord to the medulla. There the axons branch profusely and terminate in the central group of reticular nuclei. The sites of termination of the spinoreticular fibers are not uniformly distributed within the central group of nuclei; they are densest in those parts that give rise to ascending (mainly reticulothalamic) projections.

In addition to the spinoreticular input, the reticular formation receives afferent fibers from some sensory cranial nerve nuclei (the spinal trigeminal nucleus, the nucleus of the tractus solitarius, and the vestibular nuclei) and from collateral branches of ascending axons of the auditory system. Tectoreticular fibers come from the superior colliculus, which receives afferents from the visual cortex and the optic tract. Olfactory stimulation has been shown by physiological methods to evoke activity in the reticular formation, possibly mediated by corticoreticular fibers that arise from olfactory areas of the cerebral cortex.

Thus it is seen that the central group of reticular nuclei is influenced by most types of sensation. These afferent inputs are supplemented by a projection from the cortex of the parietal lobe (which includes the general somesthetic area) to the parvicellular reticular nucleus, and thence to the central group of nuclei (see Fig. 9-7).

Projections to Higher Centers

Neurons with ascending axons are present throughout the central group of nuclei, but are most abundant in the lower half of the medulla and in the lower half of the pons (see Fig. 9-7). These sites of origin are both caudal to the principal sites of origin of reticulospinal fibers, and permit maximal interaction between neurons with ascending and descending axons. The presence of neurons with branched axons projecting both rostrally and caudally has already been mentioned. The ascending fibers run in the central tegmental tract, which also contains many descending fibers destined for the inferior olivary complex. They pass rostrally into the diencephalon, where most of them end in the **intralaminar thalamic nuclei.** In humans, the **centromedian nucleus** (of the intralaminar group) is particularly well developed.

The intralaminar nuclei project to all parts of the frontal and parietal lobes of the cerebral cortex, and also to the neostriatum, which is part of the corpus striatum. The cortex also receives branches of the axons of the noradrenergic neurons of the locus ceruleus. Serotonergic neurons of the raphe nuclei project to the cortex of the limbic system.

Other ascending fibers from the reticular formation pass beneath the thalamus. Most of these terminate in the hypothalamus and in the septal area, which is a component of the limbic system and one of the regions of the brain associated with emotional responses.

Functions

The role of the reticular activating system is best understood when compared to that of the "lemniscal system" (medial, spinal, and trigeminal lemnisci). Sensory information conveyed by the latter system, when projected from the ventral posterior nucleus of the thalamus to the somesthetic cortical area, is interpreted in a specific manner with respect to the nature of the stimulus and its quantitative and discriminative aspects. The ascending reticular system is relatively nonspecific; the sensory modalities are merged as a consequence of convergence of different pathways upon the reticular formation and the thalamus, producing at best a vague awareness of any particular sensory modality. Much of the cortex is stimulated, with a profound effect on levels of consciousness and on alerting reactions to sensory stimuli. When cortical stimulation by way of the reticular formation occurs during sleep, the electrical activity of the cortex, as seen on the electroencephalogram, changes from the large-wave random pattern of sleep to the small-wave pattern of the waking state. When someone is awake, stimuli reaching the cortex through the activating system sharpen attentiveness and create optimal conditions for perception of sensory data conveyed through more direct pathways. Cutaneous stimuli appear to be especially important in maintaining consciousness whereas visual, acoustic, and mental stimuli have a special bearing on alertness and attention. Impulses from the trigeminal area of distribution have a significant influence on consciousness. This is the basis of methods found to be useful in restoring a person from a "fainting spell." To cite a once popular example, smelling salts contain ammonia or other substances that stimulate trigeminal sensory endings in the nasal mucosa.

The reticular activating system is of pharmacological interest because some general anesthetics are thought to suppress transmission through the reticular formation of the brain stem, although conduction continues along lemniscal routes. As a corollary of the above, prolonged coma results from serious damage to the pontine or mesencephalic reticular formation.

The foregoing is a much simplified account of the ascending reticular activating system, and other parts of the brain are no doubt involved as well in the sleep–arousal cycle and in related phenomena. Also, in addition to raising the level of consciousness and increasing alertness by the active process described, there may be a coexisting active process that induces sleep. Support for the existence of such a dual mechanism comes from the results of pharmacological studies and from the production of sleep in experimental animals by electrical stimulation of various parts of the brain, including the raphe nuclei.

Motor and Visceral Activities

The reticulospinal tracts constitute one of the major descending pathways involved in the control of movement. The others are the corticospinal and vestibulospinal tracts. (In many animals, but not in apes or humans, the rubrospinal tract is another major motor pathway.) Equivalent reticulobulbar connections supply the motor nuclei of cranial nerves. The **pontine reticulospinal tract,** originating in the caudal and oral pontine reticular nuclei, descends in the ventral funiculus of the same side of the spinal cord. The **medullary reticulospinal tract** arises from the gigantocellular reticular nuclei of both sides and descends in the ventrolateral funiculus. Some of the uncrossed fibers of both these tracts decussate in the ventral white commissure of the cord before terminating. The reticulospinal tracts consequently project both ipsilaterally and bilaterally to the spinal gray matter. They terminate in lamina VII and influence the motor neurons of lamina IX indirectly through synaptic relays within the spinal cord.

The regions of the central group of reticular nuclei that give rise to most of the reticulospinal fibers are located slightly rostral to the levels that send the most profuse ascending projections to the cerebral cortex (see Fig. 9-7). Because of the extensive interaction of collateral axonal branches with dendrites in the reticular formation, activity in the reticulospinal neurons is affected by activity in the rostrally projecting reticulothalamic neurons. Important afferents to the central group of reticular nuclei, with respect to the reticulospinal tracts and motor functions, are from the motor cortex of the cerebral hemispheres, cerebellar nuclei, and spinal cord. It is noteworthy that corticoreticular fibers from the motor cortex terminate principally in the parts of the central nuclear group that give rise to the greatest numbers of reticulospinal axons. The pedunculopontine nucleus in the midbrain must also be involved in motor control because of its connections with the corpus striatum and the subthalamic nucleus (see Fig. 9–7).

The **raphe spinal tract** (next section) is also a reticulospinal pathway, but it is concerned with the modulation of sensation rather than with the control of movement.

Certain regions in the reticular formation regulate visceral functions through connections with nuclei of the autonomic outflow and, in the case of respiration, with motor neurons in the phrenic nucleus and thoracic cord as well. Respiratory and cardiovascular regions, commonly referred to as "centers," have been identified by electrical stimulation within the brain stem in experimental animals. These "centers" are probably fields within the network of dendrites in the reticular formation rather than compact collections of cell bodies. Maximal inspiratory and expiratory responses are obtained from the gigantocellular reticular nucleus and the parvicellular reticular nucleus, respectively, in the medulla. A "pneumotaxic center" in the pons may influence respiratory rhythm. Stimulation of the ventral and gigantocellular reticular nuclei in the medulla has a depressor effect on the circulatory system, with slowing of the heart rate and lowering of blood pressure. The opposite effects are produced by stimulation of the parvicellular reticular nucleus in the medulla. Damage to the brain stem is life-threatening because of the presence of these centers that control vital functions.

SEROTONERGIC RAPHE NUCLEI

Afferent fibers to the raphe nuclei of the midbrain and pons come from various parts of the limbic and olfactory systems and the hypothalamus. The periaqueductal gray matter is connected to the nucleus raphe magnus in the medulla. The neurons of the raphe nuclei contain serotonin, a substance that they probably use as a neurotransmitter. Their axons are distributed to many regions of the telencephalon, diencephalon, brain stem, and spinal cord. The ascending efferents may form an important part of the ascending system that controls consciousness. Activity of the raphe nuclei induces sleep, an effect attributed to the release of serotonin from axonal endings in more rostral parts of the brain.

Interesting aspects of raphe nuclei from a clinical viewpoint are the input from the periaqueductal gray matter and the projection from the nucleus raphe magnus to the spinal dorsal horn. Electrical stimulation of either the periaqueductal gray matter or the nucleus raphe magnus results in loss of the ability to experience pain from sites of injury or disease; the former procedure has been used clinically in the management of otherwise intractable pain. Curiously, the analgesic action of a few minutes' stimulation can last for several hours.

Peptide neurotransmitters or neuromodulators known as enkephalins are released at synapses in the periaqueductal gray matter, the raphe nuclei, and the substantia gelatinosa of the dorsal horn of spinal gray matter. The enkephalins have analgesic actions similar to those of morphine and related opiate drugs, which bind to the same postsynaptic receptor molecules. The analgesic effects of stimulation of the periaqueductal gray matter and those of the medicinally used opiates require the integrity of the raphe spinal tract in the dorsolateral funiculus of the spinal cord. Drugs such as naloxone that antagonize morphine are also able to prevent the analgesia brought about by electrical stimulation of the nucleus raphe magnus or the periaqueductal gray matter. Other opiatelike peptides, the endorphins, have been found in several parts of the brain and in the pituitary gland. It is believed that the opiates produce their pharmacological effects by mimicking the actions of enkephalins and endorphins. Thus, the principal anatomical sites of the relief of pain by morphine are thought to be the periaqueductal gray matter, the nucleus raphe magnus, and the dorsal horn.

MISCELLANEOUS NUCLEI OF THE BRAIN STEM

Several nuclei in the brain stem may be considered at this time.

The **area postrema** is a narrow strip of neural tissue in the caudal part of the floor of the fourth ventricle, between the vagal triangle and the margin of the ventricle (see Fig. 6–3). It is richly vascular and contains many large sinusoids. The blood–brain barrier, which elsewhere prevents certain substances from entering nervous tissue from the blood, is lacking. Among other possible connections, the area postrema receives visceral afferents from the spinal cord, and there are reciprocal connections with the nucleus of the tractus solitarius. The area has been shown experimentally to be a chemoreceptor region for emetic drugs such as apomorphine and digoxin, and it may therefore function in the physiology of vomiting.

The **perihypoglossal nuclei** consist of three groups of neurons in the caudal medulla—the nucleus intercalatus (between the hypoglossal nucleus and the dorsal nucleus of the vagus), the nucleus of Roller (ventrolateral to the hypoglossal nucleus), and the nucleus prepositus hypoglossi (rostral to the hypoglossal nucleus), which is the largest. It is continuous at its rostral end with the paramedian pontine reticular formation (PPRF; see Fig. 8–5).

These nuclei receive afferents from several sources, including the cerebral cortex, vestibular nuclei, accessory oculomotor nuclei, and PPRF. Efferent fibers proceed mainly to the nuclei of cranial nerves III, IV, and VI, which they reach by passing in the medial longitudinal fasciculus. The perihypoglossal nuclei form part of the complex circuitry for movements of the eyes.

The **accessory oculomotor nuclei** are the interstitial nucleus of Cajal, the nucleus of Darkschewitsch, the nucleus of the posterior commissure, and the rostral interstitial nucleus of the medial longitudinal fasciculus. They are situated at the junction of the midbrain and the diencephalon, near the rostal end of the cerebral aqueduct, and are concerned with movements of the eyes. Their positions are shown in Figure 9–8. The specific connections and functions of the individual nuclei composing this group are poorly understood, so they were treated as a group in the discussion of ocular movements in Chapter 8. One of the nuclei, the interstitial nucleus of Cajal, is notable in that, together with the Edinger–Westphal nucleus, it sends some axons caudally as the interstitiospinal tract. This minor pathway probably contributes to visuomotor coordination. The rostral interstitial nucleus of the medial longitudinal fasciculus is part of the circuitry necessary for vertical eye movements.

The **periaqueductal gray matter** surrounds the cerebral aqueduct of the mid-

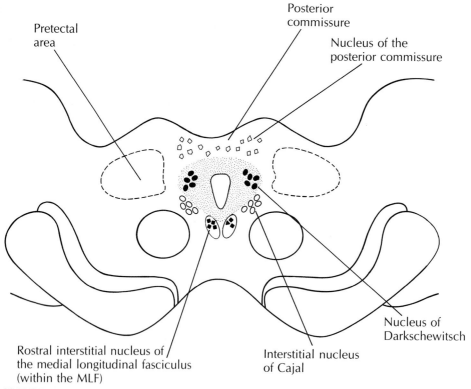

FIGURE 9-8.
Transitional zone between the midbrain and the diencephalon at the level of the posterior commissure, showing accessory oculomotor nuclei.

brain. Although afferent and efferent connections have been traced in experimental animals with regions ranging from the spinal cord to parts of the telencephalon, its physiological role is largely obscure. As mentioned earlier, electrical stimulation of the periaqueductal gray matter causes analgesia, and this effect is mediated by way of the descending projection of the nucleus raphe magnus in the medulla. The **nucleus of Darkschewitsch** is within the territory of the periaqueductal gray matter, but it probably differs in function because it is one of the accessory oculomotor nuclei.

The **interpeduncular nucleus** is in the midline ventral to the periaqueductal gray matter, and is near the roof of the most rostral part of the interpeduncular fossa. This nucleus lies on a pathway through which the limbic system projects to autonomic nuclei in the brain stem and spinal cord.

SUGGESTED READING

Amaral DG, Sinnamon HM: The locus coeruleus: Neurobiology of a central noradrenergic nucleus. Progr Neurobiol 9:147–196, 1977

Angevine JB, Cotman CW: Principles of Neuroanatomy, Chaps 11 and 14. New York, Oxford University Press, 1981

Beers RF, Bassett EF (eds): Mechanisms of Pain and Analgesic Compounds. Miles International Symposium Series, No 11. New York, Raven Press, 1979

Brodal A: Neurological Anatomy in Relation to Clinical Medicine, 3rd ed. New York, Oxford University Press, 1981

Bystrzycka EK: Afferent projections to the dorsal and ventral respiratory nuclei in the medulla oblongata of the cat, studied by the horseradish peroxidase technique. Brain Res 185:59–66, 1980

Fukushima K: The interstitial nucleus of Cajal and its role in the control of movements of the head and eyes. Prog Neurobiol 29:107–192, 1987

Kelly DD: Physiology of sleep and dreaming. Chap 40 in Kandel ER, Schwartz JH (eds): Principles of Neural Science, pp 472–485. New York, Elsevier-North Holland, 1981

Mantyh PW: Connections of the periaqueductal gray in the monkey. J Neurophysiol 49:567–594, 1983

Noback CR, Demarest RJ: The Human Nervous System, 3rd ed. New York, McGraw-Hill, 1981

Schofield BJ, Everitt BJ: The organization of catecholamine-containing neurons in the brain of the rhesus monkey (Macaca mulatta). J Anat 132:391–418, 1981

Vigier D, Portalier P: Efferent projections of the area postrema demonstrated by autoradiography. Arch Ital Biol 117:308–324, 1979

TEN

Cerebellum

Although the cerebellum has an abundant input from sensory receptors it is essentially a motor part of the brain, functioning in the maintenance of equilibrium and in the coordination of muscle action in both stereotyped and nonstereotyped movements. The cerebellum makes a special contribution to synergy of muscle action (*i.e.*, to the synchronization of muscles that make up a functional group), ensuring that there is contraction of the proper muscles at the appropriate time, each with the correct force. It follows that cerebellar lesions become manifest as disturbances of motor function without voluntary paralysis. The cerebellum increased in size in the course of vertebrate evolution. The prominent development in humans coincides with the need for synergy of muscles in learned activities that require precision.

The cerebellum consists of a **cortex,** or surface layer, of gray matter contained in transverse folds or folia, a **medullary center** of white matter, and four pairs of **central nuclei** embedded in the medullary center. The paired **inferior, middle,** and **superior cerebellar peduncles,** composed of nerve fibers, connect the cerebellum with the medulla, pons, and midbrain, respectively.

GROSS ANATOMY

The superior cerebellar surface is elevated in the midline, conforming to the dural reflection or tentorium that forms a roof for the posterior cranial fossa. The inferior surface is grooved deeply in the midline; the remainder of this surface is convex on each side and rests on the floor of the posterior cranial fossa (Fig. 10–1).

Certain terms are useful to identify regions of the cerebellar surface. The region in and near the midline is known as the

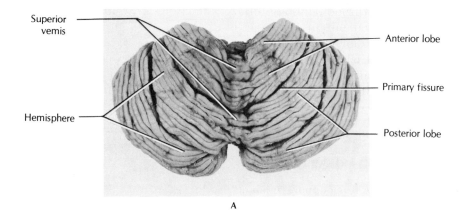

Superior vemis

Anterior lobe

Primary fissure

Hemisphere

Posterior lobe

A

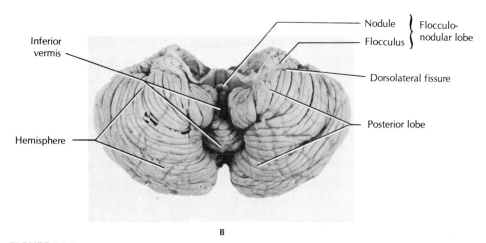

Nodule } Flocculo-
Flocculus } nodular lobe

Inferior vermis

Dorsolateral fissure

Posterior lobe

Hemisphere

B

FIGURE 10-1.
The cerebellum. **(A)** Superior surface. **(B)** Inferior surface. (× ⅔)

vermis and the remainder as the **hemispheres.** The superior vermis is not demarcated from the hemispheres, but the inferior vermis lies in a deep depression (the vallecula) and is well delineated.

Three major regions, the flocculonodular, anterior, and posterior lobes, are recognized in the horizontal plane (Fig. 10–1). The **flocculonodular lobe** (or lobule) is a small component, the oldest phylogenetically, that lies at the rostral edge of the inferior surface. The nodule is the rostral portion of the inferior vermis, and the flocculi are irregularly shaped masses on each side. The cerebellum is deeply indented by several transverse fissures. The **dorso-**

lateral fissure (also called the posterolateral fissure) along the caudal border of the flocculonodular lobe is the first of these to appear during embryonic development. The main mass of the cerebellum (all but the flocculonodular lobe) is called the **corpus cerebelli** and consists of anterior and posterior lobes. The **anterior lobe** is that part of the superior surface rostral to the **primary fissure.** This, despite its name, is the second fissure to appear during embryonic development. The remainder of the cerebellum on both surfaces constitutes the **posterior lobe.**

The roof of the rostral part of the fourth ventricle is formed by the superior cere-

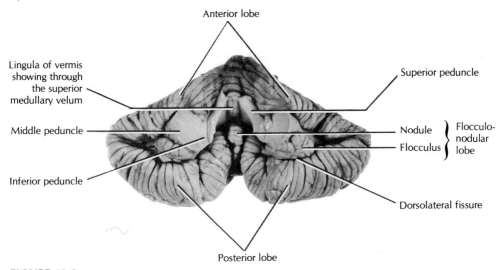

FIGURE 10-2.
Cerebellum as viewed from in front and below, showing the cut surfaces of the cerebellar peduncles. ($\times$ ⅔)

bellar peduncles and by the superior medullary velum that bridges the interval between them (Fig. 10–2). The remainder of the roof consists of the thin inferior medullary velum, formed by pia mater and ependyma. This membrane, in which a deficiency constitutes the median aperture of the fourth ventricle or foramen of Magendie (see Fig. 6–4), frequently adheres to the inferior vermis. The three pairs of peduncles are attached to the cerebellum in the interval between the flocculonodular and anterior lobes.

Other fissures outline further subdivisions or lobules, especially in the posterior lobe. The names given to these lobules by early anatomists have no functional significance; neither is there uniform acceptance of a single system of nomenclature. Figure 10–3 is inserted for reference if smaller subdivisions of the cerebellum need to be identified.

Three major divisions of the cerebellum are recognized using other criteria, based either on their order of appearance in vertebrate evolution or on the destination of different categories of afferent fibers. However, cortical histology is uni-

form throughout the cerebellum, unlike the cerebral cortex in which there are histologically different areas. The four central nuclei are likewise similar at the cellular level. The cortex and nuclei are therefore described at this point, after which the functional divisions and their individual connections will be discussed.

Cerebellar Cortex

Because of the extensive folding of the cerebellar surface in the form of thin transverse **folia,** 85% of the cortical surface is concealed. There is therefore a large cortical area, which is about three quarters as extensive as that of the much larger cerebrum.

Cortical Layers

Three layers are evident on histological section. From the surface to the white matter of the folium, these are the molecular layer, the layer of Purkinje cells, and the granule cell layer (Fig. 10–4). The **Purkinje cell layer** consists of a single row (in sections) of bodies of Purkinje cells. The

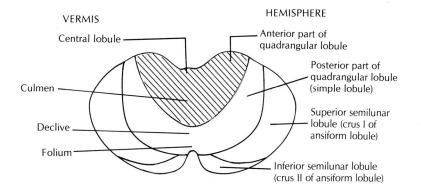

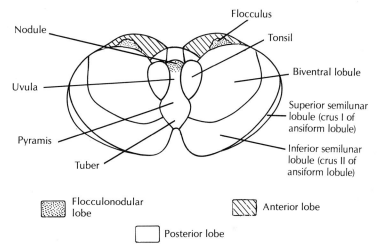

FIGURE 10-3.
Nomenclature for specific regions of the cerebellum. The lingula, not seen in these drawings, is a small flattened portion of the superior vermis beneath the central lobule and adherent to the superior medullary velum (Fig. 10–2).

molecular layer contains relatively few nerve cells; it is largely a synaptic layer, made up of profusely branching dendrites of Purkinje cells and axons of the granule cells in the deepest layer. The term *molecular* is derived from the punctate appearance of this layer in sections stained for nerve fibers. The molecular layer includes scattered stellate cells near the surface and modified stellate cells, known as basket cells, at a deeper level. The **granule cell layer** consists of closely packed small neurons, from which axons extend into the molecular layer. There are scattered neurons known as Golgi cells in the outer zone of the granule cell layer.

Of the afferent fibers to the cortex, **mossy fibers** terminate in synaptic contact with granule cells of the innermost layer, whereas **climbing fibers** enter the molecular layer and wind among the dendrites of Purkinje cells. The only fibers leaving the cortex are axons of Purkinje cells. These fibers terminate in central nuclei of

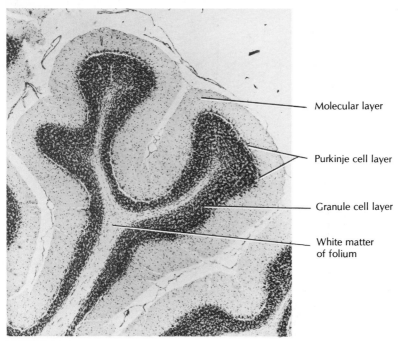

Molecular layer

Purkinje cell layer

Granule cell layer

White matter
of folium

FIGURE 10-4.
Transverse section of cerebellar folia showing the three layers of cortex and
the white matter of the folia. (Stained with cresyl violet, × 35)

the cerebellum, with the exception of some fibers from the cortex of the flocculonodular lobe that proceed to the brain stem.

Cytoarchitecture

The five neuron types in the cerebellar cortex establish a complex but remarkably regular pattern of intracortical circuits. The precise three-dimensional orientation of dendrites and axons, as shown by the Golgi staining method and by electron microscopy, has encouraged the study of cortical physiology at the cellular level by means of recording microelectrodes. The basic pattern of the neurons is indicated in Figure 10–5.

Granule Cells and Mossy Fibers. The granule cells are small and are closely packed together in the deepest cortical layer. Each cell has a spherical nucleus with a coarse chromatin pattern, and the scanty cytoplasm lacks clumps of Nissl substance. The short dendrites have clawlike endings that are contacted by mossy fibers. The unmyelinated axon enters the molecular layer, where it bifurcates and runs parallel with the folium. Because of the density of the granule cell population, the whole molecular layer contains closely arranged parallel fibers. Each granule cell axon traverses the dendritic trees of some 450 Purkinje cells, making synaptic contacts with their dendritic spines. These axons also synapse with dendrites of stellate, basket, and Golgi cells in the molecular layer.

A large proportion of the afferent fibers to the cerebellum are mossy fibers that terminate in synaptic relation with dendrites of granule cells. While still in the white matter a mossy fiber divides into several branches, which may enter the cortex of adjacent folia. On entering the granule cell layer the fiber loses its myelin sheath and

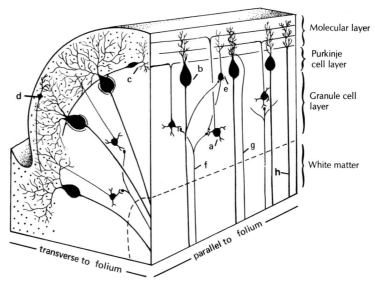

FIGURE 10-5.
Cytoarchitecture of the cerebellar cortex. (**a**) Granule cell. (**b**) Purkinje cell. (**c**) Basket cell. (**d**) Stellate cell. (**e**) Golgi cell. (**f**) Mossy fiber. (**g**) Climbing fiber. (**h**) Catecholamine fiber.

there is further terminal branching. Along the terminal portion of the fiber, and at its end, there are swellings known as rosettes, with which the dendrites of several granule cells make synaptic contact (Fig. 10–6). The synaptic configuration that includes the rosette of a mossy fiber, dendrites of granule cells, and the axon of a Golgi cell (see Stellate and Golgi Cells) is known as a **glomerulus**.

Purkinje Cells and Climbing Fibers. The number of Purkinje cells is of the order of 15 million. These cells are easily recognized by their flask-shaped cell bodies. However, their most remarkable characteristic is profuse dendritic branching in the molecular layer, in a plane transverse to the folium. The primary and secondary branches are smooth, whereas the finer branches bear regularly spaced spines. Electron micrographs show that the spines indenting parallel fibers (axons of granule cells) form synaptic junctions. The parallel

arrangement of axons of granule cells and the transverse orientation of dendrites of Purkinje cells, with respect to a folium, provide maximal opportunity for a Purkinje cell to receive stimuli from a very large number of granule cells, and also allow a granule cell to contact many Purkinje cells. The molecular layer is therefore a rich synaptic field to which stellate, basket, and Golgi cells also contribute.

Axons of Purkinje cells traverse the granule cell layer, acquire myelin sheaths, and terminate mainly in central cerebellar nuclei. Collateral branches given off by the axons synapse with adjacent Purkinje cells or, more frequently, with Golgi cells in the outer part of the granule cell layer.

As the mossy fibers have a special relationship with granule cells, so the climbing fibers have a special relationship with Purkinje cells. Climbing fibers enter the cortex from the medullary center, traverse the granule cell layer, and wind among the dendritic branches of Purkinje cells like a

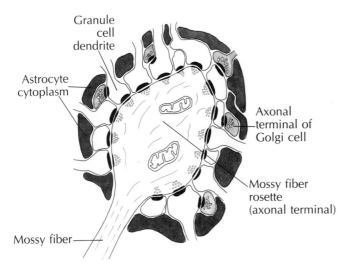

Granule cell dendrite

Astrocyte cytoplasm

Axonal terminal of Golgi cell

Mossy fiber rosette (axonal terminal)

Mossy fiber

FIGURE 10-6.
Ultrastructure of a synaptic glomerulus in the granule cell layer.

vine growing on a tree. Each climbing fiber makes synaptic contact with the smooth surface of the larger branches of a Purkinje cell dendrite. The climbing fibers probably all originate in the inferior olivary complex of nuclei.

Basket Cells. The basket cells are scattered in the molecular layer near the bodies of Purkinje cells. The dendrite of a basket cell branches in the transverse plane of the folium, receiving synaptic contacts from many granule cell axons. The axon of a basket cell is directed across the folium, and collateral branches form characteristic synapses with about 250 Purkinje cells. Each collateral branch forms a basketlike arrangement around the cell body of a Purkinje cell with the fibers concentrating around the axon hillock, where synaptic contacts are made (Fig. 10–7). Because of an overlapping arrangement, collateral branches of several basket cell axons synapse with a single Purkinje cell.

Stellate and Golgi Cells. Granule, Purkinje, and basket cells have special features, whereas stellate and Golgi cells are similar to small neurons elsewhere in the nervous system.

There are scattered stellate cells in the superficial part of the molecular layer whose dendrites are contacted by axons of granule cells. Axons of stellate cells synapse mainly with Purkinje cell dendrites; a few enter the innermost cortical layer and establish a feedback circuit by synapsing with granule cells. The Golgi cells are situated in the outer portion of the granule cell layer and their dendrites extend into the molecular layer, where they are contacted by parallel fibers. Other afferents to Golgi cells consist of collateral branches of Purkinje cell axons. Axons of Golgi cells enter glomeruli, where they synapse with the dendrites of granule cells (see Fig. 10–6).

Intracortical Circuits. Recordings from microelectrodes inserted into the cerebellar cortex have yielded information about whether synapses between specific types of neuron produce an excitatory postsynaptic potential (EPSP) or an inhibitory postsynaptic potential (IPSP). These studies show that synapses between mossy fibers and granule cells, granule cells and Purkinje cells, and climbing fibers and Purkinje cells are all excitatory. (The transmitter substance is probably glutamate.) The input to the cortex is therefore exci-

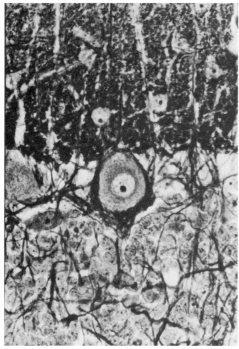

FIGURE 10-7.
Cell body of a Purkinje cell situated between the molecular layer and the granule cell layer of the cerebellar cortex. The fibers surrounding the Purkinje cell body are mostly preterminal branches of basket cell axons. (Cajal's silver nitrate method, × 450)

tatory. However, this is modified by intracortical circuits that inhibit Purkinje cells and therefore suppress transmission from cortex to central nuclei. For example, parallel fibers produce an EPSP in stellate and basket cells, but synapses between these and Purkinje cells produce an IPSP. Parallel fibers also excite Golgi cells, which inhibit granule cells. The inhibitory circuits include more synapses than do the excitatory relays. Therefore afferent volleys to the cortex first produce an EPSP in Purkinje cells, followed after 1 to 2 msec by an IPSP. The inhibitory circuits limit the area of cortex excited and the degree of excitation resulting from an incoming volley.

Aminergic Fibers. Large numbers of noradrenergic axons enter the cerebellum through its superior peduncle. These unmyelinated fibers, which come from the locus ceruleus, end by branching profusely in the molecular layer (see Fig. 10–5). The norepinephrine released from these afferent fibers may have a modulatory action at the synapses between parallel fibers and Purkinje cells. The cerebellar cortex also contains some serotonergic axons from the raphe nuclei of the reticular formation. It has been suggested that norepinephrine and serotonin may have opposing actions, the former amine enhancing, and the latter reducing, the excitatory action of the transmitter glutamate upon the dendrites of Purkinje cells.

Central Nuclei

Four pairs of nuclei are embedded deep in the medullary center; in a medial to lateral direction they are the fastigial, globose, emboliform, and dentate nuclei (Fig. 10–8). The phylogenetic development of these nuclei occurred in the same order.

The **fastigial nucleus** is nearly spherical, close to the midline, and almost in contact with the roof of the fourth ventricle. The **globose nucleus** consists of two or three small cellular masses, and the larger **emboliform nucleus** is oval or plug-shaped. In mammals as high in the phylogenetic scale as the monkey, a single nucleus (the nucleus interpositus) is situated between the fastigial and dentate nuclei. In apes and in humans, the nucleus interpositus is represented by the globose and emboliform nuclei. The **dentate nucleus** is the most prominent of the central nuclei; this mammalian nucleus is largest in primates, especially so in humans. The dentate nucleus has the irregular shape of a crumpled purse, similar to that of the inferior olivary nucleus, with the hilus facing medially. Its efferent fibers occupy the interior of the nucleus and leave through the hilus.

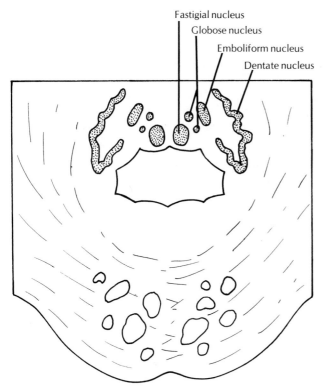

Fastigial nucleus
Globose nucleus
Emboliform nucleus
Dentate nucleus

FIGURE 10-8.
Central nuclei of the cerebellum.

The input to the cerebellar nuclei is from the Purkinje cells of the cortex and from sources outside the cerebellum. The extrinsic input consists of pontocerebellar, spinocerebellar, and olivocerebellar fibers, together with fibers from the precerebellar reticular nuclei. Most of these afferents are collateral branches of fibers proceeding to the cerebellar cortex. A few rubrocerebellar fibers end in the globose and emboliform nuclei, and the fastigial nucleus receives afferents from the vestibular nerve and nuclei. The fastigial nucleus discharges to the brain stem through the inferior cerebellar peduncle, whereas efferents from the remaining nuclei leave the cerebellum through the superior peduncle and terminate in the brain stem and in the thalamus.

Results of physiological studies have indicated that the input to the central nuclei from outside the cerebellum is excitatory, whereas the input from Purkinje cells is inhibitory. (The Purkinje cells use γ-aminobutyric acid (GABA) as their transmitter substance.) Crudely processed information in the central nuclei is refined by impulses received from the cortex. The combination of the two inputs maintains a tonic discharge from the central nuclei to the brain stem and thalamus. This discharge changes constantly according to the afferent input to the cerebellum at any given time.

Medullary Center and Cerebellar Peduncles

The white matter is scanty in the region of the vermis, where it produces a branching treelike pattern on sagittal section (Fig. 10–9). Each hemisphere, however, contains a large medullary center in which the dentate nucleus is embedded (Fig.

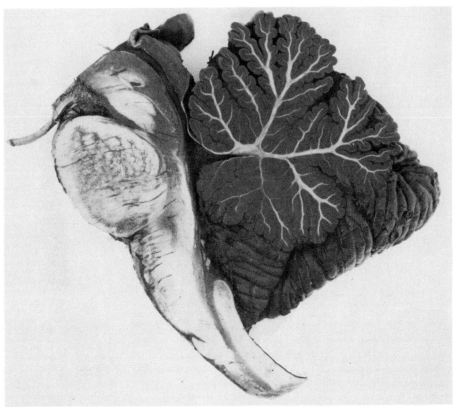

FIGURE 10-9.
Cerebellar surface in the median plane. The cut surface has been stained by a method that differentiates gray matter (*dark*) and white matter (*light*). (× 1½)

10–10). This white matter consists of afferent fibers to the cortex, axons of Purkinje cells proceeding to the central nuclei, and efferent fibers of the nuclei. The afferent and efferent systems are discussed in connection with the functional divisions of the cerebellum. They are identified at this point only as components of the cerebellar peduncles.

The **inferior cerebellar peduncle** consists mainly of fibers entering the cerebellum, with the largest component consisting of those originating in the inferior olivary complex. The other components are the dorsal spinocerebellar tract, cuneocerebellar fibers, and fibers from the vestibular nerve and nuclei, the arcuate nucleus, the nucleus of the spinal trigeminal tract, the pontine trigeminal nucleus, and the raphe and precerebellar reticular nuclei. The inferior cerebellar peduncle also contains efferent fibers that proceed from the flocculonodular lobe and fastigial nucleus to the vestibular nuclei and the central group of reticular nuclei of the medulla and pons.

The **middle cerebellar peduncle** consists of pontocerebellar fibers originating in the nuclei pontis. The **superior cerebellar peduncle** consists mainly of efferent fibers from the globose, emboliform, and dentate nuclei. The other components of the superior peduncles are afferent to the cerebellum. They include the ventral spi-

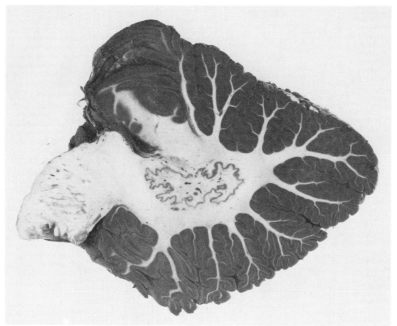

FIGURE 10-10.
Cerebellar surface in a sagittal plane through a hemisphere, stained to differentiate gray matter (*dark*) and white matter (*light*). The dentate nucleus is shown embedded in the medullary center of the white matter. (× 1½)

nocerebellar tract on the dorsolateral surface of the peduncle, fibers originating in the locus ceruleus, a few fibers from the red nucleus, and fibers from the mesencephalic nucleus of the trigeminal nerve.

FUNCTIONAL ANATOMY

Three divisions of the cerebellum are recognized on the basis of phylogenetic development (Fig. 10–11). The **archicerebellum,** which is the only component of the cerebellum in fishes and in lower amphibians, consists of the flocculonodular lobe, together with a region of the inferior vermis known as the uvula (see Fig. 10–3). The **paleocerebellum** makes its first appearance in higher amphibians and is larger in reptiles and birds. In humans it is represented by the superior vermis in the anterior lobe and by part of the inferior vermis in the posterior lobe. The cerebellar hemispheres, together with the superior vermis in the posterior lobe, constitute the **neocerebellum,** which is found only in mammals and is largest in humans.

These phylogenetic divisions of the cerebellum correspond in large part with divisions based on the major sources of afferent fibers (Fig. 10–12). Thus, the archicerebellum is identical to the **vestibulocerebellum,** which receives input from the vestibular nerve and nuclei. Those parts of the vermis that constitute the paleocerebellum, together with the adjacent (neocerebellar) medial parts of the hemispheres, make up the **spinocerebellum.** This region is the site of termination of the spinocerebellar tracts and cuneocerebellar fibers, which convey proprioceptive and other sensory information. The remainder

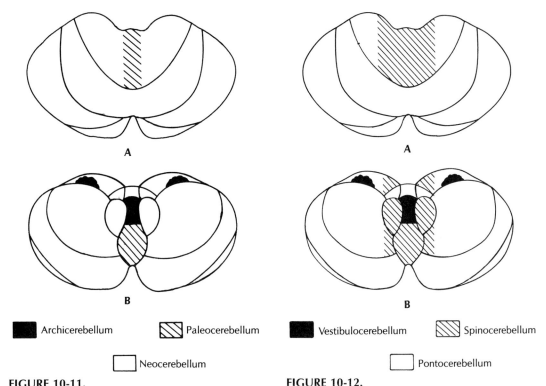

FIGURE 10-11.
Phylogenetic regions of the cerebellum.
(**A**) Superior surface. (**B**) Inferior surface.

FIGURE 10-12.
Functional regions of the cerebellum. (**A**) Superior surface. (**B**) Inferior surface.

of the neocerebellum, *i.e.*, the large lateral parts of the hemispheres and the superior vermis in the posterior lobe, constitutes the **pontocerebellum.** The contralateral pontine nuclei send afferent fibers to this area. There is some overlapping of the three divisions; for example, some ponto-cerebellar fibers terminate in the cortex of the spinocerebellum.

Vestibulocerebellum

The vestibulocerebellum receives afferent fibers from the vestibular ganglion and from the vestibular nuclei of the same side (Fig. 10–13). These enter the cerebellum in the medial part of the inferior cerebellar peduncle. Some of the afferent fibers from these sources terminate in the fastigial nu-cleus, which also receives collateral branches of the axons destined for the cortex of the vestibulocerebellum. The cortex and nucleus receive additional fibers from the accessory olivary nuclei.

A proportion of Purkinje cell axons from the vestibulocerebellar cortex proceed to the brain stem (an exception to the general rule that such fibers end in central nuclei), and the remainder terminate in the fastig-ial nucleus. Fibers from the cortex and the fastigial nucleus traverse the medial portion of the inferior cerebellar peduncle to their termination in the vestibular nuclear complex and in the central group of retic-ular nuclei. A bundle of fastigiobulbar fibers, known as the **uncinate fasciculus** (of Russell), has an aberrant course. The fasciculus crosses the midline, passes

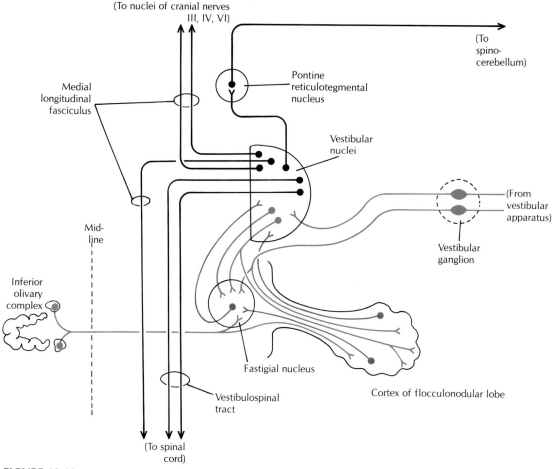

FIGURE 10-13.
Connections of the vestibulocerebellum and vestibular nuclei.

through the other fastigial nucleus, and then curves over the root of the superior cerebellar peduncle to join other efferent fibers of the vestibulocerebellum in the contralateral inferior peduncle.

The vestibulocerebellum influences motor neurons through the vestibulospinal tract, the medial longitudinal fasciculus, and reticulospinal fibers. It is concerned, as previously stated, with adjustment of muscle tonus in response to vestibular stimuli, and hence functions in maintaining equilibrium and in other motor responses to vestibular stimulation (Chap. 22).

Spinocerebellum

The following afferent systems project to the spinocerebellar cortex. The dorsal and ventral spinocerebellar tracts convey data from proprioceptive endings and from touch and pressure receptors (Fig. 10–14). The dorsal tract conveys information from the trunk and leg, whereas the ventral tract is involved mainly in conduction from the leg. Cuneocerebellar fibers from the accessory cuneate nucleus are equivalent to those of the dorsal spinocerebellar tract for the arm and neck. Data from cutaneous receptors are also carried by spinoreticular

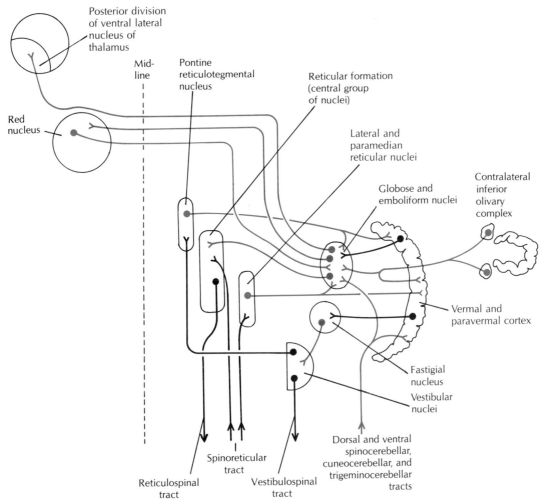

FIGURE 10-14.
Connections of the spinocerebellum.

fibers to the lateral and paramedian reticular nuclei, from which fibers project to the cerebellum. These two nuclei also receive afferent fibers from primary motor and sensory areas of the cerebral cortex. Another precerebellar reticular nucleus projecting to the vermis and medial parts of the hemispheres is the reticulotegmental nucleus in the pons. This nucleus receives afferents from the cerebral cortex and from the vestibular nuclei. Finally, the spinocerebellum receives fibers from all three sensory nuclei of the trigeminal

nerve, as well as from the accessory olivary nuclei. Some fibers from the various afferent sources terminate in the globose and emboliform nuclei, mainly as collaterals of axons proceeding to the cortex, and these nuclei also receive a small contingent of fibers from the red nucleus.

Each half of the body is represented in the ipsilateral cerebellar cortex; if fibers cross the midline from cells of origin at lower levels, they cross again in the medullary center of the cerebellum. In the monkey, and probably also in humans, the limbs are represented in two areas, one in and alongside the vermis in the anterior lobe, and the other in the medial part of the hemisphere on the inferior surface of the posterior lobe. The "head area" is in the superior vermis and in the immediately adjacent cortex in the posterior lobe. Somatotopic representation in the spinocerebellum is less clearly defined than in some areas of the cerebral cortex; there is overlap of different inputs so that trains of impulses from various sources may reach the same Purkinje cell.

The spinocerebellar cortex projects on the fastigial nucleus (from the vermis) and on the globose and emboliform nuclei (from the medial portions of the hemispheres). Synergy of muscle action and control of muscle tonus are effected in part through fastigiobulbar connections, as described for the vestibulocerebellum. Fibers from the globose and emboliform nuclei traverse the superior cerebellar peduncle and terminate in the central group of reticular nuclei. Thus, the spinocerebellum may influence motor neurons through reticulospinal fibers and a similar projection to motor nuclei of cranial nerves. Alpha and gamma motor neurons are involved in cerebellar control of muscle action, and the influence of the spinocerebellum on the skeletal musculature is ipsilateral.

Some fibers from the globose and emboliform nuclei traverse the superior cerebellar peduncle and end in the red nucleus. Others pass through or around the red nucleus and continue to the ventral lateral nucleus of the thalamus, from which fibers project to the primary motor area of the cerebral cortex. Although there is a substantial rubrospinal tract in most mammals, it is rudimentary in humans and presumably has little functional significance.

In summary, the spinocerebellum receives information from proprioceptive and exteroceptive endings and from the cerebral cortex. These data are processed in the circuitry of the cerebellar cortex, which modifies and refines the discharge of nerve impulses from the central nuclei. Motor neurons are influenced mainly through relays in the vestibular nuclei and the reticular formation. The end result is control of muscle tonus and synergy of collaborating muscles, as appropriate at any moment according to changes in posture and in many types of movement, including those of locomotion.

Pontocerebellum

Pontocerebellar fibers constitute the whole of the middle cerebellar peduncle. These fibers, originating in the nuclei pontis of the opposite side, are distributed throughout the cortex of the corpus cerebelli, *i.e.*, to all of the cortex except that of the flocculonodular lobe (Fig. 10–15). However, the greatest concentration of input from the pontine nuclei is to the large portions of the hemispheres assigned to the pontocerebellum. Through corticopontine tracts originating in widespread areas of the contralateral cerebral cortex (especially that of the frontal and parietal lobes) and the pontocerebellar projection, the cortex of a cerebellar hemisphere receives information concerning volitional movements that are about to take place or are in progress.

Purkinje cell axons from the pontocerebellar cortex terminate in the dentate nucleus, the efferent fibers of which compose most of the superior cerebellar peduncle. After traversing the decussation of the peduncles, the fibers pass through or around the red nucleus to a thalamic relay nucleus (ventral lateral nucleus), which in turn projects to the primary motor area of cortex in the frontal lobe. Through these connections the pontocerebellum can modify activity in corticospinal, corticoreticular, and corticorubral neurons. Some dentatothalamic fibers give off collateral branches that synapse in the red nucleus. In addition, on entering the mid-

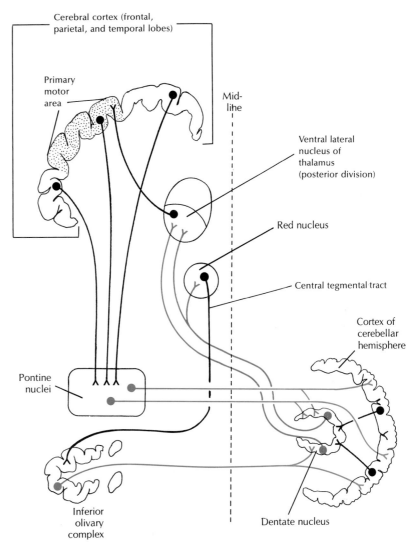

FIGURE 10-15.

Connections of the pontocerebellum.

brain, some fibers that originate in the dentate nucleus, and also in the globose and emboliform nuclei, give off collateral branches that end in the inferior olivary complex.

The output of the dentate nucleus, similar to that of the other cerebellar nuclei, fluctuates according to the excitatory input from extracerebellar sources and the refinement of discharge by the inhibitory action of Purkinje cells. Mainly through its influence on the cerebral motor cortex, the pontocerebellum ensures a smooth and orderly sequence of muscular contractions and the intended precision in the force, direction, and extent of volitional movements. A cerebellar hemisphere influences the musculature of the same side of the body because of the compensating decussations of the superior cerebellar peduncles and of the corticospinal tracts and other descending pathways.

Additional Cerebellar Connections

There is a large contingent of afferent fibers from the inferior olivary nucleus and from the dorsal and medial accessory olivary nuclei in the medulla. These cross the midline and enter the contralateral inferior cerebellar peduncle to be distributed to all parts of the cerebellar cortex. Olivocerebellar fibers also end in cerebellar nuclei. The principal inferior olivary nucleus projects to the cortex of the pontocerebellum and to the dentate nucleus, whereas the accessory olivary nuclei project to the spinocerebellar and vestibulocerebellar cortex and to the emboliform, globose, and fastigial nuclei. In addition to the rubro-olivary fibers indicated in Figure 10–15, the main afferents to the inferior olivary nucleus are cortico-olivary fibers from the sensorimotor strip of cortex of the ipsilateral cerebral hemisphere (see Fig. 7–8).

The climbing fibers from the inferior olivary complex are believed to carry instructions relating to movements that have not yet been performed. The patterns or programs concerned are stored in the cerebellum, probably as structural or functional modifications of synapses. It has been suggested that transmitters or other substances released from climbing fibers induce changes in the numbers and positions of the nearby synapses between parallel fibers and the dendrites of Purkinje cells. The execution and coordination of learned movements are mediated by the mossy fiber afferents, of which those from the pontine nuclei are the most numerous in humans. When a monkey makes an intended movement the neurons in the dentate nucleus (which receives its excitatory afferents from the pontine nuclei) are active several milliseconds before those in the primary motor area.

Data from laboratory studies, including those using monkeys, show that impulses of visual and acoustic origin reach the superior vermis of the posterior lobe through relays in the nuclei pontis. Tectopontine fibers from the superior colliculus to the dorsal region of the nuclei pontis convey acoustic data, as well as visual data, because of a connection from the inferior to the superior colliculus. Stimuli perceived by the eyes and ears are also able to influence the cerebellum through corticopontine fibers that originate in the visual and auditory areas of the cerebral cortex.

Results of animal experiments have also shown that the cerebellum has a role in visceral functions. Under certain conditions electrical stimulation of the spinocerebellar cortex produces respiratory, cardiovascular, pupillary, and urinary bladder responses. They are sympathetic in nature when the anterior lobe is stimulated and parasympathetic when the tonsils (see Fig. 10–3) of the posterior lobe are stimulated. The impulses are probably relayed to the hypothalamus through the reticular formation of the brain stem.

SIGNS OF CEREBELLAR DYSFUNCTION

Cerebellar disorders resulting from vascular occlusion, tumor growth, or other pathological conditions are classified broadly into those affecting the vestibulocerebellum (flocculonodular lobe) and those affecting the main mass of the cerebellum (corpus cerebelli).

The vestibular portion of the cerebellum may be invaded by a tumor, typically a medulloblastoma occurring in childhood, and the resulting disorder of cerebellar function is known as the **archicerebellar syndrome.** The patient is unsteady, walks on a wide base, and sways from side to side. The signs are at first limited to a disturbance of equilibrium; however, additional cerebellar signs appear if the tumor invades other parts of the cerebellum.

With respect to the corpus cerebelli, signs of cerebellar dysfunction accompany lesions that interrupt afferent pathways, cause destruction of the cortex and medullary center, or involve the central nuclei and efferent pathways in the superior cerebellar peduncle. There is considerable recovery with time because of compensation by intact regions. The motor disorder is more severe and more enduring when a lesion involves the central nuclei or the superior cerebellar peduncle. The signs of destructive lesions of the corpus cerebelli or its major afferent and efferent pathways are commonly referred to as the **neocerebellar syndrome,** although in many instances the paleocerebellum is also involved. When the lesion is unilateral, which is frequently the case, the signs of motor dysfunction are on the same side of the body as the lesion.

The following signs, in varying degrees of severity, are characteristic of the neocerebellar syndrome. Movements tend to be **ataxic** (intermittent or jerky). There is also **dysmetria;** for example, when the patient reaches out with the finger to an object, the finger overshoots the mark or deviates from it (**past-pointing**). Rapidly alternating movements such as flexion and extension of the fingers or pronation and supination of the forearm are performed in a clumsy manner (**adiadochokinesis**). **Asynergy** is reflected in the separation of voluntary movements that normally flow smoothly in sequence into a succession of mechanical or puppetlike movements (**decomposition of movements**). There may be **hypotonia of muscles,** and the muscles tire easily. Cerebellar tremor, which occurs most frequently with demyelinating lesions in the cerebellar peduncles, usually occurs at the end of a particular movement (**intention tremor**). Asynergy may involve muscles used in speech, which is then thick and monotonous. There may be **nystagmus,** especially if the lesion encroaches

on the vermis, because of involvement of projections to the oculomotor, trochlear, and abducens nuclei via the vestibular nuclei and the reticular formation. The deficits noted are superimposed on volitional movements that are themselves basically intact.

SUGGESTED READING

Brodal A: Neurological Anatomy in Relation to Clinical Medicine, 3rd ed. New York, Oxford University Press, 1981

Brooks VB: The Neural Basis of Motor Control. New York, Oxford University Press, 1986

Carpenter MB, Sutin J: Human Neuroanatomy, 8th ed. Baltimore, Williams & Wilkins, 1983

Chan-Palay V: Cerebellar Dentate Nucleus: Organization, Cytology and Transmitters. Berlin, Springer-Verlag, 1977

Colin F, Manil J, Desclin JC: The olivocerebellar system. 1. Delayed and slow inhibitory effects: An overlooked salient feature of cerebellar climbing fibers. Brain Res 187:3–27, 1980

FitzGerald MJT: Neuroanatomy Basic and Applied. London, Ballière Tindall, 1985

Ghez C, Fahn S: The Cerebellum. Chapter 30 in Kandel ER, Schwartz JH (eds): Principles of Neural Science, pp 334–346. New York, Elsevier-North Holland, 1981

Larsell O: Anatomy of the Nervous System, 2nd ed. New York, Appleton-Century-Crofts, 1951

Llinas RR: The cortex of the cerebellum. Sci Am 232:56–71, 1975

Meyer-Lohmann J, Hore J, Brooks VB: Cerebellar participation in generation of prompt arm movements. J Neurophysiol 40:1038–1050, 1977

Palay SL, Chan-Palay V: Cerebellar Cortex: Cytology and Organization. New York, Springer-Verlag, 1974

Shepherd GM: The Synaptic Organization of the Brain, 2nd ed. New York, Oxford University Press, 1979

Somjen GG: Neurophysiology—The Essentials. Baltimore, Williams & Wilkins, 1983

ELEVEN

Diencephalon

The diencephalon and telencephalon together constitute the cerebrum, of which the diencephalon forms the central core and the telencephalon the cerebral hemispheres. Because it is almost entirely surrounded by the hemispheres, only the ventral surface of the diencephalon is exposed to view in a diamond-shaped area containing hypothalamic structures (Fig. 11–1). This area is bounded in front by the optic chiasma and on each side by the optic tract and the region where the internal capsule becomes the basis pedunculi of the midbrain. The diencephalon is divided into symmetrical halves by the slit-like third ventricle. As seen in a median section (Fig. 11–2), the junction of the midbrain and diencephalon is represented by a line that passes through the posterior commissure and is immediately caudal to the mamillary body. The boundary between the diencephalon and the telencephalon is represented by a line traversing the interventricular foramen (foramen of Monro) and the optic chiasma.

GROSS FEATURES

Surfaces

The surfaces of each half of the diencephalon have the following landmarks and relations. The **medial surface** forms the wall of the third ventricle (see Fig. 11–2). A bundle of nerve fibers called the stria medullaris thalami forms an elevation along the junction of the medial and dorsal surfaces. The ependymal lining of the third ventricle is reflected from one side to the other along the striae medullares, forming the roof of the ventricle from which a small choroid plexus is suspended.

The **dorsal surface** is largely concealed by the fornix (Fig. 11–3); this robust bun-

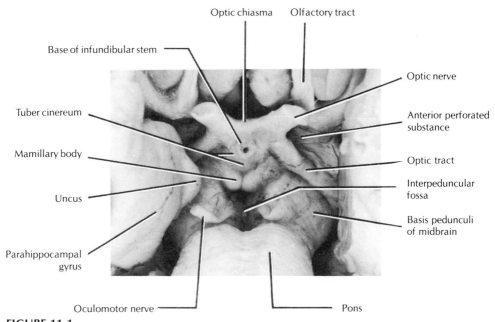

FIGURE 11-1.
An area of the ventral surface of the brain, in which the diencephalon presents to the surface. (× 1½)

dle of fibers originates in the hippocampal formation of the temporal lobe, curves over the thalamus, and ends mainly in the mamillary body. The fornices outline a triangular interval posteriorly that constitutes a rostral extension of the **transverse cerebral fissure** into the cerebrum, with the remaining part of the fissure intervening between the cerebellum and the cerebral hemispheres. Between the fornices, the transverse fissure is roofed over by the corpus callosum; its floor is formed by a small area of the diencephalon and the roof of the third ventricle. The vascular connective tissue occupying the space just delineated is known as the **tela choroidea,** and it is continuous with the vascular core of the choroid plexuses of the lateral ventricles and the third ventricle. Lateral to the fornix, the dorsal surface of the thalamus forms the floor of the central part of the lateral ventricle, much of which is concealed by the choroid plexus (Fig. 11–3).

The **lateral surface** is bounded by the thick internal capsule of white matter, which consists of fibers connecting the cerebral cortex with the thalamus and other parts of the central nervous system. The medial part of the **ventral surface** presents to the surface of the brain, as noted, and the lateral part is bounded by the internal capsule before it continues as the basis pedunculi of the midbrain.

Major Components

The diencephalon consists of four components, or regions, on each side—the thalamus, subthalamus, epithalamus, and hypothalamus. The **thalamus,** by far the largest component, is subdivided into nuclei that have different afferent and efferent connections. Certain thalamic nuclei receive sensory input for the general and special senses (except smell); these nuclei project to corresponding sensory areas of

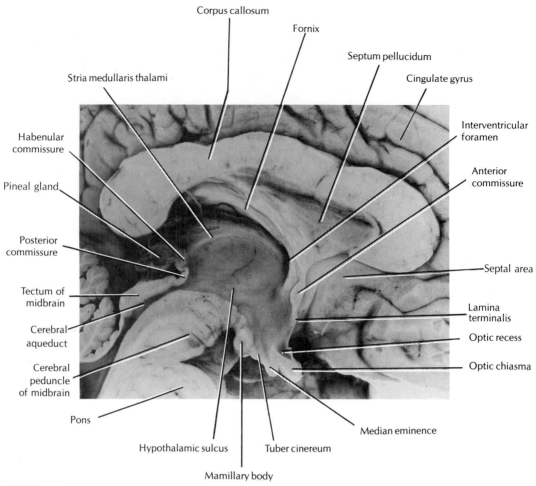

FIGURE 11-2.
Central region of the brain in median section. (× 1¼)

the cerebral cortex. Other thalamic nuclei participate in emotional aspects of brain function, are functionally related to motor and association areas of cortex, or have a role in the ascending reticular activating system. The **subthalamus** is a complex region ventral to the thalamus; it includes a nucleus with motor functions (the subthalamic nucleus), sensory tracts terminating in the thalamus, and bundles of fibers proceeding from the cerebellum and corpus striatum to the thalamus. The reticular formation, red nucleus, and substantia nigra extend from the midbrain part way into the

subthalamus. The **epithalamus,** situated dorsomedial to the thalamus and adjacent to the roof of the third ventricle, is a particularly old part of the diencephalon phylogenetically. It includes the pineal gland (also called the pineal body) and structures concerned with autonomic responses to emotional changes. The **hypothalamus** occupies the region between the third ventricle and the subthalamus; it is the main cerebral center for integrative control of the autonomic nervous system and of several endocrine glands. The neurohypophysis, which includes part of the pituitary

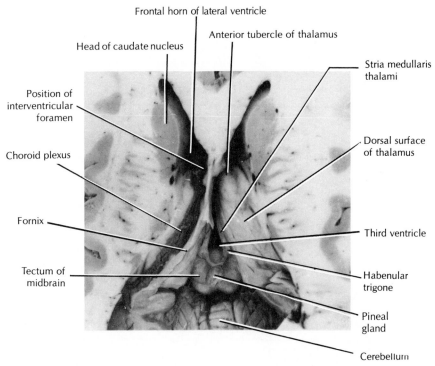

Frontal horn of lateral ventricle

Anterior tubercle of thalamus

Head of caudate nucleus

Stria medullaris thalami

Position of interventricular foramen

Dorsal surface of thalamus

Choroid plexus

Fornix

Third ventricle

Tectum of midbrain

Habenular trigone

Pineal gland

Cerebellum

FIGURE 11-3.
Dorsal aspect of the diencephalon, with the fornix and the choroid plexus removed on the right side. (× 1)

gland, is an outgrowth of the hypothalamus.

THALAMUS

The thalamus, measuring about 3 cm anteroposteriorly and 1.5 cm in the other two directions, makes up four fifths of the diencephalon. Thin laminae of white matter partially outline the thalamus; the **stratum zonale** on the dorsal surface, best developed anteriorly (see Fig. 11–12), is one such sheet of nerve fibers. The **external medullary lamina** is a thin layer of nerve fibers that covers the lateral surface of the thalamus (see Fig. 11–9). It consists of thalamocortical and corticothalamic fibers running along the surface of the thalamus briefly before entering or leaving the internal capsule. The external medullary lamina and internal capsule are separated by an attenuated layer of nerve cells that

compose the reticular nucleus of the thalamus. The **internal medullary lamina** (see Figs. 11– 4B and 11–9), consisting of fibers entering and leaving the various thalamic nuclei, divides the thalamus into three gray masses. These are a lateral nuclear mass, the medial nuclei, and the anterior nuclei, with the latter enclosed by a bifurcation of the lamina. Each mass consists of nuclei that are identified according to a pattern of thalamic organization next to be described.

Scheme of Thalamic Organization

Knowledge of the nuclei of the thalamus has come from comparative anatomy, experimental tracing of connections, and physiological study of the effects of stimulation and ablation. Notable investigators of the thalamus include Clark and Walker in the 1920s and 1930s. Their recognition

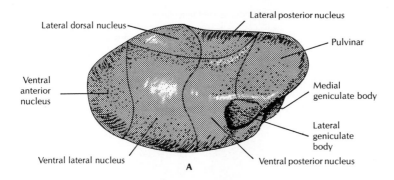

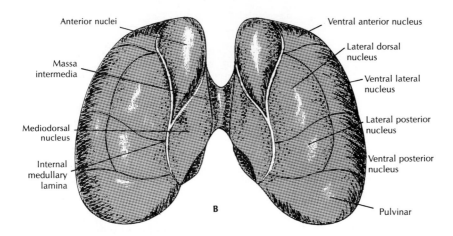

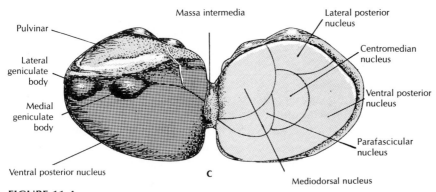

FIGURE 11-4.
A model of the thalami, showing the positions of the larger nuclei. **(A)** Lateral view.
(B) Dorsal view. **(C)** Posterior view with the posterior part of the right thalamus cut away.
(Model prepared by Dr. D. G. Montemurro)

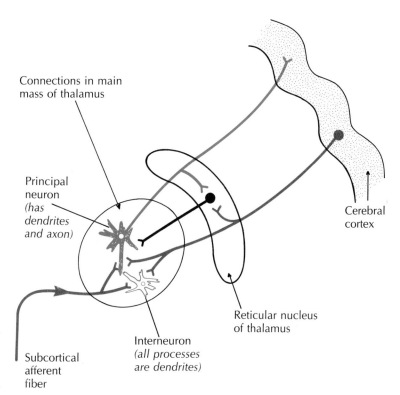

Connections in main
mass of thalamus

Principal
neuron
*(has
dendrites
and axon)*

Cerebral
cortex

Reticular nucleus
of thalamus

Interneuron
*(all processes
are dendrites)*

FIGURE 11-5.
Scheme of neuronal
connections of the thalamus.

Subcortical
afferent
fiber

of groups of "specific" and "nonspecific" nuclei is no longer tenable, but their terminology is still in use. The modern view of thalamic organization comes from numerous investigators in the 1970s and 1980s, and is derived from animal experimentation using electron microscopy, microelectrodes, and tracing methods based on axoplasmic transport.

Every nucleus of the thalamus except the reticular nucleus sends axons to the cerebral cortex, either to a sharply defined area or diffusely to a large area. Every part of the cortex receives fibers from the thalamus, probably from at least two nuclei. Every thalamocortical projection is faithfully copied, with great anatomical precision, by a reciprocal corticothalamic connection.

Both the thalamocortical and the corticothalamic axons give collateral branches to neurons in the reticular nucleus, whose neurons project to the other nuclei of the

thalamus. In addition to the two-way cortical connections, each of these nuclei receives other afferent fibers, usually from a subcortical region. The neostriatum (part of the corpus striatum) and the hypothalamus are probably the only noncortical structures to receive fibers from the thalamus. Contrary to earlier beliefs, there are no connections between the various nuclei of the main mass of the thalamus, although each individual nucleus contains interneurons. The synapses of the interneurons are inhibitory, and most are dendrodendritic. Other synapses in the thalamus are excitatory. The general plan of thalamic connections is shown in Figure 11–5.

Reticular Nucleus

As noted, the reticular nucleus consists of a thin sheet of nerve cells between the external medullary lamina and the internal capsule (see Fig. 11–9). Despite its name it is not connected with the reticular formation of the brain stem. The nucleus receives collateral branches of corticothalamic and thalamocortical fibers. The axons of cells in the reticular nucleus project into the deeper parts of the thalamus to end in the same nuclei that gave rise to afferents to those cells. All the other thalamic nuclei and all areas of the cerebral cortex are associated with corresponding regions in the reticular nucleus. The modulation by the reticular nucleus of the exchange of signals between thalamus and cortex has been studied electrophysiologically, but a simple function cannot yet be assigned to these connections.

Intralaminar Nuclei

There are six nuclei, known collectively as intralaminar nuclei, in the region of the internal medullary lamina, and partly surrounded by the lamina. Of these the **centromedian nucleus** is especially well represented in anthropoid apes and humans (see Figs. 11–4C and 11–7). A smaller **parafascicular nucleus** lies adjacent to the habenulointerpeduncular fasciculus; other intralaminar nuclei are too small in humans to merit consideration here.

The intralaminar nuclei receive afferents from the central group of nuclei of the reticular formation of the brain stem and from the locus ceruleus. Some spinothalamic and trigeminothalamic fibers also terminate in the intralaminar nuclei, although most of these fibers have the ventral posterior nucleus as their destination.

The two-way cortical connections of the intralaminar nuclei are with extensive areas of the frontal and parietal lobes. The pathway from the reticular formation through the intralaminar nuclei to the cerebral cortex is thought to provide the anatomical basis for the influence of sensory input to the brain stem and spinal cord on levels of consciousness and degrees of alertness. It also provides for vague aware-

ness of sensory stimulation without specificity or discriminative qualities but with emotional responses, especially to painful stimuli.

The intralaminar nuclei also project to the caudate nucleus and putamen, which compose the neostriatum. These connections may form part of the neuronal circuitry that controls movements, or they may indicate that the corpus striatum is involved in consciousness and arousal.

Ventral Group of Nuclei

Medial Geniculate Nucleus

The medial geniculate nucleus, located on the auditory pathway and consisting of four subnuclei, forms a swelling (the **medial geniculate body**) on the posterior surface of the thalamus beneath the pulvinar (see Figs. 7–15, 7–16, and 11–4). Afferent fibers to the medial geniculate nucleus constitute the inferior brachium coming from the inferior colliculus, which is the terminus of the lateral lemniscus. The nucleus receives data from the spiral organ (organ of Corti) of both sides, but predominantly from the opposite ear. This bilateral projection stems from the presence of some ipsilateral fibers in the lateral lemniscus and some commissural fibers passing between the inferior colliculi, and also between the nuclei of the lateral lemnisci. There is a topographical pattern in the ventral portion of the medial geniculate nucleus with respect to pitch; the pattern simulates a spiral, corresponding to the configuration of the organ of Corti.

Fibers from the medial geniculate nucleus constitute the auditory radiation, which terminates in the auditory area of the temporal lobe (see Fig. 11–13). Awareness of sounds is a function of the auditory cortex, and adjacent association cortex provides for discriminative aspects of hearing and recognition on the basis of past experience.

Lateral Geniculate Nucleus

The **lateral geniculate body** beneath the pulvinar marks the position of a main (dorsal) lateral geniculate nucleus on the visual pathway to the cerebral cortex, which is discussed here (Figs. 11–4 and 11–7), and a ventral nucleus, which is rudimentary in humans. (The medial and lateral geniculate bodies are sometimes said to compose the **metathalamus.**) The nucleus consists of 6 layers of neurons, numbered consecutively from the ventral surface. Layers 1 and 2 consist of large neurons; layers 3 through 6 are made up of small cells. The lateral geniculate nucleus is the terminus of most of the fibers of the optic tract, and it projects to the visual area of the cortex. The fibers afferent to the lateral geniculate nucleus originate in the ganglion cell layer of the retina; they are divided equally between those from the lateral half of the ipsilateral eye and those from the medial half of the contralateral eye, with the latter fibers having crossed the midline in the optic chiasma. Each nucleus therefore receives impulses related to the opposite field of vision. The crossed fibers terminate in layers 1, 4, and 6, and the uncrossed fibers end in layers 2, 3, and 5.

There is a detailed point-to-point projection of the retina on the lateral geniculate nucleus. In a more general way the superior retinal quadrants project to the medial portion of the nucleus, the inferior quadrants to the lateral portion, and the macular region for central vision to the posterior part of the nucleus. Axons of cells in the nucleus constitute the geniculocalcarine tract, which terminates in the visual area of the occipital lobe adjacent to the calcarine sulcus (see Fig. 11–13). At this site, and in the surrounding association

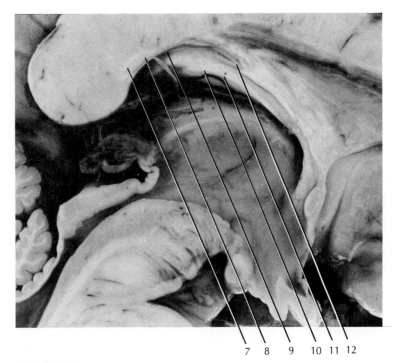

7   8   9   10 11 12

FIGURE 11-6.
Key to levels for Figures 11-7 through 11-12. See Figure 11-2 for landmarks.

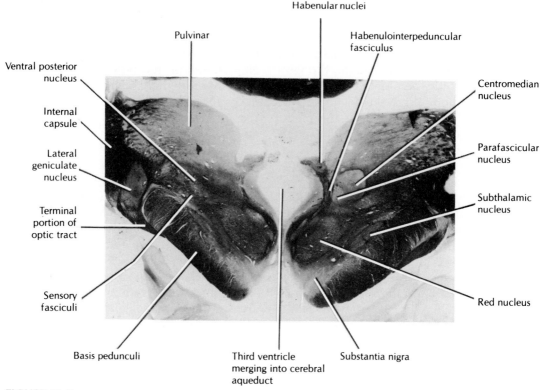

FIGURE 11-7.

Transverse section at the transition between the midbrain and the diencephalon, immediately caudal to the mamillary bodies. (Weigert stain, × 1⅕)

cortex, there is awareness of visual stimuli accompanied by discriminative and mnemonic aspects of vision.

Ventral Posterior Nucleus

The ventral posterior nucleus (Figs. 11–4, 11–7, and 11–8) is part of the pathway for conscious appreciation of sensations arising from skin, muscles, and internal parts of the body. All the fibers of the medial lemniscus and most of those of the spinothalamic and trigeminothalamic tracts terminate in this nucleus. Fibers are also received from the vestibular nuclear complex. Fibers from the contralateral lateral cervical nucleus (Chap. 5) terminate as well in the ventral posterior nucleus in the cat and monkey, but this pathway is probably smaller and less important in humans.

There is a detailed topographical projection of the opposite half of the body on the ventral posterior nucleus. The lower limb is represented in its dorsolateral part, with the upper limb in an intermediate position and the head most medially. The medial region receiving sensory data from the head is usually referred to as the **ventral posteromedial division** of the nucleus (VPm), and the larger lateral portion for the remainder of the body is referred to as the **ventral posterolateral division** (VPl). The image of the body is distorted in that the more important parts of the body with respect to sensory function, such as the hand and face, are disproportionately large. In addition, the more discriminative senses of fine touch and proprioception are represented further forward than the nociceptive senses of pain and temperature.

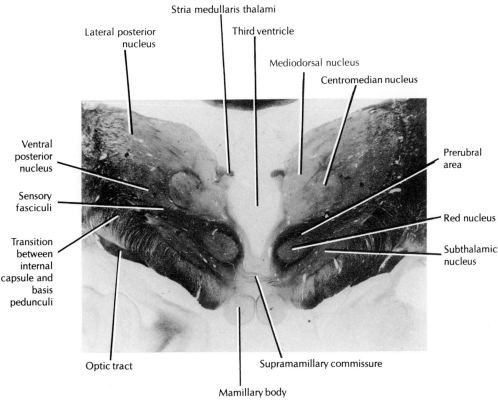

FIGURE 11-8.
Diencephalon at the level of the mamillary bodies. (Weigert stain, × 1⅘)

Nevertheless, the topographical projection of the body on the ventral posterior nucleus (and on the somesthetic area of cortex) is the basis for precise recognition of the sources of stimuli. Fibers originating in the vestibular nuclei terminate in or close to the region that receives the trigeminothalamic fibers.

Nerve fibers leave the lateral aspect of the ventral posterior nucleus in large numbers, traverse the internal capsule and medullary center of the cerebral hemisphere, and end in the first somesthetic area of cortex in the parietal lobe (see Fig. 11–13). The opposite side of the body has an inverted representation in the somesthetic cortex, with the portions assigned to the head and hand being disproportionately large. The location of the vestibular

cortical area is uncertain. It may be in the superior temporal gyrus, posterior to the auditory area.

Ventral Lateral Nucleus

The ventral lateral nucleus (VL) has posterior (VLp) and anterior (VLa) divisions (Figs. 11–4, 11–10, and 11–11). The VLp receives fibers from cerebellar nuclei, mainly the dentate nucleus, and the VLa receives fibers from the globus pallidus of the corpus striatum. Axons of neurons in both divisions enter the internal capsule and proceed to cortical areas of the frontal lobe. The VLp is connected with the primary motor area on the precentral gyrus, whereas the VLa communicates with the more anteriorly situated premotor area

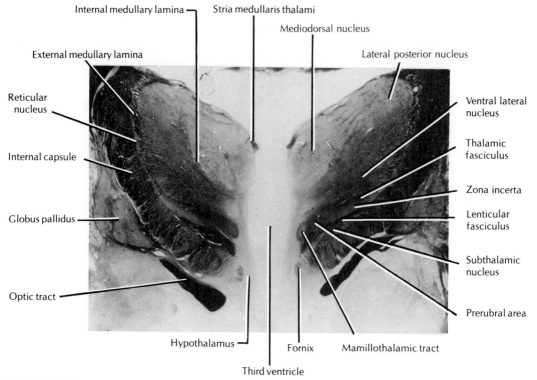

FIGURE 11-9.
Diencephalon at the level of the infundibular stem of the neurohypophysis. (Weigert stain, × 1⅖)

(see Fig. 11–13). Some symptoms of paralysis agitans (Parkinson's disease) can be ameliorated by a lesion placed in the nuclei surgically, although this form of therapy has been largely replaced by administration of L-dopa.

Ventral Anterior Nucleus

The ventral anterior nucleus is a large nucleus (Figs. 11–4 and 11–12), but little is known of its connections or functions. It projects to extensive areas of the cerebral cortex.

Ventral Medial Nuclei

There are two small ventral medial nuclei. The **principal ventromedial nucleus** receives input from the substantia nigra and also from the spinal cord. It is connected

with the cortex of the frontal lobe. The functional significance of this nucleus is not known.

The **ventral medial basal nucleus** forms part of the ascending pathway for taste. Afferent fibers are from the parabrachial nucleus, which is in the reticular formation of the midbrain. The cortical connections are with the gustatory area, which is posterior to the general sensory area for the mouth.

Posterior Group of Nuclei

In the most caudal region of the thalamus, there is a group of nuclei known as the posterior group or complex. It consists of part of the pulvinar, part of the medial geniculate body, and two small nuclei, the suprageniculate nucleus and the nucleus limitans. Some of the spinothalamic and

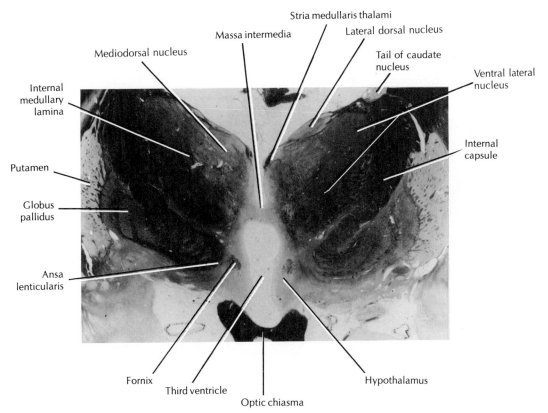

Internal medullary lamina

Putamen

Globus pallidus

Ansa lenticularis

Mediodorsal nucleus

Massa intermedia

Stria medullaris thalami

Lateral dorsal nucleus

Tail of caudate nucleus

Ventral lateral nucleus

Internal capsule

Fornix

Third ventricle

Optic chiasma

Hypothalamus

FIGURE 11-10.
Diencephalon at the level of the optic chiasma. (Weigert stain, × 1⅘)

trigeminothalamic fibers terminate in the nuclei of the posterior group, from which axons project to an area of concealed cortex called the insula, and to nearby parts of the parietal and temporal lobes, including the second somesthetic area. For the perception of pain the posterior and intralaminar nuclei are probably as important as the ventral posterior nucleus of the thalamus.

Lateral Group of Nuclei

The **lateral dorsal nucleus,** the **lateral posterior nucleus,** and the four nuclei of the **pulvinar** are all situated in the dorsal part of the lateral nuclear mass (Figs. 11–4 and 11–7 through 11–10).

The lateral dorsal nucleus is a poorly understood part of the limbic system; it receives afferent fibers from the hippocampus and projects to the cingulate gyrus in the cerebral hemisphere. The connections of this nucleus therefore have much in common with those of the anterior group of thalamic nuclei.

The lateral posterior nucleus projects to the somatosensory association cortex of the parietal lobe, but its afferent connections have yet to be determined. The nuclei of the pulvinar also project to sensory association areas in the parietal, temporal, and occipital lobes. The pulvinar receives input from the superior colliculus and the pretectal area, and a few fibers from the retina also end there. A projection of the pulvinar upon the visual cortex of the occipital lobe forms the terminal link of a series of neurons that runs in parallel with the main visual pathway. It is probably not

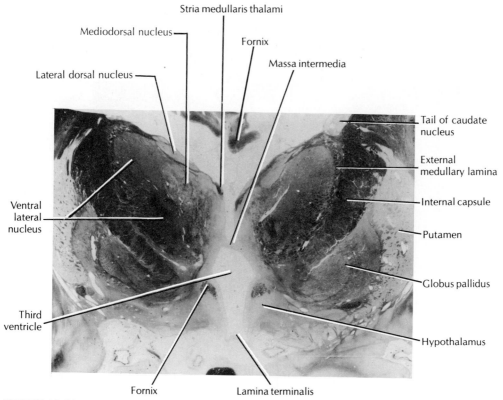

FIGURE 11-11.
Diencephalon rostral to the level of the optic chiasma. (Weigert stain, × 1⅕)

very important in humans, and it cannot take over visual functions if the pathway through the lateral geniculate nucleus is disrupted.

Medial Group of Nuclei

The medial group consists of the large mediodorsal nucleus and the smaller medioventral nucleus. The latter is also called the nucleus reuniens.

Mediodorsal Nucleus

The connections of the mediodorsal nucleus (Figs. 11–4 and 11–10) are with the olfactory and limbic systems and with the cortex of the frontal lobe. Afferent fibers come from the olfactory cortex, from the amygdaloid body (which belongs to both the olfactory and the limbic systems), and from the hypothalamus. There is a large reciprocal connection between the mediodorsal nucleus and the association cortex of the frontal lobe (prefrontal cortex) (Fig. 11–13). A bundle of fibers known as the **inferior thalamic peduncle** passes ventrally to the base of the hemisphere. This bundle provides connections between the mediodorsal thalamic nucleus and several gray areas, including orbital cortex of the frontal lobe. Through these connections, the mediodorsal nucleus constitutes part of a system that contributes to those aspects of the emotions generally considered as "moods" or "feeling tone." Depending on the nature of the present sensory input and past experience, the mood may be that of well-being or malaise, or of euphoria or mild depression. Visceral changes may

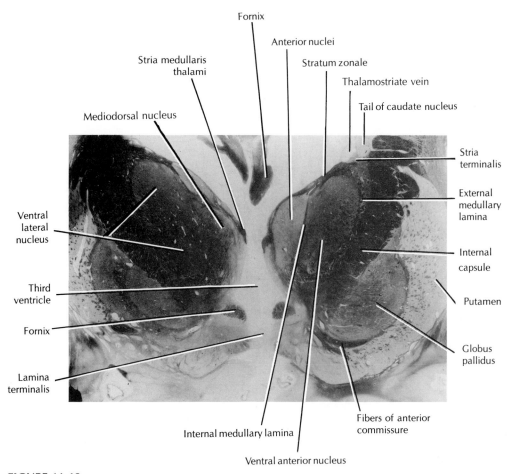

Fornix

Anterior nuclei

Stria medullaris thalami

Stratum zonale

Thalamostriate vein

Tail of caudate nucleus

Mediodorsal nucleus

Stria terminalis

External medullary lamina

Ventral lateral nucleus

Internal capsule

Third ventricle

Putamen

Fornix

Lamina terminalis

Globus pallidus

Internal medullary lamina

Fibers of anterior commissure

Ventral anterior nucleus

FIGURE 11-12.
Rostral region of the diencephalon. (Weigert stain, × 2)

accompany changes in mood through connections between the mediodorsal thalamic nucleus and the hypothalamus.

Severe anxiety states have been ameliorated by placing lesions bilaterally in the mediodorsal nuclei or, more commonly, by severing the connections between these nuclei and the prefrontal cortices (leukotomy, or prefrontal lobotomy). However, the procedure has sometimes been followed by inappropriate social behavior and by impairment of judgment and foresight, so this form of psychosurgery has been abandoned in favor of medical therapy.

In patients with intractable pain, relief has been provided by bilateral prefrontal lobotomy. This operation does not cause analgesia or any other definable sensory deficit. However, the presence of the pain is no longer distressing to the patient, who will say that the pain is still there but that it does not hurt.

The mediodorsal thalamic nucleus appears to play a role in memory. In Korsakoff's syndrome, in which amnesia is a characteristic symptom, the degenerative changes in the brain follow a variable pattern. The lesions are typically in regions surrounding the third ventricle, and the mediodorsal nucleus is reported as being most consistently affected. In addition,

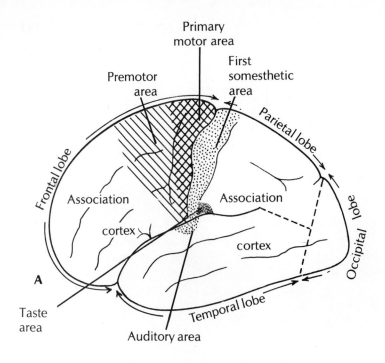

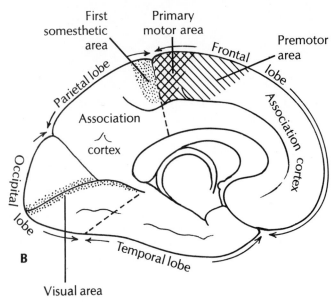

FIGURE 11-13.
Cortical areas connected with thalamic nuclei. **(A)** Lateral surface of a cerebral hemisphere. **(B)** Medial surface of a cerebral hemisphere.

memory deficits have been reported following surgical destruction of the mediodorsal thalamic nuclei.

Medioventral Nucleus

Little is known about the role of this nucleus. Its connections are with the hippocampus and parahippocampal gyrus in the temporal lobe of the cerebral hemisphere, so that it is considered to be a component of the limbic system.

Anterior Group of Nuclei

The three anterior thalamic nuclei (Figs. 11–4B and 11–12) are responsible for the anterior tubercle of the thalamus that, with the fornix, bounds the interventricular foramen, or foramen of Monro (Figs. 11–2 and 11–3). These nuclei are included in the limbic system of the brain, which is concerned with basic emotions important in the preservation of the individual and the species, and has a significant role in memory. The cortical components of the limbic system consist of the hippocampal formation in the temporal lobe and the cingulate gyrus on the medial surface of the hemisphere above the corpus callosum. The diencephalic components are the hypothalamus (especially the mamillary bodies) and the anterior, lateral dorsal, and medioventral nuclei of the thalamus. The principal fiber bundles of the limbic system are the fornix, which projects from the hippocampal formation to the hypothalamus, and the mamillothalamic fasciculus (bundle of Vicq d'Azyr), through which reciprocal connections are established between the mamillary body and the anterior thalamic nuclei. These and the lateral dorsal nucleus also have reciprocal connections with the cortex of the cingulate gyrus. (Additional components of the limbic system—*e.g.*, the amygdaloid body and its connections—are discussed in Chapter 18.)

Thalamic Syndrome

Aside from motor aspects of the ventral lateral nucleus, the thalamus is a sensory part of the brain and contributes to emotional responses to sensory experience. The thalamic syndrome is essentially a disturbance of these aspects of thalamic function, subsequent to a lesion (usually vascular in origin) involving the thalamus. The symptoms vary according to the location and extent of the lesion. The threshold for touch, pain, and temperature is usually raised on the opposite side of the body but, when the threshold is reached, the sensations are exaggerated, perverted, and exceptionally disagreeable. For example, the prick of a pin may be felt as a severe

burning sensation, and even music that is ordinarily pleasing may be disagreeable. There is spontaneous pain in some instances, which may become intractable to analgesics. There may also be emotional instability, with spontaneous or forced laughing and crying.

SUBTHALAMUS

The subthalamus contains sensory fasciculi, rostral extensions of midbrain nuclei, fiber bundles from nuclei of the cerebellum and the globus pallidus, and the subthalamic nucleus.

The **sensory fasciculi** are the medial lemniscus, spinothalamic tract, and trigeminothalamic tracts. They are spread out immediately beneath the ventral posterior nucleus of the thalamus, in which the fibers terminate (Figs. 11–7 and 11–8).

The **substantia nigra** and **red nucleus** extend from the midbrain part way into the subthalamus (Figs. 11–7 and 11–8). Dentatothalamic fibers, which have crossed the midline in the decussations of the superior cerebellar peduncles, both surround and traverse the red nucleus and then continue forward in the **prerubral area,** or **field H of Forel** (H from the German *Haube,* a cap; Figs. 11–8 and 11–9). The dentatothalamic fibers, accompanied by a few from the globose and emboliform nuclei, contribute to the thalamic fasciculus (see below) and end in the ventral lateral nucleus of the thalamus.

Efferent fibers of the globus pallidus are contained in two bundles, the lenticular fasciculus and ansa lenticularis (see Figs. 11–9, 11–10, and 12–5). The **lenticular fasciculus** consists of fibers that cut across the internal capsule to reach the subthalamus, where they form a band of white matter known as **field H$_2$ of Forel.** The fibers reverse direction in the prerubral area, enter the **thalamic fasciculus (field H$_1$ of Forel),** and terminate in the ventral lateral thalamic nucleus. At a more rostral level the **ansa lenticularis** makes a sharp bend around the medial edge of the internal capsule, continues in the thalamic fasciculus, and also ends in the ventral lateral nucleus of the thalamus. Only a few fibers from the globus pallidus turn caudally; they terminate in the pedunculopontine nucleus, which is one of the lateral group of nuclei in the reticular formation of the brain stem, situated in the midbrain.

The mesencephalic reticular formation extends into the subthalamus, where it appears as the **zona incerta** between the lenticular and thalamic fasciculi (Fig. 11–9). The connections and functions of the zona incerta are similar to those of the nearby lateral hypothalamic area. Through connections with the subfornical organ (a chemosensitive nucleus, described later in this chapter) and the hypothalamus, the zona incerta is involved in the regulation of drinking behavior.

The **subthalamic nucleus** (nucleus of Luys), a motor nucleus best developed in primates, is biconvex in shape and lies against the internal capsule (Figs. 11–7, 11–8, and 11–9). The subthalamic nucleus has reciprocal connections with the globus pallidus; these fibers constitute the **subthalamic fasciculus,** which cuts across the internal capsule. The subthalamic nucleus also receives some afferent fibers from the pedunculopontine nucleus and sends some efferents to the substantia nigra. Fibers in the supramamillary commissure (Fig. 11–8) connect one subthalamic nucleus with the other.

A lesion in the subthalamic nucleus causes a motor disturbance on the opposite side of the body known as **hemiballismus.** The condition is characterized by involuntary movements, coming on suddenly and of great force and rapidity. The movements are purposeless and generally of a throwing or flailing type, although they may be choreiform or jerky. The spontaneous movements occur most severely at proximal joints of the limbs, especially the

arms. The muscles of the face and neck are sometimes involved.

EPITHALAMUS

The epithalamus consists of the habenular nuclei and their connections and the pineal gland.

Habenular Nuclei

A slight swelling in the habenular trigone marks the position of the medial and lateral habenular nuclei (Figs. 11–3 and 11–7). Afferent fibers are received through the **stria medullaris thalami,** which runs along the dorsomedial border of the thalamus (Figs. 11–2, 11–3, and 11–9). Most of the cells of origin of the stria are situated in the septal area. This area is located on the medial surface of the frontal lobe beneath the rostral end of the corpus callosum (Fig. 11–2), and is part of the limbic system of the brain. Other strial fibers originate in the hypothalamus and the globus pallidus of the corpus striatum.

The habenular nuclei give rise to a well-defined bundle of fibers known as the **habenulointerpeduncular fasciculus** (fasciculus retroflexus of Meynert; Fig. 11–7). The main destination of the fasciculus is the interpeduncular nucleus in the roof of the interpeduncular fossa of the midbrain. Through relays in the reticular formation, the interpeduncular nucleus influences neurons in the hypothalamus and preganglionic autonomic neurons.

Pineal Gland

The pineal gland or body, also called the epiphysis, has the shape of a pine cone and is about 5×7 mm in size; it is attached to the diencephalon by the pineal stalk, into which the third ventricle extends as the pineal recess (Figs. 11–2 and 11–3). The **habenular commissure** in the dorsal wall of the stalk includes fibers of the stria medullaris thalami that terminate in the opposite habenular nuclei. The ventral wall of the pineal stalk is attached to the **posterior commissure.** The pineal gland and its stalk develop as an outgrowth from the ependymal roof of the third ventricle.

The pineal organ has undergone remarkable evolutionary changes. In some types of fish and amphibian, the distal part of the epiphysis contains light-sensitive cells, beneath a thin cranial vault. The axons of associated neurons enter the habenular commissure and then pass to undetermined sites in the diencephalon. In birds and mammals the pineal gland has the structural organization of an endocrine gland, although in some species it contains a small nucleus of neurons that are reciprocally connected with the habenular nuclei. The mammalian pineal gland receives most of its afferent nerve supply from the superior cervical ganglion of the sympathetic trunk through the nervus conarii, which runs subendothelially in the straight sinus (within the tentorium cerebelli) before penetrating the dura and distributing its branches to the pineal parenchyma.

Histologically the parenchymatous cells (pinealocytes) are arranged as cords separated by connective tissue. These cells have a granular cytoplasm and processes that end in bulbous expansions close to blood vessels at the surface of the cellular cords or in the intervening connective tissue septa. The cords contain a smaller population of neuroglial cells that resemble astrocytes. After the age of about 16 years, granules of calcium and magnesium salts appear and later coalesce to form larger particles (brain sand). The deposits may be a useful landmark in x-ray films for determining whether or not the pineal gland is displaced by a space-occupying lesion.

Clinical observations of long standing have suggested an antigonadotrophic function for the pineal gland in humans because a pineal tumor developing around the time of puberty may alter the age of onset of pubertal changes. Puberty may be precocious if the tumor is of a type that destroys parenchymatous cells, or delayed if the tumor is derived from them. Experimental work has placed these observations on a sounder basis.

Pinealectomy in experimental animals stimulates the genital system, with genital hypertrophy, precocious opening of the vagina in immature females, and changes in the estrous cycle. Administration of pineal extracts has the contrary effect through inhibition of the gonads. Chemical extraction of bovine pineal glands has produced several possible active principles including melatonin, an indoleamine related to serotonin. Melatonin causes clumping of melanin granules in the pigment-bearing cells of the skin, with concomitant lightening of overall color in lower vertebrates. In humans, the circulating level of melatonin falls sharply with the onset of puberty. In women of reproductive age there are cyclic variations, with the melatonin levels reaching minimum values at the time of ovulation.

In mammals, as in lower vertebrates, the activity of the pineal organ is influenced by light; its antigonadotrophic activity is highest when the animal is in the dark and lowest when in a light environment. The pathway is known to originate in the retina; it is also known that the sympathetic innervation has an inhibitory effect on the gland. A connection between the retina and the intermediolateral cell column in the upper thoracic segments of the spinal cord is therefore required. This connection has been shown in animals to begin as fibers leaving the optic tract near the optic chiasma, with these fibers terminating in the suprachiasmatic nucleus of the hypothalamus. Hypothalamospinal fibers traveling in the dorsal longitudinal fasciculus and terminating in the lateral horn of the upper thoracic segments of the spinal cord presumably complete the pathway.

The site of action of the pineal hormone(s) is still being investigated. The target cells may be in the gonads or in the pars distalis of the pituitary gland. Alternatively, they may be neurosecretory cells in the hypothalamus that produce releasing factors for the gonadotrophin-producing cells of the pituitary, or neurons that project to the hypothalamus. Results of some studies have implicated cells of the central nervous system, either hypothalamic cells or neurons in the reticular formation of the midbrain projecting to the hypothalamus. In addition to the antigonadotrophic function, there is some evidence that pineal hormones influence pituitary cells that produce the growth (somatotrophic) hormone (STH), the thyroid-stimulating hormone (TSH), and the adrenocorticotrophic hormone (ACTH).

HYPOTHALAMUS

The hypothalamus, occupying only a small part of the brain and weighing about 4 g, has a functional importance that is quite out of proportion to its size. The hypothalamus is at a crossroads between the thalamus and cerebral cortex (especially that of the limbic system) and ascending fiber systems from the brain stem and spinal cord. Input from the thalamus and limbic system has a special emotional significance, and the ascending fibers convey information that is largely of visceral origin. However, the hypothalamus is not influenced solely by neuronal systems; some of the constituent nerve cells respond to properties of the circulating blood, including temperature, osmotic pressure, and the levels of various hormones. Hypothalamic function becomes manifest through efferent pathways to autonomic nuclei in the brain stem and spinal cord, and through an intimate relationship with the hypophysis or pituitary gland by means of neurosecretory cells. These cells elaborate the hormones of the neurohypophysis and pro-

duce releasing factors that control the hormonal output of the adenohypophysis. By these means the hypothalamus has a major role in producing responses to emotional changes and to needs signaled by hunger and thirst, and is instrumental in maintaining a constant internal environment (homeostasis).

The hypothalamus surrounds the third ventricle ventral to the hypothalamic sulci (see Fig. 11–2). The mamillary bodies are distinct swellings on the ventral surface (see Fig. 11–1). The region bounded by the mamillary bodies, optic chiasma, and beginning of the optic tracts is known as the **tuber cinereum.** The **infundibular stem** arises from the **median eminence** just behind the optic chiasma and expands to form the **infundibular process** or pars nervosa of the pituitary gland. The median eminence, infundibular stem, and infundibular process have similar cytological and functional characteristics; together they constitute the **neurohypophysis.**

The columns of the fornix traverse the hypothalamus to reach the mamillary bodies and serve as points of reference for sagittal planes that divide each half of the hypothalamus into **medial** and **lateral zones.** The medial zone is subdivided into three regions—**suprachiasmatic, tuberal,** and **mamillary**—with ventral structures as landmarks. The medial zone consists of gray matter in which several nuclei are recognized on the basis of cellular characteristics and connections. It also includes a thin layer of fine myelinated and unmyelinated fibers beneath the ependymal lining of the third ventricle. The lateral zone or area contains fewer nerve cells but there are many nerve fibers, with most of them running in a longitudinal direction.

Hypothalamic Nuclei

The lamina terminalis represents the rostral end of the embryonic neural tube and limits the third ventricle anteriorly (Fig.

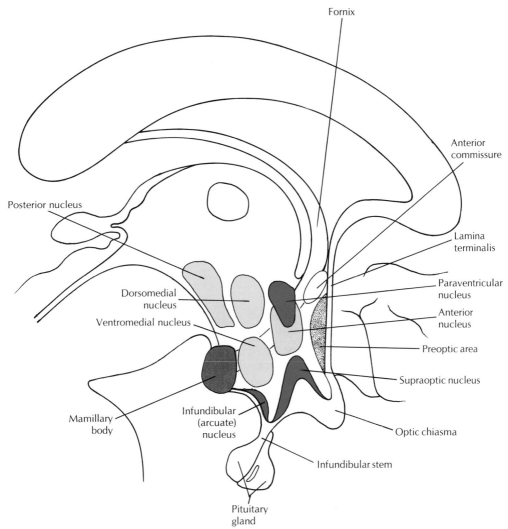

FIGURE 11-14.
Nuclei in the medial zone of the hypothalamus.

11–14). The lamina extends from the optic chiasma to the anterior commissure. The latter is a bundle of fibers connecting areas of the right and left temporal lobes, and includes some commissural fibers connecting the olfactory bulbs. The lamina terminalis and anterior commissure are telencephalic structures. So is the gray matter immediately behind the lamina terminalis (the **preoptic area**), although it is thought of as being part of the hypothalamus.

Medial Zone

Within the medial zone (Fig. 11–14) the suprachiasmatic region contains the supraoptic, paraventricular, suprachiasmatic, and anterior nuclei. The **supraoptic nucleus** consists of large cells and is best developed above the junction of the optic chiasma and optic tract. The **paraventricular nucleus** contains large cells in a matrix of smaller neurons. These two nuclei are conspicuous in Nissl-stained sections and have a plentiful supply of capillaries. The cells of the supraoptic and paraventricular nuclei elaborate neurohypophysial hormones, and secretory granules in the cytoplasm are evidence of neurosecretory activity. Axons from the nuclei constitute the hypothalamohypophysial tract, whose fibers terminate throughout the neurohypophysis where the hormones are released into capillary blood. The **suprachiasmatic nucleus** is a small cluster of neurons on each side of the midline immediately dorsal to the optic chiasma. Axons of retinal origin leave the chiasma to terminate in this nucleus. The **anterior nucleus** is similar to the preoptic area cytologically, and they are not clearly demarcated from one another.

The tuberal region contains the **ventromedial, dorsomedial,** and **infundibular (arcuate) nuclei,** with each nucleus consisting of small nerve cells. The mamillary region includes the **mamillary body** and the **posterior nucleus.** In humans the mamillary body is occupied almost entirely by a medial mamillary nucleus, and the remainder consists of an intermediate nucleus and a lateral nucleus. The cells of the lateral nucleus are large, whereas the bulk of the mamillary body is made up of small neurons. The posterior hypothalamic nucleus consists of large neurons in a background of small nerve cells.

Lateral Zone

The large nerve cells throughout the lateral zone are relatively sparse and collectively constitute the **lateral nucleus** of the hypothalamus. The cells are interspersed with longitudinally running nerve fibers that pass to or from hypothalamic nuclei or through the area. This zone includes the **lateral tuberal nucleus,** which consists of several groups of nerve cells near the surface of the tuber cinereum. The hypothalamus of humans is characterized by the large size of the medial mamillary nucleus, the well-defined lateral tuberal nucleus, and the presence of large neurons in the posterior and lateral nuclei.

Afferent Connections

As mentioned previously, the hypothalamus receives information from diverse sources in order to serve as the main integrator of the autonomic nervous system.

Ascending afferents convey data of visceral origin, and include fibers for the special visceral sense of taste. The pathways are not well defined, compared with somatic sensory tracts leading to the thalamus, and consist in part of relays through the reticular formation of the brain stem. Some of the ascending fibers are included in the dorsal longitudinal fasciculus, which also contains efferent fibers of the hypothalamus. Somatic sensory information, especially from erotogenic zones such as the nipples and genitalia, also reaches the hypothalamus.

The cells of origin of the **medial forebrain bundle** are chiefly in the septal area, with other fibers coming from the intermediate and lateral olfactory areas (Chap. 17). The bundle therefore conducts data related to basic emotional drives and the sense of smell. It runs caudally in the lateral zone of the hypothalamus, giving off fibers to hypothalamic nuclei. Other fibers of the bundle continue through the hypothalamus to the raphe nuclei of the reticular formation of the midbrain and pons. The medial forebrain bundle is small in the human brain in comparison with the brains of animals that rely heavily on their sense of smell. It also contains ascending fibers that originate in the locus ceruleus and the ventral tegmental area of the brain stem and terminate in the hypothalamus.

A second input related to smell and emotional drives comes from the amygdaloid body. This nuclear complex is situated in the temporal lobe in the region of the uncus, a small gyral configuration on the

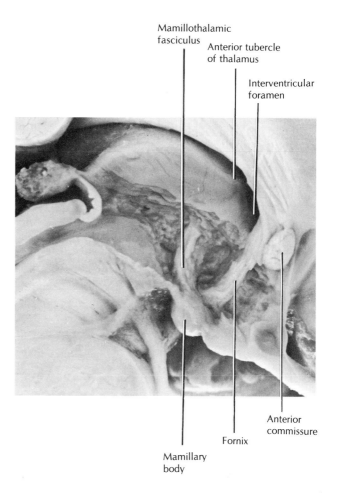

FIGURE 11-15.
Dissection showing the fornix and
mamillothalamic fasciculus on the left
side. Gray matter has been removed
piecemeal from the wall of the third
ventricle to display the bundles of
myelinated fibers. (× 2)

ventral surface (see Fig. 11–1). A slender
strand of fibers known as the **stria terminalis** arises from the amygdaloid body,
arches over the thalamus along the medial
side of the caudate nucleus (see Fig.
11–12), and terminates in part in the
preoptic area and anterior nucleus of the
hypothalamus.

The **fornix,** originating in the hippocampal formation of the temporal lobe, is
the largest of the fiber bundles that end in
the hypothalamus. As mentioned earlier,
the fornix arches over the thalamus and
into the hypothalamus, where the fibers
terminate mainly in the mamillary body
(Fig. 11–15). The mamillary body also receives fibers from the anterior thalamic
nuclei through the mamillothalamic fascic-

ulus and is therefore in communication
with the cortex of the cingulate gyrus. The
hypothalamus is an integral part of the limbic system of the brain and is essential to
the intimate relationship between basic
emotional drives and visceral function,
which is an important aspect of the physiology of the limbic system.

The hypothalamus receives fibers from
the **mediodorsal thalamic nucleus,** which
has reciprocal connections with the prefrontal cortex. It will be recalled that these
parts of the brain, among other functions,
contribute to states of mind commonly
referred to as moods. There are also direct **corticohypothalamic fibers,** especially
from cortex on the orbital surface of the
frontal lobe.

Efferent Connections

There are two principal descending pathways from the hypothalamus. The first of these begins as thinly myelinated and unmyelinated **periventricular fibers** beneath the ependyma of the third ventricle, continuing into the **dorsal longitudinal fasciculus** in the periaqueductal gray matter of the midbrain. Many of these descending fibers originate from the small cells of the paraventricular nucleus. Some end in the dorsal nucleus of the vagus nerve and, it may be presumed, in the salivatory and lacrimal nuclei. Other fibers continue into the spinal cord to terminate in the intermediolateral cell column and sacral autonomic nucleus. Thus, the hypothalamus can directly influence the preganglionic neurons of the sympathetic and parasympathetic nervous systems. Through relays in the reticular formation, and reticulobulbar and reticulospinal fibers, the hypothalamus also influences the activity of certain motor neurons supplying striated muscles. These include cells in the motor nuclei of the trigeminal and facial nerves, the nucleus ambiguus, and the hypoglossal nucleus, in connection with the role of the hypothalamus in feeding and drinking. Motor neurons of the spinal cord are influenced by the hypothalamus in temperature regulation, as in shivering to raise the body temperture.

The fibers of a second descending pathway, the **mamillotegmental fasciculus,** are collateral branches of fibers of the mamillothalamic fasciculus that turn caudally and end in nuclei of the reticular formation of the midbrain and pons. Thus, impulses originating in the mamillary body reach autonomic nuclei in the brain stem and spinal cord through synaptic relays in the reticular formation. Finally, axons of some hypothalamic neurons reach the reticular formation by way of the medial forebrain bundle, as well as through an indirect pathway that includes the stria medullaris thalami and habenular nuclei.

Activity within the hypothalamus is transmitted as well to the thalamus and cerebral cortex, where it influences affective states, both basic emotions of a primitive nature and those more closely related to moods. The large **mamillothalamic fasciculus** (bundle of Vicq d'Azyr) establishes reciprocal connections between the mamillary body and the anterior nuclei of the thalamus, which in turn have reciprocal connections with the cortex of the cingulate gyrus (see Fig. 11–15). As noted previously, the anterior thalamic nuclei and the cingulate cortex share with other components of the limbic system responsibility for those emotions and aspects of behavior that are related to preservation of the individual and of the species. The hypothalamus contributes to the subjective experience of these emotions through projections to the thalamus and cortex, and to visceral manifestations of emotions through the autonomic nervous system. A supplementary contribution to the affect, in particular to an individual's mood, derives from reciprocal connections between the hypothalamus and the mediodorsal thalamic nucleus, and between the latter and prefrontal cortex.

The hypothalamus also sends fibers to a region lateral to it called the substantia innominata. Nuclei made up of large neurons within the substantia innominata have been implicated in the pathogenesis of Alzheimer's disease, but the relationship is as yet unproven (see Chap. 12).

Functional Considerations

Autonomic and Related Aspects

Results of electrical stimulation of the hypothalamus in experimental animals have shown that some regions produce parasympathetic, and others sympathetic, responses. Parasympathetic responses are most regularly elicited by stimulation of the anterior hypothalamus, notably the preoptic area and anterior nucleus. The responses include slowing of the heart rate, vasodilation, lowering of blood pressure, salivation, increased peristalsis in the gastrointestinal tract, contraction of the urinary bladder, and sweating. Sympathetic responses, most readily elicited by stimulation in the region of the posterior and lateral nuclei, include cardiac acceleration, elevation of blood pressure, cessation of peristalsis in the gastrointestinal tract, dilation of the pupils, and hyperglycemia.

Regulation of body temperature is an instructive example of the role of the hypothalamus in maintaining homeostasis. Certain hypothalamic cells act as a thermostat, monitoring the temperature of blood flowing through the capillaries and initiating the responses necessary to maintain a normal body temperature. Thermosensitive neurons in the parasympathetic region of the anterior hypothalamus respond to an increase in temperature of the blood. Mechanisms that promote heat loss, such as cutaneous vasodilation and sweating, are activated. A lesion in the anterior hypothalamus may therefore result in hyperthermia in a hot environment or under states of high metabolic rate. Cells in the sympathetic region, especially the posterior hypothalamic nucleus, respond to a lowering of blood temperature. Responses such as cutaneous vasoconstriction and shivering are triggered for conservation and production of heat, and a lesion in the posterior hypothalamus interferes with temperature regulation in a cold environment. A lesion in the posterior part of the hypothalamus may not only destroy cells involved in conservation and production of heat but may also interrupt fibers running caudally from the heat-dissipating region. This results in a serious impairment of temperature regulation in either a cold or hot environment.

Hypothalamic regulation of food and water intake has also been demonstrated by electrical stimulation and by placing small electrolytic lesions in the hypothal-

amus. A hunger or feeding center has been located in the lateral zone, and a satiety center (inhibiting food intake) has been demonstrated in the region of the ventromedial nucleus. These centers are influenced by the glucose level of the blood, by visceral afferent fibers, by the olfactory system, and by thalamic and cortical regions concerned with the emotions. Destruction of the satiety center in an experimental animal, such as the rat, results in excessive food intake and obesity. Naturally occurring lesions affecting this center in humans may also result in obesity, and hypothalamic cells that regulate the output of gonadotrophic hormones by the adenohypophysis may be destroyed at the same time. The combination of obesity and deficiency of secondary sex characteristics is known as the adiposogenital, or Fröhlich's, syndrome. The zona incerta of the subthalamus, the lateral and ventromedial hypothalamic nuclei, and the subfornical organ are interconnected to control water intake.

Relations of the Hypothalamus to the Pituitary Gland (Hypophysis)

Neurohypophysial hormones are synthesized in the hypothalamus, and hormone production by the adenohypophysis is controlled by chemical substances produced by hypothalamic cells. The nervous system, through the neurosecretory function of hypothalamic cells, has therefore an intimate relation with the endocrine system. Only the major points concerning hypothalamic–hypophysial relationships are discussed here; the subject is a large one, comprising much of the specialty of neuroendocrinology.

Neurohypophysis. As noted previously, the neurohypophysis consists of the median eminence, infundibular stem, and infundibular process, all of which are of diencephalic origin in the embryo (Fig. 11–16). Histologically it is made up of ax-

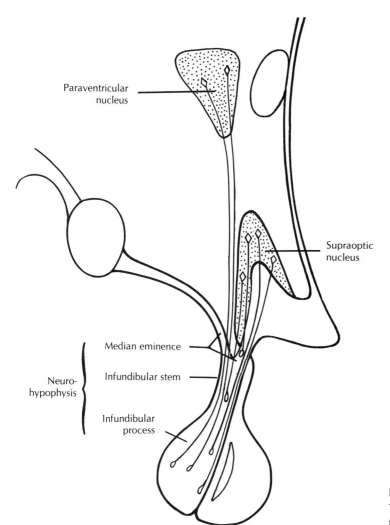

Paraventricular
nucleus

Supraoptic
nucleus

Median eminence

Infundibular stem

Neuro-
hypophysis

Infundibular
process

FIGURE 11-16.
The hypothalamohypophysial tract.

onal endings, blood vessels, and atypical astrocytes known as **pituicytes.** Although hormones enter the blood stream from the neurohypophysis they are not elaborated there, but rather are elaborated in the large neurosecretory cells of the supraoptic and paraventricular nuclei. The hormones are vasopressin and oxytocin. Vasopressin has two properties, vasoconstrictor and anti-diuretic, the former of which is of little physiological and clinical importance. Oxy-tocin causes contraction of myoepithelial cells surrounding the secretory alveoli of the mammary gland and stimulates the smooth muscle of the uterus. Results of immunocytochemical studies have shown that vasopressin-containing neurons are most abundant in the supraoptic nucleus and oxytocin-containing neurons are most abundant in the paraventricular nucleus.

The axons of cells in the supraoptic and paraventricular nuclei constitute the **hypothalamohypophysial tract** and terminate as small expansions adjacent to capillaries in the neurohypophysis (see Fig. 11–16). The secretory function of the cells is evi-dent in the secretory granules present in the cytoplasm of the cell bodies. The neurosecretions are carried distally by axoplasmic transport, and vasopressin and oxytocin enter the blood stream by way of the capillary bed throughout the neurohypophysis, but principally in the infundibular process. The neurohypophysis is the only mammalian example of a neurohemal organ, which is a structure composed of neurosecretory axons ending on capillary blood vessels. Fishes have a histologically similar organ at the caudal end of the spinal cord. Neurohemal organs are more numerous and varied in invertebrate animals. Indeed, neurosecretory cells are phylogenetically one of the oldest neuron types.

The supraoptic nucleus serves as an osmoreceptor, with the secretory activity of its cells being influenced by the osmolarity of the blood flowing through this highly vascular nucleus. A slight elevation of osmotic pressure causes the cells to propagate impulses with greater frequency. The arrival of impulses at the neurohemal terminals causes the release of the antidiuretic hormone (vasopressin) into the capillary blood of the neurohypophysis. Resorption of water from the collecting tubules of the kidney is then accelerated, and the osmolarity of the blood plasma returns to normal. A delicate mechanism is thereby provided to ensure homeostasis with respect to water balance. Destruction of the supraoptic nucleus or of the neurohypophysis results in diabetes insipidus, which is characterized by excretion of large quantities of dilute urine (polyuria) and excessive thirst and water intake to compensate (polydipsia). A lesion restricted to the infundibular process of the pituitary gland is not as a rule followed by diabetes insipidus, because some antidiuretic hormone enters the blood stream from the median eminence and infundibular stem.

The best understood actions of oxytocin are those following reflex release of the hormone induced by a suckling infant. Contraction of the myoepithelial cells of the mammary gland causes ejection of milk into the duct system while simultaneous contraction of the uterus contributes to the postpartum involution of this organ.

Pituitary Portal System. The following hormones are produced in the pars distalis of the adenohypophysis: follicle-stimulating hormone (FSH); luteinizing hormone (LH), also known as interstitial cell-stimulating hormone (ICSH) in men; prolactin; thyrotrophic or thyroid-stimulating hormone (TSH); adrenocorticotrophic hormone (ACTH); and growth or somatotrophic hormone (STH). The first three are gonadotrophic hormones. FSH promotes growth of ovarian follicles and spermatogenesis. LH promotes ovulation, converts the ruptured ovarian follicle into a corpus luteum, and, in men, stimulates interstitial cells of the testis to secrete androgens. LH also stimulates the corpus luteum to secrete progesterone, and prolactin, in concert with STH and other hormones, promotes secretion of milk in the lactating breast. Secretion of hormones by the pars distalis is under the control of the hypothalamus, but by a vascular route rather than nervous connections.

The pituitary portal system begins with the superior hypophysial artery, which arises from the internal carotid artery at the base of the brain and breaks up into capillary tufts and loops in the median eminence (Fig. 11–17). The capillaries are drained by veins that enter the adenohypophysis, where they empty into the large capillaries or sinusoids of the pars distalis. The hypothalamus contains cells that produce releasing factors, and at least two release-inhibiting factors, for prolactin and STH. There is a separate releasing factor for each hormone of the pars distalis, with the exception of FSH, which is secreted in response to the same releasing factor as for LH. There is probably a topographical pattern of cells that produce the different factors. These factors are peptides; however, the prolactin release-inhibiting factor

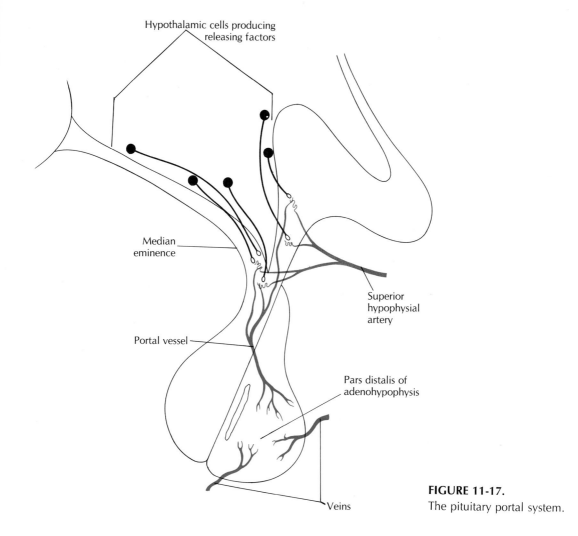

Hypothalamic cells producing releasing factors

Median eminence

Portal vessel

Superior hypophysial artery

Pars distalis of adenohypophysis

Veins

FIGURE 11-17.
The pituitary portal system.

is dopamine, a catecholamine. The releasing factors pass distally by axoplasmic transport in the axons of the cells producing them and enter the capillaries of the portal system in the median eminence to reach the pars distalis. They thereby modulate the synthesis and release of the adenohypophysial hormones. Cells producing releasing and release-inhibiting factors are influenced by the various afferent fiber connections of the hypothalamus. Their activity is also regulated by hormones of the target organs of pituitary hormones. For example, when the blood titer of estrogens or androgens is high, hypothalamic cells producing releasing factors for

gonadotrophic hormones are suppressed. Conversely, in hypogonadal conditions, these cells produce an excess of the releasing factors, and the secretion of gonadotrophins is elevated.

THIRD VENTRICLE

The diencephalic part of the ventricular system consists of the narrow third ventricle (see Fig. 11–2). The anterior wall of this ventricle is formed by the lamina terminalis; the anterior commissure crosses the midline in the dorsal part of the lamina terminalis. The rather extensive lateral wall is marked by the hypothalamic sulcus, which runs from the interventricular foramen (foramen of Monro) to the opening of the cerebral aqueduct and divides the wall of the third ventricle into thalamic and hypothalamic regions. An interthalamic adhesion (massa intermedia) bridges the ventricle in 70% of human brains. The floor of the third ventricle is indented by the optic chiasma. There is an optic recess in front of the chiasma, and behind the chiasma the infundibular recess extends into the median eminence and the proximal part of the infundibular stem. The floor then slopes upward to the cerebral aqueduct of the midbrain, with the posterior commissure forming a slight prominence above the entrance to the aqueduct. A pineal recess extends into the stalk of the pineal gland, and the dorsal wall of the stalk accommodates the small habenular commissure. The membranous roof of the third ventricle is attached along the striae medullares thalami, and a small choroid plexus is suspended from the roof.

Cerebrospinal fluid enters the third ventricle from each lateral ventricle through the interventricular foramen (foramen of Monro). The foramen is bounded by the fornix and by the anterior tubercle of the thalamus, and is closed posteriorly by a reflexion of ependyma between the fornix and the thalamus. The **subfornical organ**, mentioned earlier in this chapter, is a small eminence on the medial side of the column of the fornix, above the interventricular foramen. It is a nucleus of nerve cells containing blood vessels that are permeable to circulating macromolecules, unlike the vessels of most parts of the brain. The nucleus responds to circulating levels of angiotensin II, a peptide whose concentration in plasma varies with circulating levels of sodium and potassium ions, and with changes in blood volume. The neurons of the subfornical organ project to the zona incerta and hypothalamus.

Cerebrospinal fluid leaves the third ventricle by way of the cerebral aqueduct of the midbrain, through which it reaches the fourth ventricle and then the subarachnoid space surrounding the brain and spinal cord.

SUGGESTED READING

Boivie J: An anatomical reinvestigation of the termination of the spinothalamic tract in the monkey. J Comp Neurol 186:343–370, 1979

Braak H, Braak E: The hypothalamus of the human adult: Chiasmatic region. Anat Embryol (Berl) 176:315–330, 1987

Carpenter MB, Carleton SC, Keller JT, Conte P: Connections of the subthalamic nucleus in the monkey. Brain Res 224:1–29, 1981

Collins P, Woollam DHM: The circumventricular organs. Chapter 5 in Harrison RJ, Holmes RL (eds): Progress in Anatomy, Vol 1, pp 123–139. Cambridge, Cambridge University Press, 1981

Cooper KE: The neurobiology of fever: Thoughts on recent developments. Ann Rev Neurosci 10:297–324, 1987

Crosby EC, Humphrey T, Lauer EW: Correlative Anatomy of the Nervous System. New York, Macmillan, 1962

Haywood JN: Functional and morphological aspects of hypothalamic neurons. Physiol Rev 57:574–658, 1977

Jones EG: The Thalamus. New York, Plenum Press, 1985

Kelly DE: Pineal organs: Photoreception, secretion and development. Am Sci 50:597–625, 1962

Kordon C: Neural mechanisms involved in pituitary control. Neurochem Int 7:917–925, 1985

LuQui IJ, Fox CA: The supraoptic nucleus and the supraopticohypophysial tract in the monkey (Macaca mulatta). J Comp Neurol 168:7–40, 1976

Mark MH, Farmer PM: The human subfornical organ: An anatomic and ultrastructural study. Ann Clin Lab Sci 14:427–442, 1984

Morgane PJ, Panksepp J (eds): Handbook of the Hypothalamus, Vol 1: Anatomy of the Hypothalamus. New York, Marcel Dekker, 1979

O'Riordan JLH, Malan PG, Gould RP: Essentials of Endocrinology. Oxford, Blackwell Scientific Publications, 1982

Reiter RJ: Pineal function in the human: Implications for reproductive physiology. J Obstet Gynaecol 6 (Suppl 2):577–581, 1986

Saper CB: Anatomical substrate for the hypothalamic control of the autonomic nervous system. In Brooks CMcC, Koizumi K, Sato A (eds): Integrative Functions of the Autonomic Nervous System, Chap 24. Amsterdam, Elsevier-North Holland, 1979

Swanson LW, Mogenson GJ: Neural mechanisms for the functional coupling of autonomic, endocrine and somatomotor responses in adaptive behavior. Brain Res Rev 3:1–34, 1981

Swanson LW, Sawchenko PO: Paraventricular nucleus: A site for the integration of neuroendocrine and autonomic mechanisms. Neuroendocrinology 31:410–417, 1980

von Euler C: Physiology and pharmacology of temperature regulation. Pharmacol Rev 13:361–398, 1961

TWELVE

Corpus Striatum

The corpus striatum is a substantial region of gray matter near the base of each cerebral hemisphere. It consists of the **caudate nucleus** and the **lentiform nucleus,** with the latter divided into the **putamen** and the **globus pallidus.** The corpus striatum, claustrum, and amygdaloid body are sometimes referred to as the basal "ganglia" of the telencephalon. The claustrum is a thin sheet of gray matter of obscure significance situated lateral to the putamen, and the amygdaloid body in the temporal lobe is a component of the olfactory and limbic systems. Clinically the term *basal ganglia* is usually applied to the corpus striatum, subthalamic nucleus, and substantia nigra. The three nuclei are grouped under the common heading because they share an importance in motor disturbances called dyskinesias, characterized by involuntary purposeless movements.

PHYLOGENETIC DEVELOPMENT

The topography of the corpus striatum of humans is best understood against a phylogenetic background. In amphibians the telencephalon is formed into two tubular "hemispheres," each with a central ventricular cavity. The dorsal wall of the ventricle is the pallium, the forerunner of all the cortical structures of the mammalian cerebrum. The medial wall is the septum, which persists in mammals as the septal area, a component of the limbic system. The ventrolateral wall is the corpus striatum. In reptiles the corpus striatum forms a thickening that bulges into the floor of the lateral ventricle. In birds and mammals the large corpus striatum has two distinct zones. They are the **paleostriatum** (homologous with the whole corpus striatum of amphibians and reptiles) and the

neostriatum. The expansion of the pallium to form the extensive cerebral cortex in mammals caused the corpus striatum to be displaced from the ventrolateral wall of a tubular structure into the center of the hemisphere, where it still bulges into the floor of the lateral ventricle. In mammals the neostriatum is much larger than the paleostriatum.

The development of an extensive cerebral cortex is also responsible for a partial separation of the neostriatum into two components. Fibers connecting the cortex with subcortical centers traverse the neostriatum and run along the medial side of the smaller paleostriatum (globus pallidus) as the internal capsule. The neostriatum is thereby divided into the caudate nucleus on the medial side of the itinerant fibers, and the putamen lateral to the globus pallidus (Fig. 12–1). The globus pallidus and the putamen constitute the lentiform nucleus.

The neostriatum is also called the **striatum,** and the globus pallidus is then referred to as the **pallidum.** The shorter forms are useful in naming afferent and efferent connections (*e.g.,* corticostriate and pallidothalamic fibers). The following correlations may be helpful in understanding the use of terms:

neostriatum = striatum = putamen + caudate nucleus

paleostriatum = pallidum = globus pallidus

lentiform nucleus = globus pallidus + putamen

LENTIFORM AND CAUDATE NUCLEI

It is helpful to understand the configuration and relations of the lentiform and caudate nuclei, even though the division of the corpus striatum into paleostriatum and neostriatum has a greater relevance to the

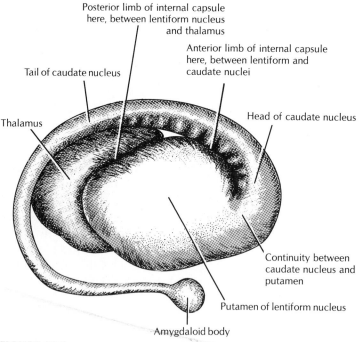

Posterior limb of internal capsule here, between lentiform nucleus and thalamus

Anterior limb of internal capsule here, between lentiform and caudate nuclei

Tail of caudate nucleus

Head of caudate nucleus

Thalamus

Continuity between caudate nucleus and putamen

Putamen of lentiform nucleus

Amygdaloid body

FIGURE 12-1.
Lateral aspect of the right corpus striatum. The globus pallidus of the lentiform nucleus is concealed by the larger putamen.

afferent and efferent connections of this part of the brain.

Lentiform Nucleus

The lentiform nucleus is wedge-shaped, and has been described as having the approximate size and shape of a Brazil nut (Figs. 12–2 and 12–3). The narrow part of the wedge facing medially is occupied by the **globus pallidus,** which is divided into medial and lateral parts by a lamina of nerve fibers. The globus pallidus of humans may have three divisions. The **putamen** forms the lateral portion of the lentiform nucleus and extends beyond the globus pallidus in all directions except at

the base of the nucleus. The two components of the lentiform nucleus are separated by another lamina of nerve fibers.

The lentiform nucleus is bounded laterally by a thin layer of white matter that constitutes the **external capsule** (see Figs. 12–2 and 12–3). This is followed by the **claustrum,** which is a thin sheet of gray matter coextensive with the lateral surface of the putamen. Its functional significance is unknown. The best documented connections of the claustrum are reciprocal connections with the cortices of the frontal, parietal, and temporal lobes. The **extreme capsule** separates the claustrum from the **insula** (island of Reil), an area of cortex buried in the depths of the lateral

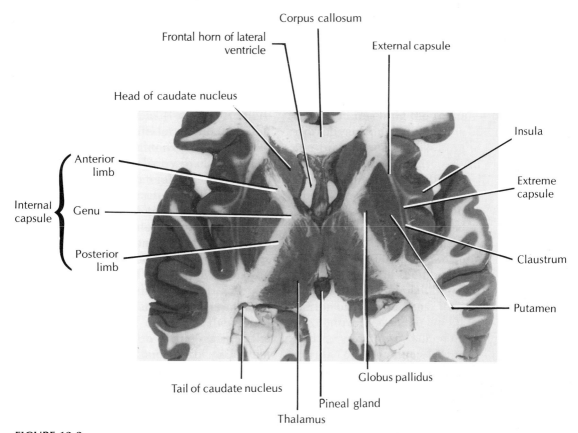

FIGURE 12-2.
Horizontal section of the cerebrum, stained by a method that differentiates gray matter (*dark*) and white matter (*light*), showng the components and relations of the corpus striatum. (× ⅘)

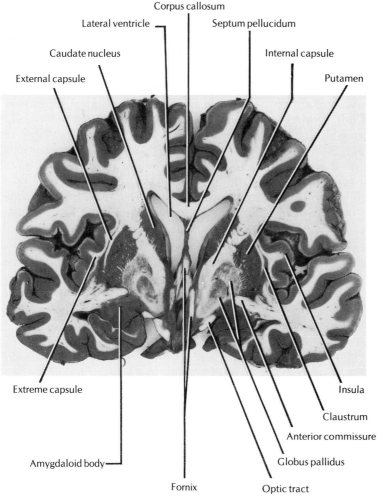

FIGURE 12-3.
Coronal section of the cerebrum anterior to the thalamus, stained by a method that differentiates gray matter (*dark*) and white matter (*light*), showing the components and relations of the corpus striatum. (× ⅕)

sulcus of the cerebral hemisphere, also known as the fissure of Sylvius. The medial surface of the lentiform nucleus lies against the internal capsule. The ventral surface is close to structures at the base of the hemisphere, such as the anterior perforated substance, optic tract, and amygdaloid body (see Fig. 12–3).

Caudate Nucleus

The caudate nucleus consists of an anterior portion or **head,** which tapers into a

slender **tail** extending backward and then forward into the temporal lobe (see Fig. 12–1). The extension of the caudate nucleus into the temporal lobe terminates at the amygdaloid body, with which the caudate nucleus has no functional relationship, and consists of an attenuated interrupted strand of gray matter in some human brains.

The head of the caudate nucleus bulges into the frontal horn of the lateral ventricle, and the first part of the tail lies along the lateral margin of the central part of the ventricle (see Figs. 12–2 and 11–12). The tail follows the contour of the lateral ventricle into the roof of its temporal horn. Two structures lie along the medial side of the tail of the caudate nucleus. These are the **stria terminalis,** a slender bundle of fibers originating in the amygdaloid body, and the **thalamostriate vein (vena terminalis),** which drains the caudate nucleus, thalamus, internal capsule, and nearby structures (see Fig. 11–12).

The anterior limb of the internal capsule intervenes between the head of the caudate nucleus and the lentiform nucleus, and the tail of the caudate nucleus is medial to the internal capsule as the latter merges with the medullary center of the hemisphere. However, the cortical afferent and efferent fibers constituting the internal capsule do not completely separate the two components of the neostriatum. The head of the caudate nucleus and the putamen are continuous with one another through a bridge of gray matter beneath the anterior limb of the internal capsule (Fig. 12–1). In addition, numerous strands of gray matter joining the head and tail of the caudate nucleus with the putamen cut across the internal capsule. The most ventral part of the neostriatum in this region is called the **nucleus accumbens septi,** although it is not part of the septal area. Ventral to the nucleus accumbens is the substantia innominata, which is described at the end of this chapter.

CONNECTIONS

Neostriatum

The caudate nucleus and the putamen are similar histologically, as is to be expected. They consist mainly of small neurons that form intranuclear connections or project to the globus pallidus. Only about one cell in twenty is of relatively large size; these cells send fibers to the globus pallidus and to the substantia nigra.

The neostriatum receives fibers from the cerebral cortex, thalamus, and substantia nigra (Fig. 12–4). **Corticostriate** fibers originate in widespread areas of cortex, including that of all four lobes, but especially the frontal and parietal lobes. Most of the fibers enter the neostriatum from the internal capsule, although a substantial number enter the putamen from the external capsule. **Thalamostriate** fibers originate in the intralaminar nuclei of the thalamus, especially the centromedian nucleus. **Nigrostriate** fibers from the pars compacta of the substantia nigra constitute a particularly important afferent connection of the corpus striatum. The nigral neurons use dopamine as a transmitter so that in Parkinson's disease, which involves degeneration of neurons in the pars compacta, the neostriatum is deprived of its dopaminergic input.

The fibers leaving the neostriatum are **striopallidal,** bringing the globus pallidus under the influence and control of the neostriatum, and **strionigral,** terminating in the substantia nigra.

Paleostriatum

The globus pallidus, which is the principal efferent part of the corpus striatum, consists of moderately large, multipolar neurons. Their axons are well myelinated, accounting for the pallor of the nucleus in fresh sections and for the name "globus pallidus." Conversely, the globus pallidus is darker than the putamen and the caudate nucleus in Weigert-stained sections.

The **striopallidal** fibers noted previously are the principal afferents to the globus pallidus. Many of these are collateral branches of the strionigral axons, which pass through the globus pallidus on their way to the substantia nigra.

Efferent fibers of the globus pallidus take either of two routes initially (Fig. 12–5). Some fibers cross the internal capsule and appear as the **lenticular fasciculus** (field H_2 of Forel) in the subthalamus, dorsal to the subthalamic nucleus. Other fibers curve around the medial edge of the

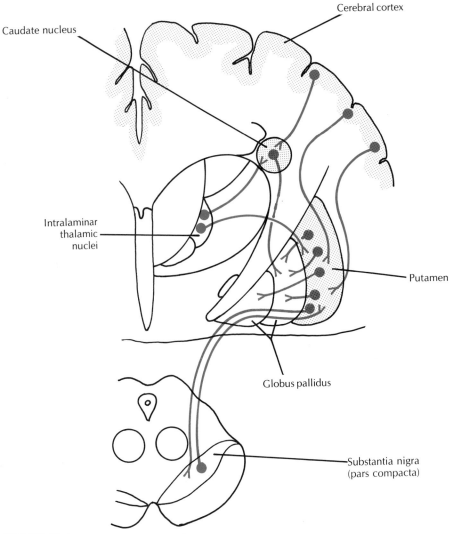

FIGURE 12-4.
Afferent and efferent connections of the neostriatum. The connections of the caudate nucleus are similar to those of the putamen.

internal capsule, forming the **ansa lenticularis.** These fasciculi consist mainly of **pallidothalamic** fibers. They enter the prerubral area of the subthalamus (field H of Forel), turn laterally into the thalamic fasciculus (field H$_1$ of Forel), and terminate in the anterior division of the ventral lateral nucleus of the thalamus. This nucleus projects to the premotor area of cortex in the frontal lobe, including the portion of the area on the medial surface of the hemisphere that is designated the supplementary motor area. A few pallidofugal fibers accompany the main outflow to the thalamus but continue into the stria medullaris thalami and terminate in the habenular nuclei. Through this connection the corpus striatum is potentially able to modify the descending output of the limbic system.

Some of the relatively few fibers of the

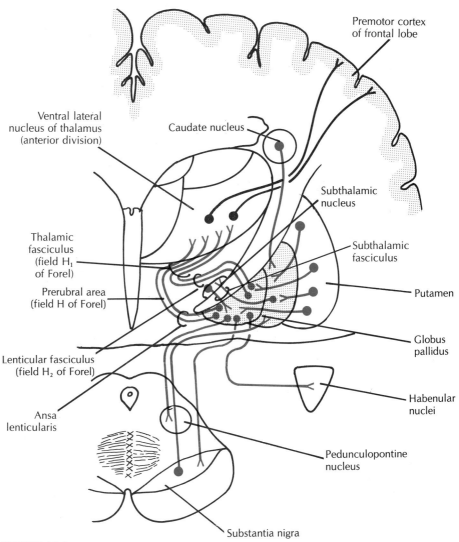

FIGURE 12-5.
Afferent and efferent connections of the paleostriatum (globus pallidus).

efferent fasciculi of the globus pallidus that turn caudally end in the substantia nigra. There are also reciprocal connections with the pedunculopontine nucleus, which is one of the lateral group of reticular nuclei in the brain stem. Fibers from the pedunculopontine nucleus proceed to the subthalamic nucleus, and there are probably additional projections that have not yet been determined. The globus pallidus has an important direct connection

with the subthalamic nucleus; it consists of fibers that pass in both directions across the internal capsule, with these fibers forming the **subthalamic fasciculus** (Fig. 12–5).

The striatum inhibits the pallidum, and the pallidum inhibits the thalamocortical neurons. In both cases the inhibitory transmitter is γ-aminobutyric acid (GABA). Electrical recordings in animals indicate that the neurons of the striatum are quiescent and those of the pallidum active when no movements are being made. Shortly before and during a movement, the situation is reversed. Removal of pallidal inhibition allows the ventral lateral thalamic nucleus to be stimulated by other afferent fibers, most of which come from the premotor area of the cerebral cortex. The thalamocortical neurons are excitatory to the premotor cortex. The nigrostriatal dopaminergic neurons are active all the time, though their rates of firing increase with activity of the contralateral musculature.

DYSKINESIAS AND THE CORPUS STRIATUM

The involuntary movements seen in the dyskinesias related to the corpus striatum take various forms. **Choreiform** movements are brisk, jerky, and purposeless, resembling fragments of voluntary movements. They are most pronounced in the axial and proximal limb musculature; the facial muscles and the tongue are involved at times, and there may be hypotonia of the affected muscles. There are two diseases in which choreiform movements are a cardinal sign. Sydenham's chorea (St. Vitus' dance) is typically a disease of childhood; it occurs more frequently in girls than in boys, and often follows an infectious disease caused by hemolytic streptococci. Because the disease is seldom fatal the pathology of Sydenham's chorea is not well understood. The most common findings are scattered minute hemorrhages and capillary emboli in the corpus striatum. Huntington's chorea is a dominant hereditary disorder with onset of clinical signs in middle life, in which there is neuronal degeneration in the corpus striatum, most marked in the neostriatum. Concurrent loss of neurons in the cerebral cortex leads to progressive mental deterioration.

Athetoid movements are slow, sinuous, and aimless, especially involving the distal musculature of the limbs. The movements blend together in a continuous mobile spasm and are usually associated with varying degrees of paresis and spasticity. The muscles of the face, neck, and tongue may be affected, with grimacing, protrusion and writhing of the tongue, and difficulty in speaking and swallowing. Athetosis is often part of a congenital complex of neurological signs (including those of cerebral palsy) that result from disordered development of the brain, birth injury, or other etiological factors. Athetoid movements are most frequently associated with pathological changes in the neostriatum and the cerebral cortex, although lesions are sometimes also present in the globus pallidus and in the thalamus.

Wilson's disease (hepatolenticular degeneration) is caused by a genetically determined error in copper metabolism. The signs of Wilson's disease usually appear between the ages of 10 and 25 years; they include muscular rigidity, tremor, impairment of voluntary movements (including those of speech), and loss of facial expression. There may be uncontrollable laughing or crying without apparent cause. The degenerative changes are most pronounced in the putamen and progress to cavitation of the lentiform nucleus. There may also be cellular degeneration in the cerebral cortex, thalamus, red nucleus, and cerebellum. In addition to these neurological abnormalities, patients also have cirrhosis of the liver. Dystonia musculorum deformans is a particularly disabling motor disturbance in which degenerative changes involve the corpus striatum, along with other parts of the brain. The slow, writhing, involuntary movements of the axial and limb musculature are sustained, which may lead to contracture of muscles.

SUBSTANTIA INNOMINATA

The substantia innominata is the territory ventral to the internal capsule, nucleus accumbens, and anterior commissure, dorsal to the anterior perforated substance, medial to the amygdala, and lateral to the hypothalamus. The region contains three groups of large neurons: the **nucleus basalis of Meynert,** the **nucleus of the diagonal band,** and part of the **septal area.** These groups of cells receive afferent fibers from the cortex of the limbic system and from the hypothalamus. The large neurons, which are cholinergic, project to all areas of the cerebral neocortex, and also to the hippocampus and the amygdaloid body. They constitute the sole source of cholinergic innervation of the cortex, perhaps providing an important link between the limbic system and the neocortex.

The magnocellular neurons in the substantia innominata have been implicated in the pathogenesis of **Alzheimer's disease.** This disorder is the commonest cause of mental deterioration (senile dementia) in the elderly. The large cholinergic neurons at the base of the forebrain degenerate in this disease, and the cortex loses its cholinergic afferent fibers. Severe degenerative changes are also seen in the hippocampus and in the locus ceruleus. In advanced Alzheimer's disease there is also considerable neuronal loss, with shrinkage of gyri, throughout the cerebral cortex. There are fibrillary tangles in neuronal somata in all affected parts of the brain, and also large deposits of fibrillary material known as senile plaques. It has been suggested that the primary abnormality in Alzheimer's disease is degeneration of the cholinergic neurons of the substantia innominata, the other changes being due to transneuronal degeneration, which sometimes occurs in deafferented neurons. To date, however, there is little evidence to support or refute the hypothesis.

SUGGESTED READING

Alexander GE, DeLong MR, Strick PL: Parallel organization of functionally segregated circuits linking basal ganglia and cortex. Annu Rev Neurosci 9:357–381, 1986

Carpenter MB: Anatomy of the corpus striatum and brain stem integrating systems. In Handbook of Physiology, 2nd ed. The Nervous System, Part II, Chap 19, pp 947–995. Bethesda, American Physiological Society, 1981

Crosby EC, Schnitzlein HN (eds): Comparative Correlative Neuroanatomy of the Vertebrate Telencephalon. New York, Macmillan, 1982

Doucette R, Fisman M, Hachinski VC, Mersky H: Cell loss from the nucleus basalis of Meynert in Alzheimer's disease. Can J Neurol Sci 13:435–440, 1986

Dray, A: The physiology and pharmacology of mammalian basal ganglia. Progr Neurobiol 14:221–235, 1980

Hedreen JC, Struble RG, Whitehouse PJ, Price DL: Topography of the magnocellular basal forebrain system in the human brain. J Neuropathol Exp Neurol 43:1–21, 1984

Heimer L: The Human Brain and Spinal Cord. New York, Springer-Verlag, 1983

Kemp JM, Powell TPS: The connections of the striatum and globus pallidus: Synthesis and speculation. Philos Trans R Soc Lond [Biol] 262:441–457, 1971

Mesulam M-M, Mufson EJ: Neural inputs into the nucleus basalis of the substantia innominata (Ch 4) in the rhesus monkey. Brain 107:253–274, 1984

Northcutt RG: Evolution of the telencephalon in non-mammals. Annu Rev Neurosci 4:301–350, 1981

Penney JB, Young AB: Speculations on the functional anatomy of basal ganglia disorders. Annu Rev Neurosci 6:73–84, 1983

Perry RH, Candy JM, Perry EK, Thompson J, Oakley AE: The substantia innominata and adjacent regions in the human brain: Histochemical and biochemical observations. J Anat 138:713–732, 1984

Price DL: New perspectives on Alzheimer's disease. Annu Rev Neurosci 9:489–512, 1986

Sarnat HB, Netsky MG: Evolution of the Nervous System, 2nd ed. New York, Oxford University Press, 1981

THIRTEEN

Topography of the Cerebral Hemispheres

The complicated folding of the surface of the cerebral hemispheres substantially increases the surface area and therefore the volume of cerebral cortex. The folds or convolutions are called **gyri,** and the intervening grooves are called **sulci.** About two thirds of the cortex forms the walls of the sulci and is therefore hidden from surface view. Although some gyri are constant features of the cerebral surface, others vary from one brain to another and even between the two hemispheres of the same brain.

A sulcus is a groove on the surface of a cerebral hemisphere, whereas a **fissure** is a cleft that separates large components of the brain. Despite the different definitions of sulci and fissures, the two terms are often used interchangeably for the deepest sulci.

MAJOR SULCI AND THE FISSURES

The lateral and parieto-occipital sulci appear early in fetal development, and are especially deep in the mature brain. These, together with the central and calcarine sulci, are the boundaries for division of the cerebral hemisphere into the frontal, parietal, temporal, and occipital lobes (Figs. 13–1 and 13–2).

The **lateral sulcus** (fissure of Sylvius) begins as a deep furrow on the inferior surface of the hemisphere. This is the **stem** of the sulcus, which extends laterally between the frontal and temporal lobes and divides into three rami on reaching the lateral surface. The **posterior ramus** is the main part of the sulcus on the lateral surface of the hemisphere, whereas the **anterior** and **ascending rami** project for only

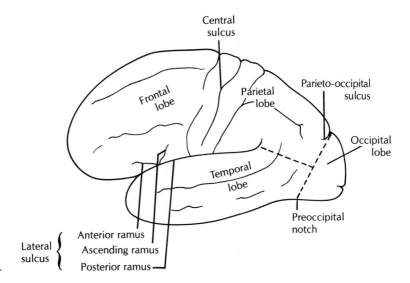

FIGURE 13-1.
Lobes of the cerebral hemisphere (lateral surface).

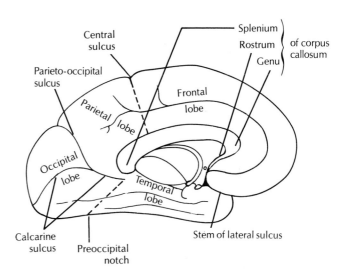

FIGURE 13-2.
Lobes of the cerebral hemisphere (medial and inferior surfaces).

a short distance into the frontal lobe. An area of cortex called the **insula** (island of Reil) lies at the bottom of the lateral sulcus and is hidden from surface view. This cortex appears to have been bound to the underlying corpus striatum during fetal development; growth of the surrounding cortex would then produce the deep lateral sulcus.

The **central sulcus** (sulcus of Rolando) is an important landmark for the sensori-motor cortex because the general sensory area is immediately behind the sulcus and the motor area is immediately in front of it. The central sulcus indents the superior border of the hemisphere about 1 cm behind the midpoint between the frontal and occipital poles. The sulcus slopes downward and forward at an angle of 70 degrees to the vertical, stopping just short of the lateral sulcus, and there are usually two bends along its course. The central sulcus is about 2 cm deep, and its walls therefore constitute much of the sensorimotor cortex.

The **calcarine sulcus** on the medial surface of the hemisphere begins under the posterior end of the corpus callosum and follows an arched course to the occipital pole. In some brains the sulcus continues over the pole for a short distance on the lateral surface. The calcarine sulcus is an important landmark for the visual cortex, most of which lies in the walls of the sulcus.

The **parieto-occipital sulcus** extends from the calcarine sulcus to the superior border of the hemisphere, intersects the border about 4 cm from the occipital pole, and continues for a short distance on the lateral surface.

The longitudinal and transverse cerebral fissures are external to the hemispheres, and are therefore in a different category from the foregoing surface markings. The **longitudinal cerebral fissure** separates the hemispheres, and a dural partition called the falx cerebri extends into the fissure. The corpus callosum, which constitutes the main cerebral commissure, crosses from one hemisphere to the other at the bottom of the longitudinal fissure. The **transverse cerebral fissure** intervenes between the cerebral hemispheres above and the cerebellum, midbrain, and diencephalon below. The posterior part of the fissure is between the cerebral hemispheres and the cerebellum; it contains a dural partition known as the tentorium cerebelli. The anterior part of the transverse fissure intervenes between the corpus callosum and the diencephalon. It is triangular in outline, tapering anteriorly, and contains the tela choroidea, which consists of vascular connective tissue derived from the pia mater that covers the brain. The tela choroidea is continuous with the connective tissue core of the choroid plexuses of the lateral ventricles and the third ventricle, and the plexuses are completed by

choroid epithelium derived from the ependymal lining of the ventricles.

LOBES OF THE CEREBRAL HEMISPHERES

Each cerebral hemisphere has lateral, medial, and inferior surfaces on which the extent of the lobes of the hemisphere will now be defined (see Fig. 13–1 and 13–2).

The **frontal lobe** occupies the entire area in front of the central sulcus and above the lateral sulcus on the lateral surface. The medial surface of the frontal lobe envelops the anterior part of the corpus callosum and is bounded posteriorly by a line drawn between the central sulcus and the corpus callosum. (Such lines are drawn elsewhere; they have no functional significance and can be ignored after serving their initial purpose.) The inferior surface of the frontal lobe rests on the orbital plate of the frontal bone.

The natural boundaries of the **parietal lobe** on the lateral surface are the central and lateral sulci. The other boundaries consist of two lines; the first of these is drawn between the parieto-occipital sulcus and the preoccipital notch, and the second line runs from the middle of the one just established to the lateral sulcus. (The preoccipital notch is an inconspicuous landmark, consisting of a shallow indentation of the brain formed by the petrous portion of the temporal bone.) On the medial surface the parietal lobe is bounded by the frontal lobe, corpus callosum, calcarine sulcus, and parieto-occipital sulcus.

The **temporal lobe** is outlined on the lateral surface by the lateral sulcus and the lines previously noted. The inferior surface of the temporal lobe extends to the temporal pole from a line drawn between the anterior end of the calcarine sulcus and the preoccipital notch. Most of the **occipital lobe** appears on the medial surface of the hemisphere, where it is separated from the temporal lobe as already described and from the parietal lobe by the parieto-occipital sulcus. On the lateral surface, the occipital lobe consists of the small area posterior to the line that joins the parieto-occipital sulcus and preoccipital notch.

The portion of the great cerebral commissure in and near the midline is known as the **trunk of the corpus callosum,** and the fibers of the commissure that spread out within the medullary centers of the hemispheres constitute the **radiations of the corpus callosum.** Names are assigned to certain regions of the trunk of the commissure (see Fig. 13–2), and these regions are used as reference points further on. The enlarged posterior portion of the trunk is called the **splenium.** The anterior portion, or **genu,** thins out to form the **rostrum.** This is continuous with the lamina terminalis, which limits the third ventricle anteriorly.

GYRI AND SULCI

Some surface markings of the hemisphere are landmarks for important functional areas—the central sulcus for the sensorimotor cortex and the calcarine sulcus for the visual cortex are examples. For the most part, however, the sulci and gyri serve only as a rough frame of reference for cortical areas whose functions may or may not be known. The markings can be identified according to lobes for the lateral surface, but this is not practicable for the medial and inferior surfaces.

Lateral Surface

Frontal Lobe

The **precentral sulcus** (often broken into two or more parts) runs parallel to the central sulcus; these sulci outline the **precentral gyrus,** which is a landmark for the primary motor area of the cerebral cortex (Fig. 13–3). The remainder of the lateral surface of the frontal lobe is divided into **superior, middle,** and **inferior frontal gyri** by the **superior** and **inferior frontal sulci.** The anterior and ascending rami of the lateral sulcus divide the inferior frontal gyrus into **opercular, triangular,** and **orbital portions.** In the left hemisphere the opercular and triangular portions consist of cortex of the motor speech area. In the frontal lobe, as in the other lobes of the hemisphere, there are secondary gyri and sulci that contribute to the variable topography of different brains.

Parietal Lobe

The **postcentral sulcus** runs parallel to the central sulcus; these sulci bound the **postcentral gyrus,** which is the landmark for the first general sensory area of cortex. The **intraparietal sulcus** extends posteriorly from the postcentral sulcus and divides that part of the surface not occupied by the postcentral gyrus into **superior** and **inferior parietal lobules.** Those portions of the inferior parietal lobule that surround the upturned ends of the lateral sulcus and superior temporal sulcus are called the **supramarginal gyrus** and the **angular gyrus,** respectively. In the left hemisphere these gyri consist of cortex included in the area for perception and interpretation of spoken and written language.

Temporal Lobe

Superior and **inferior temporal sulci** divide the lateral surface of the temporal lobe into **superior, middle,** and **inferior temporal gyri.** Among variations in the temporal lobe the inferior temporal sulcus may be discontinuous, making it difficult to identify. The superior temporal gyrus has a large surface that forms the floor of the lateral sulcus. On this surface **transverse temporal gyri** (also known as **Heschl's convolutions**) extend to the bottom of the lat-

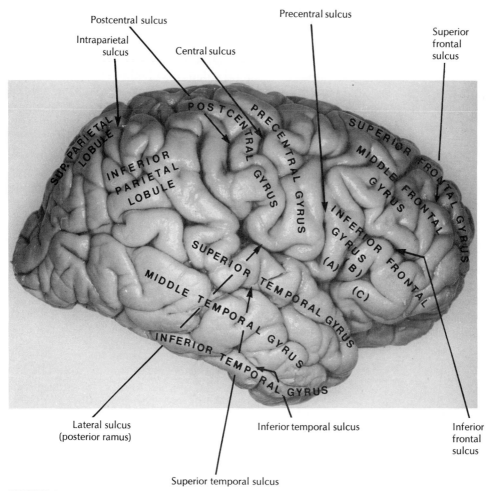

FIGURE 13-3.
Gyri and sulci on the lateral surface of the right cerebral hemisphere. **(A)**, **(B)**, and **(C)** indicate the opercular, triangular, and orbital portions of the inferior frontal gyrus, respectively. ($\times$ ⅝)

eral sulcus and mark the location of the auditory area of cortex.

Occipital Lobe

In the brains of primates other than humans, and in some human brains, the calcarine sulcus continues for a short distance over the occipital pole. There is then a curved **lunate sulcus** around the end of the calcarine sulcus. Except for this inconstant marking, the small area of the occipital lobe on the lateral surface has minor grooves and folds of no special significance.

Insula

It is customary to consider the insula (island of Reil) separately from the four main lobes of the hemisphere. The regions that conceal the insula are known as the **frontal, parietal,** and **temporal opercula;** they must be spread apart or cut away in order

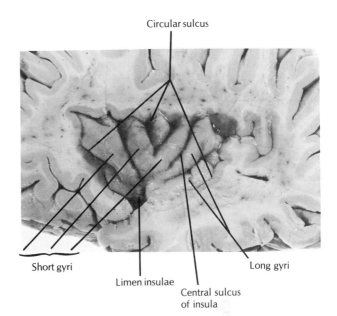

Circular sulcus

Short gyri

Limen insulae

Central sulcus of insula

Long gyri

FIGURE 13-4.
The insula (island of Reil) of the left cerebral hemisphere, exposed by cutting away the frontal, parietal, and temporal opercula. ($\times$ 1⅖)

to expose the insula (Fig. 13–4). The insula is outlined by a circular sulcus, and is divided into two regions by a central sulcus. Several short gyri lie in front of the central sulcus, and one or two long gyri lie behind it. The inferior part of the insula in the region of the stem of the lateral sulcus is known as the **limen insulae.**

Medial and Inferior Surfaces

The **cingulate gyrus** begins beneath the genu of the corpus callosum and continues above the corpus callosum as far back as the splenium (Fig. 13–5). The gyrus is separated from the corpus callosum by the **sulcus of the corpus callosum** (callosal sulcus). The superior surface of the corpus callosum is covered by an attenuated layer of cortical gray matter known as the **indusium griseum.** The **cingulate sulcus** intervenes between the cingulate gyrus and the **medial frontal gyrus,** which is continuous with the superior frontal gyrus on the lateral surface of the hemisphere. The cingulate sulcus gives off a **paracentral sulcus** and then divides into **marginal** and **subparietal sulci** in the parietal lobe. The

region bounded by the paracentral and marginal sulci, which surrounds the indentation made by the central sulcus on the superior border, is called the **paracentral lobule.** The anterior and posterior parts of the paracentral lobule are extensions of the precentral and postcentral gyri, respectively, of the lateral surface of the hemisphere. The area above the subparietal sulcus is called the **precuneus,** and is continuous with the superior parietal lobule on the lateral surface. The parieto-occipital and calcarine sulci bound the **cuneus** of the occipital lobe.

On the medial surface of the frontal lobe, underneath the rostrum of the corpus callosum, is the **subcallosal gyrus,** also known as the parolfactory area. This is not cortex but is part of the septal area, a component of the limbic system.

On the inferior surface of the hemisphere (Figs. 13–5 and 13–6) a convolution extends from the occipital pole almost to the temporal pole. The posterior part of the convolution consists of the **lingual gyrus;** the anterior part forms the **parahippocampal gyrus,** which hooks sharply backward on its medial aspect as the **un-**

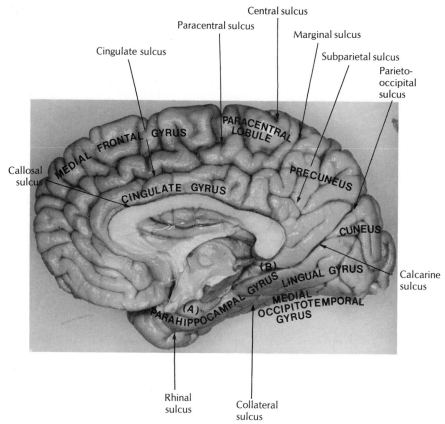

FIGURE 13-5.
Gyri and sulci on the medial and inferior surfaces of the right cerebral hemisphere.
(A) Uncus. **(B)** Isthmus connecting the cingulate and parahippocampal gyri. (× ⅝)

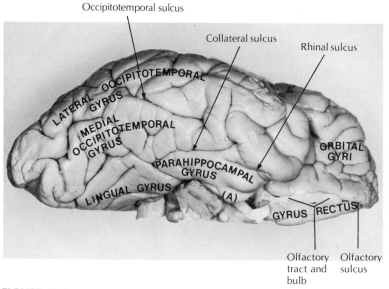

FIGURE 13-6.
Gyri and sulci on the inferior surface of the right cerebral hemisphere.
(A) Uncus. (× ⅝)

cus. The **collateral sulcus** defines the lateral margin of the lingual and parahippocampal gyri, and the short **rhinal sulcus** is situated at the lateral edge of the parahippocampal gyrus anteriorly. The **medial occipitotemporal gyrus,** which is inconstant in morphology and is broken up by irregular sulci, lies along the lateral side of the collateral sulcus. The **occipitotemporal sulcus** intervenes between the medial occipitotemporal gyrus and the **lateral occipitotemporal gyrus.** The latter is continuous with the inferior temporal gyrus on the lateral surface of the hemisphere.

The **olfactory bulb** and **olfactory tract** on the orbital surface of the frontal lobe (Fig. 13–6) conceal most of the **olfactory sulcus.** The **gyrus rectus** is medial to the olfactory sulcus, and the large area lateral to the olfactory sulcus consists of irregular **orbital gyri.** The cingulate and parahippocampal gyri are connected by a narrow **isthmus** (retrosplenial cortex) beneath the splenium of the corpus callosum and form the **limbic lobe** of the cerebral hemisphere, in which the hippocampus is also included. The limbic lobe is part of the limbic system of the brain, which incorporates several additional structures, most prominently the dentate gyrus and amygdaloid body (both in the temporal lobe), hypothalamus (especially the mamillary bodies), septal area, and anterior and some other nuclei of the thalamus.

SUGGESTED READING

Montemurro DG, Bruni E: The Human Brain in Dissection. Philadelphia, WB Saunders, 1981

Nieuwenhuys R, Voogd J, van Huijzen C: The Human Central Nervous System. A Synopsis and Atlas, 2nd ed. Berlin, Springer-Verlag, 1981

FOURTEEN

Histology of the Cerebral Cortex

Each cerebral hemisphere has a mantle of gray matter, the cortex or pallium, with a characteristic structure that consists of nerve cells and nerve fibers arranged in layers. There are three types of cortex according to phylogenetic development and histological characteristics.

In amphibians the pallium constitutes the dorsal surface of each tubular "hemisphere" of the telencephalon and does not have the layered structure of cerebral cortex. The pallium consists of two regions; the lateral one receives afferent fibers from the olfactory bulb, and the medial region receives most of its afferents from the septum or medial wall of the hemisphere. Because of their great phylogenetic ages the layered cortices that have evolved from the lateral and medial pallial regions are called the **paleocortex** and **archicortex**, respectively. Their locations in the human brain are described in subsequent chap-

ters dealing with the olfactory and limbic systems.

In the reptilian brain there are three cortical zones because of the first appearance of an area of **neocortex** between the paleocortex and archicortex. The amount of neocortex increased during mammalian evolution, culminating in neocortex that constitutes most of the cortex in the human brain. In addition to its important sensory and motor functions, the abundant neocortex has an important bearing on the intellectual capabilities of humans.

The number of layers evident histologically in paleocortex and archicortex varies according to region. There may be as many as five layers in paleocortex, although the more superficial ones are indistinct, and the largest number in archicortex is three. In the neocortex, which is the subject of this chapter, six layers are always recognizable at some stage in its development.

The six-layered structure is transient in some areas, and in these certain layers are absent in the adult brain because of merging of adjoining layers. Paleocortex and archicortex are sometimes referred to as **allocortex,** in contrast to **isocortex,** which is a synonym for neocortex.

CORTICAL NEURONS

Values obtained for the number of nerve cells in the human cerebral cortex vary widely because of the technical difficulties in their enumeration. They range from 2.6 $\times$ 10^9 to 14 $\times$ 10^9, and the number of cortical neurons is therefore enormous. The five most conspicuous types are **pyramidal cells, fusiform cells, stellate cells, cells of Martinotti,** and **horizontal cells of Cajal** (Fig. 14–1). The pyramidal and fusiform neurons are principal cells with widely spreading dendrites and long axons. The other types are interneurons.

Pyramidal cells range in height from 10 to 50 μm for most cells. The others are giant pyramidal cells, also known as **Betz cells,** with cell bodies up to 100 μm high. These are present only in the primary motor area of the frontal lobe. Fusiform cells are located in the deepest layer of the cortex. Of the interneurons, stellate cells (also known as granule cells) are by far the most numerous. The identifying feature of the cell of Martinotti is that the axon is directed toward the surface of the cortex. Horizontal cells of Cajal are restricted to the most superficial layer, and their axons run tangentially to the cortical surface.

Cortical neurons connect with other neurons in three ways. **Projection neurons** transmit impulses to subcortical centers such as the corpus striatum, thalamus, brain stem, or spinal cord. **Association neurons** establish connections with cortical nerve cells elsewhere in the same hemisphere. Axons of **commissural neurons** proceed to the cortex of the opposite hemisphere. Most of the commissural fibers constitute the corpus callosum; smaller

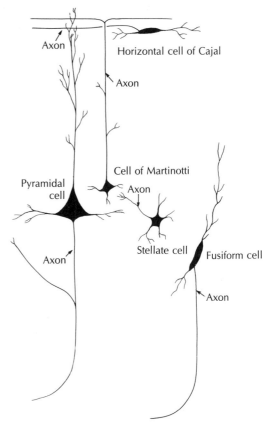

FIGURE 14-1.
Main types of cortical neuron.

numbers connect cortical areas of the temporal lobes through the anterior commissure.

CORTICAL LAYERS

The thickness of the neocortex varies from 4.5 mm in the primary motor area of the frontal lobe to 1.5 mm in the visual area of the occipital lobe. The cortex is generally thicker over the crest of a gyrus than in the depths of a sulcus. The six layers, which differ in the density of cell population and in the size and shape of constituent neurons, can be recognized by about the seventh month of intrauterine life. The layers, starting at the surface and omitting regional differences for the present, are as follows (Fig. 14–2A):

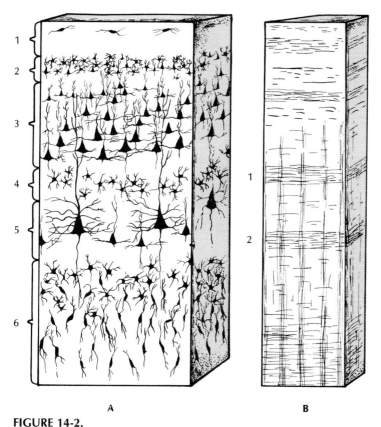

FIGURE 14-2.
Cortical histology.   **(A)** Golgi method: *(1)* molecular layer;
(2) external granular layer; *(3)* external pyramidal layer; *(4)* internal
granular layer; *(5)* internal pyramidal layer; *(6)* multiform layer.
(B) Weigert method: *(1)* outer line of Baillarger; *(2)* inner line of
Baillarger.

1. **Molecular layer.** The superficial layer consists predominantly of delicate neuronal processes, both dendrites and axons, which give it a punctate or "molecular" appearance in sections stained for nerve fibers. Most of the dendritic branches come from pyramidal cells. The axons originate in cortex elsewhere in the same hemisphere, in that of the opposite hemisphere, and in the thalamus. Cells of Martinotti in any deeper layer also contribute axons to layer 1. The infrequent horizontal cells of Cajal and scattered stellate cells intervene between some axons and dendrites. The molecular layer is essentially a synaptic field of the cortex.

2. **External granular layer.** This layer contains a great many small neurons, both small pyramidal cells and stellate cells. The dendrites of many of these cells extend into the molecular layer; most of the axons terminate in deeper layers, and the remainder enter the medullary center. The external granular layer makes an important contribution to the complexity of intracortical circuits.

3. **External pyramidal layer.** The neurons

are typical pyramidal cells that increase in size from the external to the internal borders of the layer. Apical dendrites extend into the synaptic field of layer 1; axons of the pyramidal cells enter the white matter and proceed to their destinations as projection, association, or commissural fibers.

4. **Internal granular layer.** This consists of closely arranged stellate cells, many of which receive stimuli from fibers originating in the thalamus. The short axons of the stellate cells synapse with dendrites passing through the layer from cells in layers 5 and 6, with other stellate cells, and with cells of Martinotti. As in any nervous tissue that includes large numbers of interneurons, the connections and circuits involving the stellate cells of layer 4 are numerous and complex.

5. **Internal pyramidal layer.** This layer contains pyramidal cells intermingled with scattered stellate cells and cells of Martinotti. The giant pyramidal cells (cells of Betz) in the primary motor area of cortex in the frontal lobe are situated in layer 5.

6. **Multiform layer.** Although fusiform cells predominate, there are also neurons of various shapes. Axons of the neurons in this layer are included among the projection, commissural, and association fibers in the white matter of the hemisphere.

Layers 5 and 6 are considered to be phylogenetically older than the more superficial layers, which contain many small neurons that provide for complex intracortical circuitry. Layers 5 and 6 are sometimes referred to as the infragranular layers, and layers 1 through 4 as the supragranular layers. Layers 5 and 6 are also ontogenetically older—they are derived from the first cortical neuroblasts to migrate out from the germinative epithelium of the neural tube of the telenceph-

alon. The neuroblasts destined to form layers 2, 3, and 4 migrate through the infragranular layers to take up their more superficial positions.

The layers described are evident in sections stained by the Nissl and Golgi techniques. When silver staining methods for axons or the Weigert method for myelin sheaths are used, nerve fibers within the neocortex are seen to accumulate in radial bundles and in tangential bands (Fig. 14-2B). The radial bundles are close together; they include axons of pyramidal and fusiform cells leaving the cortex, together with afferent fibers from the thalamus and from cortex elsewhere. The tangential bands consist largely of collateral and terminal branches of afferent fibers. They leave the radial bundles and run parallel to the surface for some distance, branching again and making synaptic contacts with large numbers of cortical neurons. The most prominent tangential bands are the **outer** and **inner lines of Baillarger,** located in layer 4 and in the deep portion of layer 5, respectively. Fibers originating in the thalamic nuclei of sensory pathways contribute heavily to the lines of Baillarger, especially the outer one, and they are therefore prominent in sensory cortical areas. In the visual area in the walls of the calcarine sulcus, the outer line of Baillarger on the cut surface is thick enough to be just visible to the unaided eye. In this location it is known as the **line of Gennari** (Fig. 14–3), having been first described by Francesco Gennari, an eighteenth century Italian medical student. Because of the presence of the line of Gennari, the visual cortex is known alternatively as the striate area.

VARIATIONS IN CYTOARCHITECTURE

The foregoing description of cortical histology establishes the general pattern. Six layers can be identified throughout most of the neocortex, which is said to be hom-

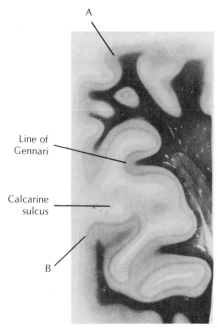

FIGURE 14-3.
Vertical section through the medial surface of the occipital lobe at the site of the calcarine sulcus. The line of Gennari, extending from *A* to *B,* identifies the visual area of cortex—the striate area. (Weigert stain, × 2)

otypical cortex. However, in some areas, known as **heterotypical** cortex, it is not possible to identify six layers. For example, in the visual area and in part of the auditory and general sensory areas, the stellate cells of layer 4 overflow into adjoining layers. Layers 2 through 5 therefore merge into a single layer of small cells, many of which receive thalamocortical fibers. This type of heterotypical cortex is called **granular cortex** or **koniocortex** (from the Greek *konis,* dust). The opposite extreme is found in the primary motor and premotor areas of the frontal lobe. Layers 2 through 5 again appear as a single, well-developed layer that consists mainly of efferent pyramidal cells (**agranular cortex**).

The cerebral cortex has been divided into cytoarchitectural areas based on differences in the thickness of individual layers, neuronal morphology in the layers, and the details of nerve fiber lamination. Such studies require infinite patience and attention to detail. The few investigators who have undertaken meticulous analyses of cortical cytoarchitecture hoped to establish bases for structural and functional correlations. The attempt has been only partially successful because of differing histological criteria and an incomplete understanding of the functional significance of many parts of the cerebral cortex. Different investigators have divided the cortex into 20 to 200 areas, depending on the cytoarchitectural criteria used. Brodmann's map, which was published in 1909 and consists of 52 areas, remains the most widely used map of cortical cytoarchitectural areas.

Results of more recent studies agree that heterotypical areas may be easily identified. For example, the anterior portion of the general sensory cortex in the postcentral gyrus is granular heterotypical cortex (area 3 of Brodmann); the visual cortex around the calcarine sulcus (area 17) and the central part of the auditory cortex in the superior temporal gyrus (area 41) also consist of granular cortex. The primary motor and premotor areas of the frontal lobe (areas 4 and 6) are agranular heterotypical cortex. Area 4 is distinguished by the presence of giant pyramidal (Betz) cells. In view of the obvious difficulties in establishing boundaries between areas with rather subtle histological differences, it is not surprising that the cytoarchitectural areas described for the large expanse of association cortex have met with some skepticism. However, the concept has considerable appeal and has resulted in the widespread use of the numbering system based on cortical histology. Areas of Brodmann's map referred to later in the text are shown in Figures 15–1 and 15–2.

INTRACORTICAL CIRCUITS

Results of studies of cortical neurons using the Golgi technique, combined with elec-

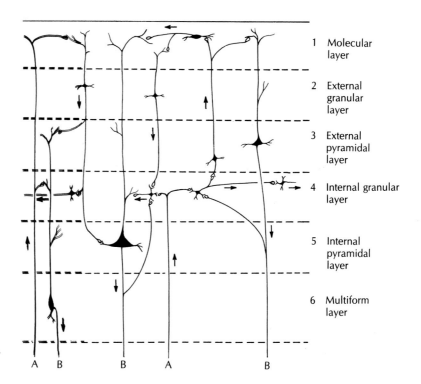

1 Molecular layer

2 External granular layer

3 External pyramidal layer

4 Internal granular layer

5 Internal pyramidal layer

6 Multiform layer

FIGURE 14-4.
A simplified scheme of intracortical circuits.
(A) Afferent cortical fibers.
(B) Efferent cortical fibers.

A   B   B   A   B

trical recording from microelectrodes placed in the cortex, have yielded information concerning intrinsic circuits. These are suggested in Figure 14–4; in reality the circuits are much more complex than the figure indicates.

Afferent fibers entering the cortex originate in cortex elsewhere in the same hemisphere and in the opposite hemisphere, or they come from the thalamus. Thalamocortical fibers originate in either the ventral group of nuclei or in other groups of nuclei. The axons from the ventral nuclei divide into branches that synapse with cortical neurons mainly in the region of the outer line of Baillarger. Fibers from elsewhere in the thalamus and from other regions of cortex terminate in all cortical layers, with an emphasis on layers 1 through 3. Cortical efferent fibers are axons of the larger neurons, notably pyramidal and fusiform cells. They enter the white matter for distribution as projection, association, or commissural fibers.

The histology of the neocortex is basi-cally the same in all mammals, but the population of interneurons having short axons increases the higher the mammal is in the phylogenetic scale. The principal attribute of the neocortex of humans is the presence of an especially large population of these small neurons, notably the small pyramidal cells of layer 2 and the stellate cells of layer 4. An afferent fiber may establish synaptic contact directly with an efferent neuron, but usually differing numbers of interneurons intervene between afferent fibers and efferent neurons. In addition, collateral branches of axons of efferent cells establish synaptic contact with interneurons and contribute to the reverberating circuits in the cortex.

Recordings from microelectrodes inserted into the cortex have shown that it is organized functionally as minute vertical units that include nerve cells of all layers. This has been demonstrated best in sensory areas. All neurons in the unit are activated selectively by the same peripheral stimulus, whether it originates in a particular type of cutaneous receptor at a particular location or in a specific point on the retina. Each unit resembles a barrel 200 to 500 μm in diameter whose height is the thickness of the cortex. It represents the piece of cortex supplied by a single axon from one of the ventral group of thalamic nuclei. Vertically organized functional units corresponding to those detected with microelectrodes can also be defined by autoradiography. To do this, a labeled amino acid is injected into the appropriate thalamic nucleus, or labeled 2-deoxyglucose is given systemically while a sensory system is receiving stimuli. Columnar organization of the neocortex is established in fetal life, but maturation occurs postnatally in response to external sensory stimuli.

The columnar organization of cortical neurons has been most intensively studied in the primary visual cortex of the occipital lobe. There, distinct columns of neurons respond to neural input associated with one or both eyes (ocular dominance columns), and to meaningful features in the observed image, such as edges, horizontal lines, and right angles. Populations of the different kinds of cell column form stripes that extend across the surface of the calcarine cortex. The Nobel Prize for Medicine and Physiology was awarded in 1981 to D. H. Hubel and T. N. Wiesel for their discovery of the distribution and development of columnar functional units in the primate visual cortex.

SUGGESTED READING

Braak H: Architectonics of the Human Telencephalic Cortex. Berlin, Springer-Verlag, 1980

Crosby EC, Humphrey T, Lauer EW: Correlative Anatomy of the Nervous System. New York, Macmillan, 1962

Hubel TH, Wiesel TN: Functional architecture of macaque monkey visual cortex. Proc R Soc Lond [Biol] 198:1–59, 1977

Jones EG, Friedman DP, Endry SHC: Thalamic basis of place- and modality-specific columns in monkey somatosensory cortex: A correlative anatomical and physiological study. J Neurophysiol 48:545–568, 1982

Rockel AJ, Hiorns RW, Powell TPS: The basic uniformity in structure of the neocortex. Brain 103:221–244, 1980

FIFTEEN

Functional Localization in the Cerebral Cortex

Results of clinicopathological studies and animal experiments conducted over more than a century have provided information concerning functional specialization in different regions of the cerebral cortex. For example, three main sensory areas have been found; they are for general sensation, vision, and hearing, to which may be added gustatory and vestibular areas. There are also motor areas from which contraction of the skeletal musculature can be elicited by electrical stimulation. The remainder of the neocortex is usually referred to as association cortex, which may be closely related functionally to the sensory areas or to more complex levels of behavior and the intellect. The trend in mammalian evolution has been toward increasing amounts of association cortex.

DEVELOPMENT OF THE CONCEPT OF CORTICAL LOCALIZATION

The first indications of functional localization came from clinical observations. Broca (1861) examined postmortem the brain of a patient who had suffered from a speech defect (expressive aphasia). A lesion was found in the inferior frontal gyrus, and the region is still known as Broca's motor speech area. On the basis of clinicopathological findings, Hughlings Jackson (1864) concluded that a form of localized epilepsy, now known as jacksonian epilepsy, was caused by focal irritation of the precentral gyrus. This study drew attention to the probability of the existence of a motor area. An area from which motor responses could be elicited on weak electrical stimulation was demonstrated by Fritsch and Hitzig (1870) in the dog, and by Ferrier (1875), Horsley and Beevor (1894), and Sherrington and Grünbaum (1901) in the monkey and chimpanzee.

The identification of sensory areas has a similar history. In 1870 Gudden showed that removal of the eyes from young animals interfered with full development of the occipital lobes, and in 1873 Ferrier found that an animal's ears would rise on stimulation of a particular region of the temporal lobe. The latter region included the auditory area, and stimulation produced a normal response to a sound. Similarly, Dusser de Barenne (1916) showed that application of strychnine to a small area of the monkey's postcentral gyrus resulted in scratching of the skin in one place or another depending on the precise point at which cortical neurons were stimulated. He was able to map the somesthetic cortex of the monkey with this technique. (Strychnine, a convulsant poison, is now known to block postsynaptic receptors that respond to glycine, an inhibitory transmitter.) Head's meticulous study of patients who received brain injuries during World War I aided greatly in understanding the sensory areas of the human cerebral cortex.

Studies on subhuman primates were extended to the human brain by neurosurgeons, notably Cushing, Foerster, and Penfield. In certain neurosurgical procedures it is essential to identify the motor area, a sensory area, or even a particular region within these areas. Identification of sensory areas requires operating on a conscious patient under local anesthesia, a procedure made possible because the brain itself is insensitive to procedures that are painful elsewhere in the body. Electrical stimulation of the brain under these circumstances has provided important information with respect to functional localization in the human cerebral cortex.

PARIETAL, OCCIPITAL, AND TEMPORAL CORTEX

General Sensation

The **first somesthetic area** (general sensory area) occupies the postcentral gyrus on the lateral surface of the hemisphere and the posterior part of the paracentral lobule on the medial surface (Figs. 15–1 and 15–2). It consists of areas 3, 1, and 2 of the Brodmann cytoarchitectural map. Area 3, most of which is in the posterior wall of the central sulcus, is granular heterotypical cortex, whereas areas 1 and 2 are homotypical cortex. Electrical stimulation of the general sensory area elicits modified forms of the tactile sense, such as a tingling sensation. It is possible to elicit motor responses by stimulating the first somesthetic area, as well as eliciting sensory responses from the motor area in the precentral gyrus. The functions of the two areas therefore overlap to some extent, and they should be considered as a **sensorimotor strip** that surrounds the central sulcus. The postcentral gyrus and its extension in the paracentral lobule are designated as the first sensory area because they have the highest density of points that produce localized sensations on electrical stimulation.

The ventral posterior nucleus of the thalamus is the main source of afferent fibers for the first sensory area. This thalamic nucleus is the site of termination of all the fibers of the medial lemniscus and of most of the fibers of the spinothalamic and trigeminothalamic tracts. The thalamocortical fibers traverse the internal capsule and medullary center, conveying data for the various modalities of general sensation. Fibers for cutaneous sensibility end preferentially in the anterior part of the area, and those for deep sensibility in the posterior part.

The contralateral half of the body is represented as inverted. The pharyngeal

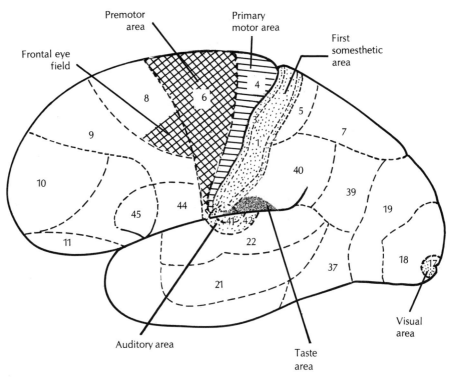

FIGURE 15-1.
Areas of functional localization of the lateral surface of the cerebral hemisphere. Areas of the Brodmann cytoarchitectural map shown here and in Figure 15-2 are those referred to in the text.

region, tongue, and jaws are represented in the most ventral part of the somesthetic area, followed by the face, hand, arm, trunk, and thigh. The area for the remainder of the leg and the perineum is in the extension of the somesthetic cortex on the medial surface of the hemisphere. The size of the cortical area for a particular part of the body is determined by the functional importance of the part and its need for sensitivity. The area for the face, especially the lips, is therefore disproportionately large, and a large area is assigned to the hand, particularly the thumb and index finger.

When this somesthetic cortex is the site of a large destructive lesion, a crude form of awareness persists for the nociceptive sensations of pain, heat, and cold on the affected opposite side of the body. There is poor localization of the stimulus, for which qualitative and quantitative interpretations are diminished or absent. The somesthetic cortex must be intact for any appreciation of the more discriminative sensations of fine touch and position and movement of the parts of the body.

In addition to the main or first somesthetic area, the existence of a **second somesthetic area** has been demonstrated in primates, including humans. This small area is situated in the dorsal wall of the lateral sulcus in line with the postcentral gyrus, and may extend onto the insula. The parts of the body are represented bilaterally, although contralateral representation predominates. The second sensory area receives input from the intralaminar nuclei and from the posterior group of nuclei of the thalamus. The afferent fibers to these

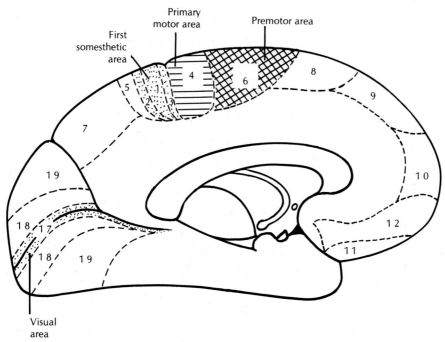

FIGURE 15-2.
Areas of functional localization on the medial surface of the cerebral hemisphere.

nuclei come, respectively, from the reticular formation, and from the spinothalamic and trigeminothalamic tracts. Consequently, the area is involved mainly in the less discriminative aspects of sensation. An intact second somesthetic area probably explains such residual sensibility as exists following a destructive lesion that includes the first sensory area. No clinical disorder has been ascribed to selective destruction of the second somesthetic area.

The **somesthetic association cortex** is mainly in the superior parietal lobule on the lateral surface of the hemisphere and in the precuneus on the medial surface. Much of it coincides with areas 5 and 7 of the Brodmann cytoarchitectural map. This association cortex receives fibers from the first somesthetic area. Data pertaining to the general senses are integrated, permitting, for example, a comprehensive assessment of the characteristics of an object held in the hand and its identification without visual aid. When there is a lesion

in the somesthetic association cortex, leaving the somesthetic area itself intact, awareness of the general senses persists but the significance of the information received on the basis of previous experience is elusive. A defect in understanding the significance of sensory information is called **agnosia;** there are several types, depending on the sense that is most affected. A lesion that destroys a large portion of the somesthetic association cortex causes tactile agnosia and astereognosis, which are closely related. They combine when a person is unable to identify a common object, such as a pair of scissors, held in the hand while the eyes are closed. It is impossible to correlate the surface texture, shape, size, and weight of the object or to compare the sensations with previous experience. Astereognosis includes a loss of awareness of the spatial relations of parts of the contralateral side of the body. The most extreme form of the condition is "cortical neglect," in which the patient ignores and even denies the existence of one side of the body and of the corresponding visual field. The condition is most often due to large lesions in the superior part of the right parietal lobe.

Vision

The **visual area** surrounds the calcarine sulcus on the medial surface of the occipital lobe, extending over the occipital pole in some brains (see Fig. 15–2). The area is more extensive than the illustration suggests because most of it is in the walls of the deep calcarine sulcus, on which there are secondary folds. The visual cortex is thin granular heterotypical cortex, corresponding to area 17 of the Brodmann map. The visual area is also called the **striate area** because the cortex here contains the line of Gennari, which is just visible to the unaided eye.

The chief source of afferent fibers to area 17 is the lateral geniculate nucleus of the thalamus by way of the geniculocalcarine tract. Part of this tract passes forward in the medullary center of the temporal lobe and then swings back (Meyer's loop) to the striate area. A lesion that causes a defect in the visual field may therefore be located in the temporal lobe, far removed from the visual area of cortex.

The visual cortex, through a synaptic relay in the lateral geniculate nucleus, receives data from the temporal half of the ipsilateral retina and the nasal half of the contralateral retina. The dividing line runs vertically through the fovea centralis, a specialized region of the macula lutea of the retina, at the posterior pole of the eye. The left half of the field of vision is therefore represented in the visual area of the right hemisphere, and vice versa. There are spatial patterns within the striate area. The lower retinal quadrants (upper field of vision) project on the lower wall of the calcarine sulcus, and the upper retinal quadrants (lower field of vision) project on the upper wall of the sulcus. Another pattern is related to central and peripheral vision. The macula lutea is represented at the occipital pole, in the posterior part of area 17; the remaining retina, proceeding from the macula to the ora serrata (anterior limit of the functional retina), is represented progressively more anteriorly. The macula is responsible for central vision of maximal discrimination. Consequently, the part of area 17 that receives data for central vision accounts for a disproportionately large amount (one third) of the visual cortex.

A lesion that involves the visual cortex of a hemisphere causes an area of blindness in the opposite visual field. The size and location of the defect are determined by the extent and location of the lesion. Examination of the visual fields may show that central vision is intact following a unilateral lesion in the occipital lobe (*e.g.*, an infarction caused by a thrombus in the posterior cerebral artery). This clinical observation, known as "macular sparing," cannot be explained on the basis of bilateral cortical representation of the macula. It has been suggested that anastomoses between branches of the middle and posterior cerebral arteries may partially maintain the large part of area 17 concerned with central vision following occlusion of the posterior cerebral artery. It has also been suggested that macular sparing is an artifact of testing, caused by slight movements of the patient's eyes during examination of the visual fields.

The **visual association cortex** corresponds to areas 18 and 19 of Brodmann, which surround the visual area on the medial and lateral surfaces of the hemisphere (see Figs. 15–1 and 15–2). These areas receive fibers from area 17 and have reciprocal connections with other cortical areas and with the pulvinar of the thalamus. The role of this association cortex includes, among other complex aspects of vision, the relating of present to past visual experience, with recognition of what is seen and appreciation of its significance. A substantial lesion involving areas 18 and 19 therefore results in visual agnosia. Bilateral lesions involving the superior parts of area 19 cause visual disorientation, loss of coordination of eye movements, and inability to carry out visually guided movements of the hands.

The inferolateral surface of the temporal lobe (inferior temporal and lateral occipitotemporal gyri) is also visual association cortex. Electrical stimulation of this region evokes vivid hallucinations of scenes from the past, indicating a role of this cortex in the storage or recall of visual memories. Bilateral destruction of the inferior surfaces of the occipital and temporal lobes can cause **prosopagnosia,** a rare condition in which there is impaired recognition of previously known familiar faces.

Corticotectal fibers connect the visual cortex and visual association cortex with the superior colliculus of the midbrain, which, through indirect connections, controls the oculomotor, trochlear, and abducens nuclei. This is part of a pathway for fixation of gaze and for tracking of a moving object in the field of vision. It also functions in the accommodation–convergence reaction on directing attention to a near object. These motor aspects of the occipital cortex are related to those of the frontal eye field, to be described later in the chapter.

Hearing

Most of the **auditory area** (acoustic area) is concealed because it is in the ventral wall of the lateral sulcus (Figs. 15–1 and 15–3). The surface of the superior temporal gyrus forming the floor of the sulcus is marked by transverse temporal gyri. The two most anterior of these, called **Heschl's convolutions,** are landmarks for the auditory area, which corresponds to areas 41 and 42 of Brodmann. Area 41 is granular heterotypical cortex, whereas area 42 is homotypical.

The medial geniculate nucleus of the thalamus is the principal source of fibers ending in the auditory cortex, with these fibers constituting the auditory radiation in the medullary center. There is a spatial representation in the auditory area with respect to the pitch of sounds. Impulses for low frequencies impinge on the anterolateral part of the area and impulses for high frequencies impinge on the posteromedial part. Although the medial geniculate nucleus receives information that originates mainly in the spiral organ (organ of Corti) of the opposite side, some ipsilateral conduction ensures a substantial input from the ear of the same side. A unilateral lesion involving the auditory area causes diminution in the acuity of hearing in both ears, and the loss is greater in the opposite ear. However, the impairment is slight because of the bilateral projection to the cortex and the deficit is difficult to detect by clinical tests.

The **auditory association cortex** for more elaborate perception of acoustic information occupies the floor of the lateral sulcus behind the auditory area (the region labeled "planum temporale" in Fig. 15–3) and the posterior part of Brodmann's area 22 on the lateral surface of the superior temporal gyrus. The region of cortex thus defined is also known as **Wernicke's area** and is of major importance in language functions.

Taste

The **taste area** (gustatory area) is located in the inferior part of the parietal lobe, posterior to the general sensory area for the mouth (Fig. 15–1). Nerve impulses from taste buds reach the gustatory nucleus in the brain stem (*i.e.,* the rostral portion of the nucleus of the tractus solitarius). Fibers from the gustatory nucleus go to the parabrachial nucleus in the midbrain reticular formation, from which fibers proceed to the ventral medial basal

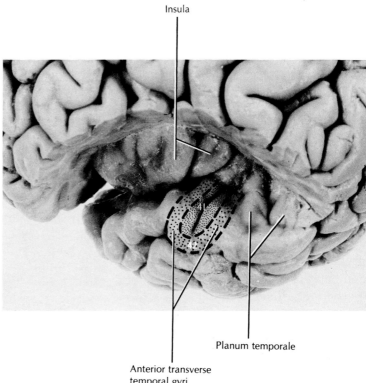

Insula

Planum temporale

Anterior transverse
temporal gyri
(Heschl's convolutions)

FIGURE 15-3.
The auditory area of cortex after being exposed by removing part of the hemisphere dorsal to the lateral sulcus. (× ⅘)

nucleus of the thalamus. The pathway is completed by thalamocortical fibers.

Vestibular Representation

The location of a vestibular cortical area is still uncertain. In monkeys electrical stimulation of the vestibular nerve has been shown to evoke potentials in a cortical area that corresponds to the inferior parietal lobule of the human brain. Electrical stimulation of this same region in conscious patients has occasionally produced dizziness and vertigo. However, examination of regional cortical blood flow in the human brain does not support the idea of a primary vestibular area in the parietal lobe.

When the kinetic labyrinth is stimulated by warm water in the external ear (see Chap. 22), increased blood flow is detected only in the superior temporal gyrus, posterior to the auditory area. Some earlier clinical observations had indicated a vestibular function for the anterior end of the superior temporal gyrus. The cortical projection from the vestibular labyrinth, wherever directed, presumably contributes information for motor regulation and awareness of spatial orientation. The ascending fibers from the vestibular nuclei are almost entirely crossed and travel near the medial lemniscus. The thalamic relay is thought to be in or near the part of the ventral posterior nucleus that receives fibers for general sensation for the head.

Association Cortex

Areas of association cortex adjacent to the main sensory areas and closely related functionally to them have already been described. There is additional association cortex in the parietal lobe and in the posterior part of the temporal lobe. Data reaching the sensory areas and analyzed in the adjacent association cortex are presumably correlated in this intervening region to yield a comprehensive assessment of the immediate environment. The association cortex of the three "sensory" lobes has abundant connections with cortex of the frontal lobe through fasciculi in the medullary center. Complex and flexible behavioral patterns are formulated on the basis of experience, emotional tones are added, and overt expression may follow through the motor system.

The anterior part of the temporal lobe, like the area for visual memory on its inferolateral surface, appears to have special properties related to thought and memory. Electrical stimulation of this region in the conscious subject may elicit recall of objects seen, music heard, or other experiences in the recent or distant past. A patient with a temporal lobe tumor may have auditory or visual hallucinations that sometimes reproduce earlier events.

The total expanse of association cortex in the parietal, occipital, and temporal lobes is responsible (along with association cortex in the frontal lobe) for many of the unique qualities of the human brain. Engrams or memory traces are laid down over the years, possibly as macromolecular changes in neurons throughout the cerebral cortex. These form the basis of learning at an intellectual level. The complex neuronal circuitry of the cortex permits the coalescence of memory traces in the form of ideas and conceptual, abstract thinking. Recently acquired information is not consolidated into long-term memory when the forebrain is extensively damaged, as in Alzheimer's disease, or if there are bilateral lesions involving the limbic system. However, there is probably no disease that causes loss of established memories, indicating that the engram is contained in many parts of the brain. (Rare instances of permanent amnesia that follow head injury are probably due to failure of the recalling mechanisms, because most amnesic patients recover their memories eventually.)

FRONTAL CORTEX

The neocortex of the frontal lobe has a special role in motor activities, in the attributes of judgment and foresight, and in determining mood or "feeling tone."

Motor Areas

The **primary motor area** has been identified on the basis of elicitation of motor responses at a low threshold of electrical stimulation. The area is located in the precentral gyrus, including the anterior wall of the central sulcus, and in the anterior part of the paracentral lobule on the medial surface of the hemisphere (see Figs. 15–1 and 15–2). This cortex (area 4 of Brodmann) is thick agranular heterotypical cortex, in which giant pyramidal cells of Betz are present in layer 5.

The main sources of input to area 4 are the premotor cortex (area 6), somesthetic cortex, and the posterior division of the ventral lateral thalamic nucleus, which in turn receives input from the cerebellum. Although area 4 contributes fibers to several motor pathways, the efferents that give it a special significance are those that are included in the pyramidal motor system (corticospinal and corticobulbar tracts). About 30% of these fibers arise in area 4; another 30% come from area 6. The remainder arise in the parietal lobe, with the largest proportion having their cell bodies in the first somesthetic area. These include fibers that are not motor in function but that terminate in relay nuclei of general sensory pathways and thereby modulate transmission of sensory data to the thalamus and cortex.

There is agreement between the number of Betz cells in the region of area 4 that contributes fibers to the corticospinal tract and the number of large, thickly myelinated axons (about 10 μm in diameter) in the tract. The number is about 30,000, which accounts for some 3% of the fibers in the medullary pyramid. These axons of Betz cells conduct particularly rapidly.

Electrical stimulation of the primary motor area elicits contraction of muscles that are mainly on the opposite side of the body. Although cortical control of the skeletal musculature is predominantly contralateral, there is some ipsilateral control of most of the muscles of the head and of the axial muscles of the body. The body is represented in the motor area as inverted, with the pattern being similar to that of the somesthetic cortex. The sequence from below upward is pharynx, larynx, tongue, and face; the region for muscles of the head comprises about one third of the whole of area 4. Continuing dorsally, there is a small region for muscles of the neck, followed by a large area for muscles of the hand; this is consistent with the importance of manual dexterity in humans. Next in order are areas for the arm, shoulder, trunk, and thigh, continuing with an area on the medial surface of the hemisphere for the remainder of the leg and for the perineum.

The primary motor area has a low threshold of excitability as compared with other areas from which contraction of voluntary muscles can be elicited by electrical stimulation. Contractions of contralateral muscles are usually elicited, as has been noted, and the muscles responding depend on the particular part of area 4 that is stimulated. The response usually involves muscles that make up a functional group, although occasionally there is contraction of a single muscle. In experimental animals small clusters of neurons that control individual muscles have been recognized in the primary motor cortex.

Destructive lesions of area 4 result in voluntary paresis of the affected part of the body. The muscles involved are flaccid; spastic voluntary paralysis characteristically follows lesions that spread beyond area 4 or that interrupt projection fibers in the medullary center or internal capsule. There is considerable recovery with time, with the residual deficit being most evident as impairment of movement in the distal part of the limbs. Destruction of part of the motor area without involvement of adjacent cortex or the underlying white matter is rarely encountered clinically. Deficits resulting from damage to area 4 are inferred from results of experiments on subhuman primates and from isolated instances in which a region of area 4 was removed in humans as a therapeutic procedure, as in the treatment of epilepsy.

A **second** and a **supplementary motor area** have been identified by cortical stimulation in primates, including humans. The second motor area is ventral to the sensorimotor strip in the dorsal wall of the lateral sulcus, overlapping the second somesthetic area. The supplementary motor area is in the part of area 6 that lies on the medial surface of the hemisphere, and it is therefore a part of the premotor area that has special properties. In both areas, contraction of muscles on both sides of the body can be elicited by electrical stimulation. Results of experiments in monkeys indicate that loss of function of the supplementary motor area may cause the spasticity of muscles paralyzed as the result of an "upper motor neuron" lesion. In humans, there is increased blood flow in the supplementary motor area during the mental processes that precede the execution of a movement. Bilateral lesions involving this area cause profound paralysis, as well as mutism.

Premotor Area

The premotor area, which coincides with Brodmann's area 6, is situated anterior to the primary motor area on the lateral and medial surfaces of the hemisphere (see Figs. 15–1 and 15–2). The cytoarchitecture of area 6 is similar to that of area 4, except that Betz cells are lacking. In addition to connections with other cortical areas, the premotor cortex receives fibers from the anterior division of the ventral lateral nucleus of the thalamus, which in turn receives input from the corpus striatum.

The premotor area contributes to motor function by its direct contribution to the pyramidal and other descending motor pathways, and by its influence on the primary motor cortex. With respect to the latter, area 6 (including the supplementary motor area) elaborates programs for motor routines necessary for skilled voluntary action, both when a new program is established and when a previously learned program is altered. In general, the primary motor area is the cortex through which commands are channeled for the *execution* of movements. In contrast, the premotor area programs skilled motor activity and thus *directs* the primary motor area in its execution.

The term **apraxia** refers to the result of a cerebral lesion characterized by impairment in the performance of learned movements in the absence of paralysis. One form of apraxia follows a lesion involving the premotor area. The disability includes functional impairment of muscles that work on the shoulder and hip joints. The ability to carry out tasks at arm's length is then severely impaired. Another form of apraxia is caused by a lesion involving the somesthetic association cortex, proprioception being a necessary background for motor proficiency. When the disability affects writing it is called **agraphia.**

The **frontal eye field** is in the lower part of area 8 on the lateral surface of the hemisphere, extending slightly beyond that area. It controls voluntary conjugate movements of the eyes, and electrical stimulation of the frontal eye field causes deviation of the eyes to the opposite side. Destruction of the frontal eye field causes conjugate deviation of the eyes toward the side of the lesion. The patient cannot voluntarily move the eyes in the opposite direction, but this movement occurs involuntarily when an object is observed moving across the field of vision. Convergence of the eyes can also be accomplished without the frontal eye fields. The involuntary tracking movement and convergence are directed by the visual and visual association cortex of the occipital lobe.

Prefrontal Cortex

The large expanse of cortex in the frontal lobe from which motor responses are not elicited on stimulation falls under the heading of association cortex. This region envelops the frontal pole and is called the prefrontal cortex. Corresponding to areas 9, 10, 11, and 12 in Brodmann's cytoarchitectural map, it is well developed only in primates, especially so in humans. The prefrontal cortex has extensive connections through fasciculi in the medullary center with cortex of the parietal, temporal, and occipital lobes, thus gaining access to contemporary sensory experience and to the repository of data derived from past experience. There are also reciprocal connections with the mediodorsal thalamic nucleus, forming a system that determines affective reactions to present situations on the basis of past experience. The prefrontal cortices also monitor behavior and exercise control based on such higher mental faculties as judgment and foresight.

LANGUAGE AREAS

The use of language is a peculiarly human accomplishment, requiring special neural mechanisms in association areas of the cerebral cortex. Areas of cortex that have particular roles with respect to language have been identified by the study of patients in whom these areas were damaged by occlusion of blood vessels. Until recently the most reliable information was based on the results of long-term studies of patients with deficits in the use of language, whose brains were subjected to careful postmortem examination. In recent years it has been possible to localize infarcted regions of the brain accurately by scanning to detect the distribution of an intravenously injected tracer and by computed tomography.

Two cortical areas have specialized language functions (Fig. 15–4). The **sensory language area** consists of the auditory association cortex (Wernicke's area) and of adjacent parts of the parietal lobe, notably the supramarginal and angular gyri. The **motor speech area** (Broca's area) occupies the opercular and triangular portions of the inferior frontal gyrus, corresponding to areas 44 and 45 of Brodmann. The integrity of the supplementary motor area on the medial surface of the hemisphere is also necessary for normal speech. The language areas are situated in the left hemisphere, with few exceptions, and this is therefore the dominant hemisphere as a rule with respect to language. The sensory and motor language areas are in communication with one another through the superior longitudinal (arcuate) fasciculus in the medullary center.

A lesion involving the language areas or their connections results in aphasia; there are several types, depending on the location of the lesion. **Receptive aphasia** (Wernicke's aphasia), in which auditory and visual comprehension of language, naming of objects, and repetition of a sentence spoken by the examiner are all defective, is caused by a lesion in the sensory language area, notably in Wernicke's area. A lesion involving Wernicke's area and the superior longitudinal or arcuate fasciculus

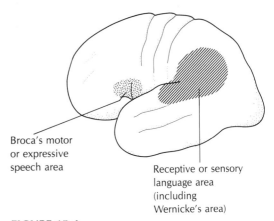

Broca's motor or expressive speech area

Receptive or sensory language area (including Wernicke's area)

FIGURE 15-4.
The language areas.

results in **jargon aphasia,** with fluent but unintelligible jargon. Interruption of the arcuate fasciculus connecting Wernicke's and Broca's areas causes **conduction aphasia,** in which there is poor repetition of a sentence spoken by the examiner, but relatively good comprehension and spontaneous speech. Infarcts that isolate the sensory language area from surrounding parietal and temporal cortex may cause **anomic aphasia** (isolation syndrome), characterized by fluent but circumlocutory speech caused by word-finding difficulties. **Alexia** refers to the loss of the ability to read, and occurs with or without other aspects of aphasia. "Pure alexia" may result from a lesion involving the white matter of the occipital lobe of the dominant hemisphere and the splenium of the corpus callosum. Such a lesion severs connections between both visual cortices and the unilaterally located language areas. **Dyslexia** is incomplete alexia, and is characterized by an inability to read more than a few lines with understanding. **Expressive aphasia** (Broca's aphasia), caused by a lesion in Broca's area of the frontal lobe, is characterized by hesitant and distorted speech with relatively good comprehension. The term **global aphasia** refers to a virtually complete loss of the ability to communicate, which occurs when there is destruction of the cortex on both sides of the lateral sulcus.

There is usually some recovery of function, even in severe cases of aphasia. This is attributed to assumption of linguistic functions by the intact contralateral cerebral hemisphere.

HEMISPHERAL DOMINANCE

Memory traces established in one hemisphere (e.g., in the cortex of the left hemisphere as a result of some particular activity involving the right hand) are in general transferred to the cortex of the other hemisphere through the corpus callosum. There are therefore bilateral cortical memory patterns for previous experience. This does not pertain to language, for which there is no adequate explanation. In right-handed persons, and in most of those who are left-handed, language is a function of the left hemisphere. The "talking" hemisphere is said to be dominant relative to the "nontalking" hemisphere. A left-sided cerebral lesion is therefore more serious than one in the right hemisphere, because aphasia may be added to other neurological deficits. The reverse is true for those few whose right hemisphere is dominant.

Although factors that determine hemispheral dominance for speech are not well known, heredity is almost certainly involved to some extent. The planum temporale posterior to the auditory area on the dorsal surface of the superior temporal gyrus (see Fig. 15–3) is larger in the left than the right hemisphere in 65% of human brains, and larger on the right side in only 11% of human brains. This indicates that the dominance with respect to language may be reflected in cerebral asymmetry because the planum temporale constitutes a large part of Wernicke's area.

About 75% of the population is right-handed, preferring the right hand for skilled tasks. In these the right hand is controlled by the left cerebral hemisphere, which is also the dominant hemisphere for language. However, handedness is not always correlated with linguistic dominance, because 70% of those who are left-handed have their language areas in the left hemisphere, rather than in the one controlling the left hand.

For some activities the right hemisphere is the dominant one in most people. The most notable faculty residing in the right hemisphere is three-dimensional, or spatial, perception. The evidence is derived from the results of a study of patients in whom the corpus callosum had been sectioned as a therapeutic measure in severe epilepsy. Following commissurotomy these patients were able to copy drawings and to arrange blocks in a desired position more efficiently with the left hand than with the right hand. The right hemisphere is therefore better equipped to direct such acts. Another ability for which the right hemisphere dominates is singing and the playing of musical instruments. Musical skills are commonly lost following vascular occlusions in the right hemisphere, and it is not unusual for a patient severely aphasic from a lesion in the left hemisphere to retain the ability to sing.

SUGGESTED READING

Asanume H: Recent developments in the study of the columnar arrangement of neurons within the motor cortex. Physiol Rev 55:143–156, 1975

Beaton A: Left Side, Right Side. A Review of Laterality Research. London, Batsford Academic & Educational, 1985

Damasio AR: Prosopagnosia. Trends Neurosci 8:132–135, 1985

Damasio AR, Damasio H: The anatomic basis of pure dyslexia. Neurology 33:1573–1583, 1983

Damasio H, Damasio AR: The anatomical basis of conduction aphasia. Brain 103:337–350, 1980

Damasio AR, Geschwind N: The neural basis of language. Annu Rev Neurosci 7:127–147, 1984

Friberg L, Olsen IS, Roland PE, Paulson OB, Lassen NA: Focal increase of blood flow in the cerebral cortex of man during vestibular stimulation. Brain 108:609–623, 1985

Geschwind N: Specializations of the human brain. Sci Am 241:180–199, 1979

Kertesz A: Aphasia and Associated Disorders. Taxonomy, Localization and Recovery. New York, Grune & Stratton, 1979

Penfield W, Rasmussen T: The Cerebral Cortex of Man: A Clinical Study of Localization of Function. New York, Macmillan, 1950

Powell TPS: The somatic sensory cortex. Br Med Bull 33:129–135, 1977

Roland PE, Larsen B, Lassen NA, Skinhøj E: Supplementary motor area and other cortical areas in organization of voluntary movements in man. J Neurophysiol 43:118–136, 1980

Roland PE, Skinhøj E, Lassen NA, Larsen B: Different cortical areas in man in organization of voluntary movements in extrapersonal space. J Neurophysiol 43:137–150, 1980

Schwarz DWF, Frederickson JM: Rhesus monkey vestibular cortex: A bimodal primary projection field. Science 172:280–281, 1971

Springer SP, Deutsch G: Left Brain, Right Brain, rev ed. San Francisco, WH Freeman & Co, 1985

Wada JA, Clarke R, Hamm A: Cerebral hemisphere asymmetry in humans. Arch Neurol 32:239–246, 1975

SIXTEEN

Medullary Center, Internal Capsule, and Lateral Ventricles

Each cerebral hemisphere includes a large volume of white matter that constitutes the medullary center and accommodates the vast number of fibers running to and from all parts of the cortex. The medullary center is bounded by the cortex, lateral ventricle, and corpus striatum. Nerve fibers that establish connections between the cortex and subcortical gray matter continue from the medullary center into the internal capsule. The lateral ventricles, one in each hemisphere, are the largest of the four ventricles of the brain, and are important in the dynamics of the cerebrospinal fluid system.

MEDULLARY CENTER

The nerve fibers of the medullary center are of three types, depending on the nature of their connections (Fig. 16–1). **Association fibers** are confined to a hemi-sphere and connect one cortical area with another. Many of these fibers accumulate in longitudinally running bundles that can be displayed by dissection, and that have been assigned names. **Commissural fibers** connect the cortices of the two hemispheres; most of the neocortical commissural fibers comprise the corpus callosum, with the remainder included in the anterior commissure. **Projection fibers** establish connections between the cortex and such subcortical structures as the corpus striatum, thalamus, nuclei of the brain stem, and spinal cord. They are afferent (corticipetal) or efferent (corticofugal) with respect to the cortex; the former originate in the thalamus.

Association Fasciculi

Association fibers are the most numerous of the three types of fiber noted. Operative

244

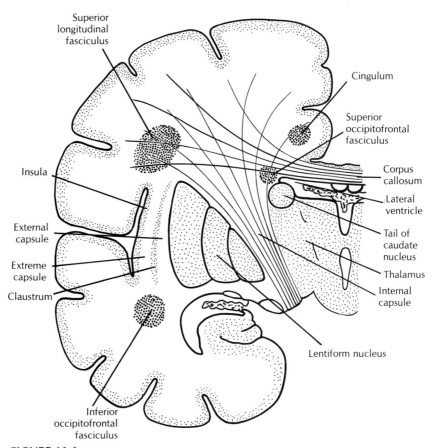

FIGURE 16-1.
Coronal section through a cerebral hemisphere, indicating the positions of the association, commissural, and projection fibers.

procedures, vascular accidents, or other lesions involving the fasciculi may lead to dysfunction by disconnecting functionally related regions of the cerebral cortex.

The **cingulum,** which is most easily displayed by dissection in the cingulate gyrus (Figs. 16–2 and 16–3), is an association fasciculus of the limbic lobe. The fibers of this longitudinal bundle run in both directions and interconnect the cingulate gyrus, parahippocampal gyrus of the temporal lobe, and septal area below the genu of the corpus callosum.

The **superior longitudinal fasciculus** (Figs. 16–2 and 16–3), also known as the **arcuate fasciculus,** runs in an anteroposterior direction above the insula, and many

of the fibers turn downward into the temporal lobe. This fasciculus, in common with other association bundles, consists of fibers of various lengths that enter or leave the fasciculus at any point along its course. The superior longitudinal fasciculus provides an important communication between cortex of the parietal, temporal, and occipital lobes and cortex of the frontal lobe, including the sensory and motor language areas. An **inferior longitudinal fasciculus** has been described as running superficially beneath the lateral and ventral surfaces of the occipital and temporal lobes. This thin sheet of association fibers is difficult to demonstrate by dissection or to distinguish from other fibers at a deeper

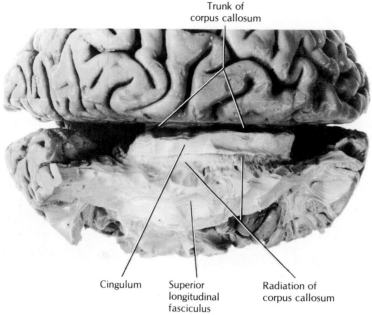

Trunk of
corpus callosum

Cingulum   Superior   Radiation of
               longitudinal   corpus callosum
               fasciculus

FIGURE 16-2.
Dissection of the right cerebral hemisphere, dorsal view. (× ⅔)

level, in particular from projection fibers of the geniculocalcarine tract.

The **inferior occipitofrontal fasciculus** and **uncinate fasciculus** are components of a single association system (Figs. 16–4 and 16–5). The fibers are compressed into a well-defined bundle between the stem of the lateral sulcus below and the insula and lentiform nucleus above. The longer part of the fiber system, extending the length of the hemisphere, is the inferior occipitofrontal fasciculus. The uncinate fasciculus is the part that hooks around the stem of the lateral sulcus to connect the frontal lobe, especially cortex on its orbital surface, with cortex in the region of the temporal pole.

The **superior occipitofrontal fasciculus,** also called the **subcallosal bundle,** is located deep in the hemisphere and therefore cannot be dissected from a lateral approach. The fasciculus is compact in the midregion of the hemisphere, where it is bounded by the corpus callosum, internal capsule, tail of the caudate nucleus, and

lateral ventricle (see Fig. 16–1). The fibers spread out to cortex of the frontal lobe and to cortex in the posterior part of the hemisphere.

Large numbers of **arcuate fibers** connect adjacent gyri. These short subcortical association fibers are oriented at right angles to the gyri and bend sharply under the intervening sulci. Spread of activity along a gyrus is provided by other subcortical association fibers and by the wealth of interneurons within the cortex.

Commissures

Corpus Callosum

Most of the neocortical commissural fibers constitute the **corpus callosum;** the remainder are included in the anterior commissure, along with fibers of other than neocortical origin. The number of fibers in the corpus callosum is of the order of 300 million; however, the commissure normally varies considerably in size. The pos-

Cingulum

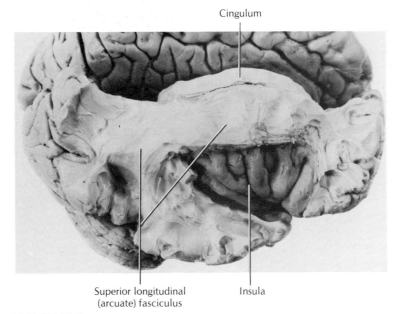

Superior longitudinal
(arcuate) fasciculus

Insula

FIGURE 16-3.
Dissection of the right cerebral hemisphere, dorsolateral view. ($\times$ $\frac{2}{3}$)

Corona radiata

External capsule

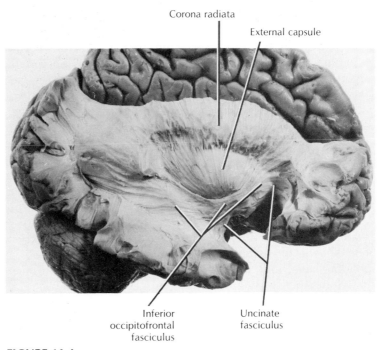

Inferior
occipitofrontal
fasciculus

Uncinate
fasciculus

FIGURE 16-4.
Medullary center of the right cerebral hemisphere after removal of the superior longitudinal fasciculus, insula, and underlying structures down to the external capsule. ($\times$ $\frac{2}{3}$)

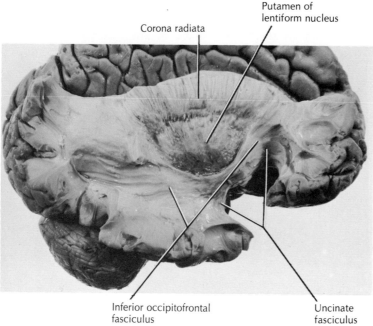

Corona radiata

Putamen of
lentiform nucleus

Inferior occipitofrontal
fasciculus

Uncinate
fasciculus

FIGURE 16-5.

Dissection illustrated in Figure 16-4 continued by removal of the
external capsule to expose the putamen of the lentiform nucleus. (× ⅔)

terior part of the corpus callosum (the splenium) is reported to be generally larger in human females than in human males when viewed in sagittal section.

The **trunk** of the corpus callosum is the compact portion of the commissure in and near the midline (see Fig. 16–2). On entering the medullary center, the fibers constitute the **radiation** of the corpus callosum, which intersects association bundles and projection fibers. In experimental animals, commissural fibers from an area of cortex in one hemisphere have been shown to terminate in the corresponding area, and in cortex closely related functionally with that area, in the other hemisphere.

The trunk of the corpus callosum is considerably shorter than the hemispheres; this accounts for the enlargement of each end, which are the **splenium** posteriorly and the **genu** anteriorly (see Fig. 13–2). The splenium and the radiations that con-

nect the occipital lobes comprise the **forceps occipitalis** (forceps major) (Fig. 16–6), and the genu and the radiations connecting the frontal lobes form the **forceps frontalis** (forceps minor). The genu tapers into the **rostrum** of the corpus callosum, which is continuous with the lamina terminalis forming the anterior wall of the third ventricle. Some fibers of the radiation form a thin sheet, called the **tapetum,** over the temporal horn of the lateral ventricle (Fig. 16–6). These fibers aid in communication between the cortex of the temporal lobes, especially cortex on the ventral surface of these lobes.

Certain relations of the corpus callosum are partly the result of invasion of phylogenetically older parts of the brain by this neocortical commissure. The dorsal surface of the trunk of the corpus callosum is clothed by the **indusium griseum,** a thin layer of gray matter in which two delicate strands of fibers on each side called the

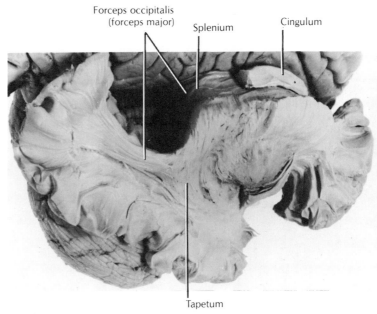

FIGURE 16-6.
Dissection of portions of the corpus callosum in the right hemisphere, dorsolateral view. (× ⅔)

medial and **lateral longitudinal striae** (of Lancisi) are embedded. The indusium griseum is a remnant of archicortex. The longitudinal striae consist of fibers that proceed from the septal area on the medial surface of the frontal lobe to the hippocampus in the temporal lobe.

The ventral surface of the corpus callosum forms the roof of the lateral ventricles and has relations with the fornix and septum pellucidum in the midline. The **fornix,** consisting of symmetrical halves, is a robust fiber system that connects the hippocampal formation of each temporal lobe with the hypothalamus, especially the mamillary bodies (see Fig. 18–2). The crura of the fornix begin at the posterior end of each hippocampus; they curve forward and merge to form the body of the fornix, which is in contact with the undersurface of the trunk of the corpus callosum. The body of the fornix divides into two columns that turn ventrally away from the corpus callosum; they form the anterior boundaries of the interventricular foram-

ina and continue to the hypothalamus. The resulting interval between the fornix and corpus callosum is bridged by the **septum pellucidum** (see Fig. 11–2), a thin sheet of tissue that contains scattered groups of neurons at its anterior end and is covered on each side by ependyma. The septum pellucidum separates the frontal horns of the lateral ventricles; it is a double membrane containing a slitlike cavity, the cavum septi pellucidi, which does not communicate with the ventricular system or with the subarachnoid space. A hole in the septum pellucidum is often present in the brains of professional boxers. No functional disability is known to result from this perforation, but boxers commonly have numerous other small lesions in their cerebral hemispheres.

Anterior Commissure

The **anterior commissure** is a bundle of fibers that crosses the midline in the lamina terminalis; it traverses the anterior

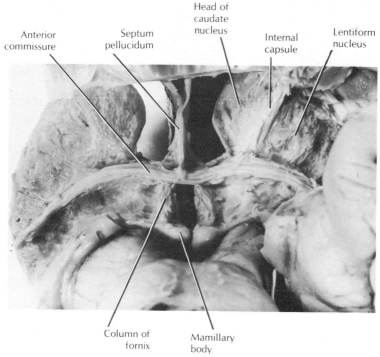

Anterior commissure   Septum pellucidum   Head of caudate nucleus   Internal capsule   Lentiform nucleus

Column of fornix   Mamillary body

FIGURE 16-7.
Dissection exposing the anterior commissure, anteroventral view.
(× 1⅔)

parts of the corpora striata and provides for additional communication between the temporal lobes (Fig. 16–7). The anterior commissure includes fibers that connect the middle and inferior temporal gyri of the two sides; this is a neocortical component similar to the corpus callosum. Other fibers run between olfactory cortex of the temporal lobes (the lateral olfactory areas), for which the uncus is a landmark. There are also fibers that connect the olfactory bulbs, but these are a minor component of the anterior commissure in man.

Role of the Cerebral Commissures

The interhemispheric connections provided by the corpus callosum and anterior commissure contribute to the bilaterality of memory traces. The role of the neocortical commissures in interhemispheric transfer has been studied by assessing the effect of section of the corpus callosum and anterior commissure in the monkey and chimpanzee (split-brain preparation). In normal unoperated animals a training exercise learned with one hand is performed efficiently by the other hand because of interhemispheric transfer of the neural basis of learning. In the case of the split-brain monkey or chimpanzee, however, a previously unfamiliar task learned by use of one hand can not be performed by the other hand unless training in the exercise is repeated with that hand.

Similar observations, with an extension in the area of language, are available for humans. These were made on those who suffered from severe epilepsy and in whom the corpus callosum was sectioned in order to confine the epileptic discharge to one hemisphere. There are no significant changes in intellect, behavior, or emotional responses that can be attributed to commissurotomy. However, a task learned postoperatively with one hand is no longer transferable to the other hand, as is to be expected from the results of experiments on other primates.

A particularly significant result of commissurotomy in humans is related to language. Let us say that the linguistic faculties reside in the left hemisphere, as is usually the case. After section of the corpus callosum the patient is unable to describe an object held in the left hand (with the eyes closed) or seen only in the left visual field, although the nature of the object is understood. There is no such difficulty when the sensory data reach the left hemisphere. After commissurotomy the right hemisphere is rendered mute and agraphic because it has no access to memory for language in the left hemisphere. However, the subordinate hemisphere with respect to language is superior in certain other activities. These include copying drawings that include perspective and arranging blocks in a prescribed manner. The nonlinguistic hemisphere is therefore the more proficient side of the brain in functions requiring special competence in three-dimensional perspective. Another activity dependent on the right cerebral hemisphere is the production of music, as when singing or playing an instrument.

The Nobel Prize for Medicine and Physiology in 1981 was shared by Hubel and Wiesel (see Chap. 15) with R.W. Sperry. The latter award was made chiefly for studies of the functions of the cerebral commissures.

INTERNAL CAPSULE AND PROJECTION FIBERS

The projection fibers are concentrated in the internal capsule and fan out as the **corona radiata** in the medullary center (Fig. 16–5). The internal capsule consists of an **anterior limb,** a **genu,** a **posterior limb,** a **retrolentiform part,** and a **sublentiform part,** all of which have topographic relations with adjacent gray masses (Fig. 16–8). The anterior limb is bounded by the lentiform nucleus and by the head of the caudate nucleus. The genu is medial to the apex of the lentiform nucleus, and the posterior limb intervenes between the lentiform nucleus and thalamus. The retrolentiform part of the internal capsule occupies the region behind the lentiform nucleus, and the sublentiform part consists of fibers that pass beneath the posterior part of the lentiform nucleus.

Thalamic Radiations

Many of the projection fibers establish reciprocal connections between the thalamus and cerebral cortex. The **anterior thalamic radiation,** which is included in the anterior limb of the internal capsule, consists mainly of fibers connecting the mediodorsal thalamic nucleus and prefrontal cortex. The **middle thalamic radiation** is a component of the posterior limb of the internal capsule. This radiation includes the projection from the ventral posterior thalamic nucleus to the somesthetic area in the parietal lobe; these fibers run in the posterior part of the posterior limb, where they are partly intermingled with motor projection fibers. Other fibers of the middle thalamic radiation establish reciprocal connections between the thalamus and the association cortex of the parietal lobe. Fibers from the ventral lateral nucleus of the thalamus reach the motor and premotor areas of the frontal lobe by traversing the genu and adjacent region of the posterior limb of the internal capsule.

The **posterior thalamic radiation** establishes connections between the thalamus and cortex of the occipital lobe. The geniculocalcarine tract that ends in the visual cortex is a particularly important component of this radiation. Originating in the lateral geniculate nucleus, the geniculocalcarine tract first traverses the retrolen-

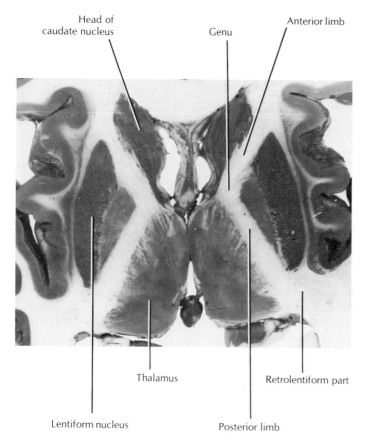

Head of
caudate nucleus   Genu   Anterior limb

Thalamus   Retrolentiform part

Lentiform nucleus   Posterior limb

FIGURE 16-8.
Horizontal section of the cerebrum stained by a method that differentiates gray matter *(dark)* and white matter *(light)* illustrating regions of the internal capsule. The sublentiform part lies ventral to the plane of this section, below the posterior part of the lentiform nucleus. (× 1)

tiform and sublentiform parts of the internal capsule. The constituent fibers then spread out into a broad band bordering the lateral ventricle and turn backward into the occipital lobe. Some of the fibers, constituting Meyer's loop, proceed forward for a considerable distance into the temporal lobe above the temporal horn of the lateral ventricle before turning back into the occipital lobe (see Fig. 20–7). The posterior thalamic radiation also contains fibers that establish reciprocal connections between the pulvinar of the thalamus and the cortex of the occipital lobe. The **inferior thalamic radiation** consists of fibers directed horizontally in the sublentiform part of the internal capsule that connect thalamic nuclei with cortex of the temporal lobe. Most of the fibers are included in the auditory radiation that originates in the medial genic-

ulate nucleus and terminates in the auditory area, for which Heschl's convolutions are a landmark on the superior surface of the superior temporal gyrus.

Motor Projection Fibers

The remaining projection fibers are corticofugal, and most of them have motor functions. (The exceptions are fibers proceeding from the somesthetic cortex to relay nuclei on general sensory pathways.) The **corticobulbar (corticonuclear)** and **corticospinal tracts,** which together constitute the pyramidal motor system, originate in the motor and premotor areas in the frontal lobe and in the parietal lobe. The fibers converge as they traverse the corona radiata and enter the anterior half of the posterior limb. In their passage through the internal capsule, the pyramidal fibers are shifted into the posterior half of the posterior limb by frontopontine fibers that have already traversed the anterior limb. Corticobulbar fibers are most anterior, followed in sequence by corticospinal fibers related to the upper limb, trunk, and lower limb. However, there is considerable overlap of the territories occupied by fibers for the major regions of the body.

Corticopontine fibers originate in widespread areas of cortex, but in greatest numbers in the frontal and parietal lobes. They terminate in the nuclei pontis, in the basal portion of the pons. Fibers of the **frontopontine tract** traverse the anterior limb of the internal capsule and the anterior portion of the posterior limb. Most of the fibers of the **parietotemporopontine tract** originate in the parietal lobe and traverse the retrolentiform part of the internal capsule.

Corticostriate fibers originate in all parts of the neocortex, most profusely in the sensorimotor strip, and end in the neostriatum. The caudate nucleus and putamen receive these fibers from the internal capsule and the putamen receives some from the external capsule as well. Other projection fibers pass to the red nucleus, reticular formation, and inferior olivary complex. **Corticorubral fibers** arise from the motor and premotor areas of the frontal lobe; some of them are collateral branches of corticospinal axons. The **corticoreticular fibers** begin in the motor cortex and in cortex of the parietal lobe, especially the somesthetic area. They terminate in the central and lateral groups of reticular nuclei. **Cortico-olivary fibers,** mainly from the motor area, terminate in the nuclei of the inferior olivary complex. These descending pathways accompany the fibers of the pyramidal system through the internal capsule and basis pedunculi into the pons and medulla. Along with the corticospinal and corticobulbar tracts, they are severed by destructive lesions in the internal capsule. Such lesions also involve the thalamocortical fibers from the ventral lateral thalamic nucleus to the motor and premotor areas of the cortex.

An infarction in the posterior part of the internal capsule results in especially serious neurological deficits. These include the effects of an "upper motor neuron lesion" caused mainly by interruption of pyramidal and corticoreticular fibers. The same lesion causes general sensory deficits by involvement of the thalamocortical projection to the somesthetic area, and a visual field defect caused by interruption of geniculocalcarine fibers.

The composition of the **external capsule** is incompletely understood, but it is known that this thin layer of white matter between the putamen and claustrum consists mainly of projection fibers. These include some of the corticostriate fibers that end in the putamen and some of the corticoreticular fibers.

LATERAL VENTRICLES

The lateral ventricles, one in each cerebral hemisphere, are roughly C-shaped cavities lined by ependyma and filled with cerebrospinal fluid. Each lateral ventricle consists of a central part in the region of the parietal lobe from which horns extend into the frontal, occipital, and temporal lobes. The principal features of the ventricular walls are shown in Figures 16–9 and 16–10. The configuration of the entire ventricular system of the brain is illustrated in Figure 16–11.

The **central part** of the lateral ventricle has a flat roof that is formed by the corpus callosum. The floor includes part of the dorsal surface of the thalamus, of which the anterior tubercle is a boundary of the interventricular foramen (foramen of Monro) that leads to the third ventricle. The tail of the caudate nucleus forms a ridge along the lateral border of the floor. The stria terminalis, a slender bundle of fibers originating in the amygdaloid body in the temporal lobe, lies in the groove

Fornix

Cut surface of
corpus callosum

Choroid plexus

Foramen of Monro

Thalamus

Septum
pellucidum

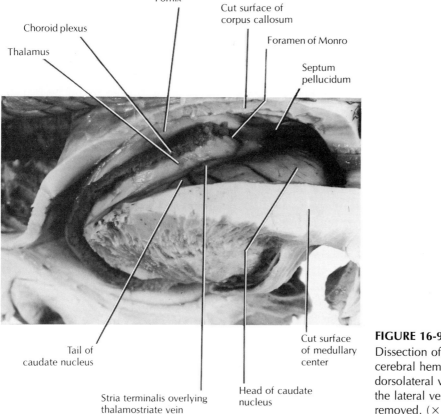

Tail of
caudate nucleus

Cut surface
of medullary
center

Stria terminalis overlying
thalamostriate vein

Head of caudate
nucleus

FIGURE 16-9.
Dissection of the right
cerebral hemisphere,
dorsolateral view. The roof of
the lateral ventricle has been
removed. ($\times$ 1¼)

Calcar avis

Bulb of posterior horn

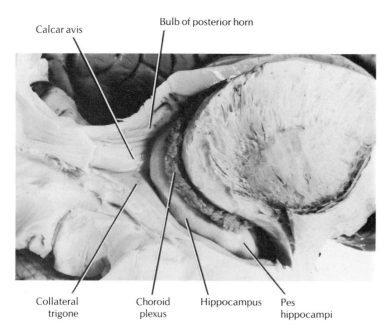

Collateral
trigone

Choroid
plexus

Hippocampus

Pes
hippocampi

FIGURE 16-10.
Dissection of the right
cerebral hemisphere (lateral
view), exposing the occipital
and temporal horns of the
lateral ventricle. ($\times$ 1¼)

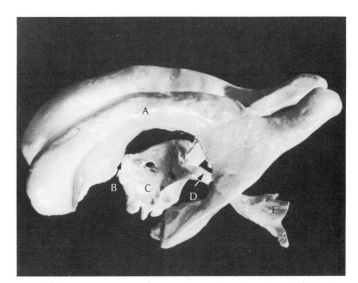

FIGURE 16-11.
Cast of the ventricular system of the brain. **(A)** Lateral ventricle, consisting of a central part and frontal, temporal, and occipital horns. **(B)** Interventricular foramen (foramen of Monro). **(C)** Third ventricle. **(D)** Cerebral aqueduct (aqueduct of Sylvius) **(E)** Fourth ventricle. (Prepared by Dr. D. G. Montemurro)

between the tail of the caudate nucleus and thalamus, along with the thalamostriate vein (vena terminalis). The fornix completes the floor medially, and the choroid plexus is attached to the margins of the **choroid fissure,** which intervenes between the fornix and thalamus.

The **frontal horn** extends forward from the region of the interventricular foramen. The corpus callosum continues as the roof, and the genu of the corpus callosum limits the frontal horn in front. The septum pellucidum bridges the interval between the fornix and corpus callosum in the midline, separating the frontal horns of the two lateral ventricles. The **occipital horn,** which is of variable length, is surrounded by the medullary center. There are two elevations on the medial wall of the occipital horn. The more dorsal prominence, for which the forceps occipitalis is responsible, is referred to as the **bulb of the occipital horn;** the lower prominence, formed by the calcarine sulcus, is called the **calcar axis.**

The **temporal horn** extends to within 3 to 4 cm of the temporal pole. There is a triangular area, called the collateral trigone, in the floor of the ventricle where the occipital and temporal horns diverge

from the central part of the ventricle. The collateral sulcus on the external surface of the hemisphere is at the site of the trigone and may produce a **collateral eminence.** The tail of the caudate nucleus, now considerably attenuated, extends forward in the roof of the temporal horn as far as the amygdaloid body. This latter nucleus is situated above the anterior end of the temporal horn, which places it close to the uncus on the external surface. The stria terminalis and thalamostriate vein run along the medial side of the tail of the caudate nucleus.

The floor of the temporal horn includes an important structure, the **hippocampus** (see Fig. 16–10). The hippocampus may be visualized as an extension of the parahippocampal gyrus on the external surface that has been "rolled into" the floor of the temporal horn. The slightly enlarged anterior end of the hippocampus is known as the **pes hippocampi** because it resembles an animal's paw. Efferent fibers from the hippocampus (and from part of the parahippocampal gyrus) form a ridge, the **fimbria,** along it medial border. The fimbria continues as the **crus of the fornix** after the hippocampus terminates beneath the splenium of the corpus callosum. The choroid plexus of the central part of the ventricle continues into the temporal horn, where it is attached to the margins of the choroid fissure above the fimbria of the hippocampus.

IMAGING TECHNIQUES FOR THE BRAIN

The brain, ventricles, and subarachnoid space are not seen in ordinary x-ray pictures but can be demonstrated by special methods, which are important diagnostic tools in clinical neurology.

Radiographic Methods

In **pneumoencephalography,** some of the cerebrospinal fluid is replaced by air (Fig. 16–12). However, this technique has certain disadvantages, and it has been almost completely replaced by the use of **computed tomography** (CT scan). This new application of x-ray imaging is based on scanning the head with a narrow moving beam of x-rays and measuring the attenuation of the emerging beam. The density readings from thin "sections" of the head are processed by computer to generate an image whose brightness depends on the absorption value of the tissues (Fig. 16–13). The CT scan is so sensitive that the information obtained extends beyond that provided by air studies. The technique is valuable in clinical diagnosis because the density of many cerebral lesions is greater or less than the density of normal brain tissue.

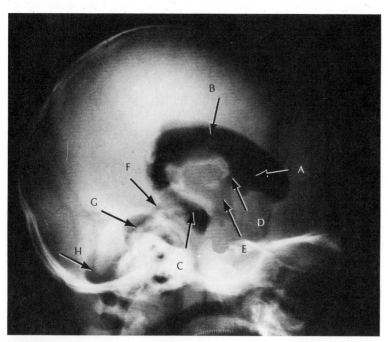

FIGURE 16-12.
Pneumoencephalogram of a 9-month-old child (lateral view). The head was in the brow-up position, so the occipital horn of the lateral ventricle contains cerebrospinal fluid. **(A)** Frontal horn of lateral ventricle. **(B)** Central part of lateral ventricle. **(C)** Temporal horn of lateral ventricle. **(D)** Interventricular foramen. **(E)** Third ventricle. **(F)** Cerebral aqueduct. **(G)** Fourth ventricle. **(H)** Cisterna magna. (Courtesy of Dr. J. M. Allcock)

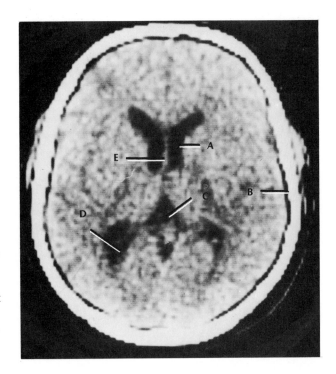

FIGURE 16-13.
CT scan at a level showing portions of the ventricular system. **(A)** Frontal horn of lateral ventricle. **(B)** Subarachnoid space. **(C)** Subarachnoid cistern (of great cerebral vein). **(D)** Occipital horn of lateral ventricle. **(E)** Septum pellucidum. (Courtesy of Dr. R. H. Coates and Dr. H. W. K. Barr)

For technical reasons the plane of the "sections" pictured by computed tomography is oblique, being somewhat closer to horizontal than to coronal. Special neuroanatomical atlases are available in which CT scans are compared with photographs of slices of the brain cut in the same plane.

Nuclear Magnetic Resonance Imaging

Nuclear magnetic resonance imaging (NMRI) was developed from a physical method used in chemical analysis. In a strong magnetic field, the nuclei of atoms absorb radiofrequency energy. The absorbed frequency is characteristic of the element, and of the immediate molecular environment of its atoms. In diagnostic NMRI, a frequency is chosen that is absorbed mainly by the nuclei of the hydrogen atoms of water. The patient's head is put into a magnetic field and irradiated with the radiofrequency radiation for protons. The measured energy absorptions are integrated in a computer, which generates a series of pictures of sections through the head. The sections may be reconstructed in the same plane as that used for CT, and also in and parallel to the midline.

The advantages of NMRI are that no potentially harmful radiation is used, and that the anatomical resolution is greatly superior to that obtainable with x-rays. The chief disadvantage is that NMRI is a slow process, requiring more than an hour to obtain information that CT can provide in a few minutes. The disadvantage of NMRI and CT in comparison to positron emission tomography, discussed in the following section, is that the two former techniques fail to distinguish living from dead tissue.

Positron Emission Tomography

Positrons are emitted by certain short-lived radioactive isotopes, of which ^{15}O, ^{13}N, ^{11}C, and ^{18}F are the most useful clinically. Positron emission tomography

(PET) is a computerized scanning procedure for building pictures of the brain based on the detection of emitted positrons. The isotopes have half-lives of less than 2 hours, during which time they must be made, incorporated into suitable compounds, and administered to the patient. This technique can be used only in a hospital equipped with a cyclotron and a laboratory for radiochemical syntheses. Images produced by PET show the distribution of metabolic processes such as the utilization of glucose or the binding of drugs to receptors on the surfaces of cells. These pictures, some of which display the distributions of neurons that use or respond to particular synaptic transmitters, can be more informative to the physician than the purely anatomical images obtained with CT and NMRI.

Regional Cerebral Blood Flow Monitoring

For regional cerebral blood flow monitoring, a radioactive tracer such as ^{133}Xe that circulates in the blood is administered, and the intensities of the emitted gamma rays are measured at the surface of the patient's head. The intensity of the radiation at any point varies with the rate of vascular perfusion of the underlying tissues. The method is most valuable for examining different parts of the cerebral cortex. Although the flow of blood through the whole brain does not change much, there are transient but conspicuous local increases in flow associated with activity of the cortical neurons. Computerized synthesis of the measurements of radioactivity provides anatomical pictures of the functioning areas, although the resolution is inferior to that obtained with radiological methods. Clinicians use this method to identify regions in which the circulation is inadequate. Regional cerebral blood flow can also be studied by PET, using [^{15}O]carbon dioxide as the tracer.

Angiography, another clinical investigative technique that can yield anatomical information, is mentioned in Chapter 25.

SUGGESTED READING

Bleier R, Houston L, Byne W: Can the corpus callosum predict gender, age, handedness, or cognitive differences? Trends Neurosci 9:391–394, 1986

de Lacoste-Utamsing C, Holloway RL: Sexual dimorphism in the human corpus callosum. Science 216:1431–1432, 1982

Gawler J, Bull JWD, Du Bourlay GH, Marshall J: Computerized axial tomography: The normal EMI scan. J Neurol Neurosurg Psychiatry 38:935–947, 1975

Gazzaniga MS, Sperry RW: Language after section of the cerebral commissures. Brain 90:131–148, 1967

Hardy TL, Bertrand G, Thompson CJ: The position and organization of motor fibers in the internal capsule found during stereotactic surgery. Appl Neurophysiol 42:160–170, 1979

Lammertsma AA: Positron emission tomography of the brain: Measurement of regional cerebral function in man. Clin Neurol Neurosurg 86:1–11, 1984

Lufkin RB: Magnetic resonance imaging of the central nervous system: Interpretation and normal anatomy. Semin Neurol 6:1–7, 1986

Sperry RW: The great cerebral commissure. Sci Am 210:42–52, 1964

Springer SP, Deutsch G: Left Brain, Right Brain, rev ed. San Francisco, WH Freeman & Co, 1985

Stahl SM, Leenders KL, Bowery NG: Imaging neurotransmitters and their receptors in living human brain by positron emission tomography. Trends Neurosci 9:241–245, 1986

Tredici G, Pizzini G, Bogliun G, Tagliabue M: The site of motor corticospinal fibres in man. A computerized tomographic study of restricted lesions. J Anat 134:199–208, 1982

SEVENTEEN

Olfactory System

The olfactory system consists of the olfactory epithelium, bulbs, and tracts, together with the cerebral olfactory areas.

Lower vertebrates and many mammals rely heavily on the sense of smell. They are said to be "macrosmatic"; in the mammalian class the dog is a familiar example. Humans are "microsmatic," with smell being much less important than the other senses, especially sight and hearing. The study of comparative anatomy contributes much to an understanding of those parts of the brain involved in olfaction, which constitute the **rhinencephalon.** Thus, in macrosmatic animals the rhinencephalic structures are large and prominent, whereas in humans they are small by comparison with the remainder of the brain. However, even in humans olfaction is a significant sense that conjures up memories and arouses emotions. Smell also contributes to alimentary pleasures. Those

who have lost their sense of smell complain of impairment of "taste," stating that everything is bland and tastes alike, and they may be unaware of their inability to smell. Much of our enjoyment of "taste" is in fact an appreciation of aromas through the olfactory system. Nevertheless, loss of smell is not a serious disability. Anosmia is the technical word for loss of the sense of smell, but there is no word in everyday use comparable to blindness and deafness.

The olfactory system has few clinical applications as compared with other sensory systems; it is discussed here only briefly in the context of the cerebral hemispheres, of which it forms an integral part.

OLFACTORY EPITHELIUM AND OLFACTORY NERVES

The olfactory epithelium (Fig. 17–1) covers an area of 2.5 cm^2 in the roof of each nasal cavity and extending for a short distance on the lateral wall of the cavity and the nasal septum. The sensory olfactory cells are contained in a pseudostratified columnar epithelium, which is thicker than that lining the respiratory passages elsewhere. Olfactory glands (glands of Bowman) beneath the epithelium bathe the surface with a layer of mucous fluid, in which odoriferous substances are dissolved. The **olfactory neurosensory cells,** the functional cells with respect to smell, are bipolar neurons that are modified to serve as sensory receptors as well as conducting neurons. The major modification consists of specialization of the dendrite; this process extends to the surface of the epithelium, where it ends as an exposed bulbous enlargement known as an olfactory vesicle, bearing cilia that are exceptional in that they may be up to 100 μm long.

Unmyelinated axons of the olfactory cells constitute the olfactory nerves, which pass through the foramina of the cribriform plate of the ethmoid bone and enter the olfactory bulb. The axons form a superficial fibrous stratum in the olfactory bulb, then continue more deeply, and terminate in specialized synaptic configurations, the **glomeruli.** The olfactory neurosensory cell is a primitive type of receptor, similar to neuroepithelial cells of invertebrates. This is the only instance in humans in which the effective stimulus has direct access, without the intervention of nonnervous tissue, to a neuron that is specialized to serve as a receptor cell. The few neurosensory cells shown in Figure 17–1 represent some 25 million such cells in each half of the olfactory epithelium. A corresponding number of axons of neurosensory cells constitute about 20 olfactory nerve bundles on each side.

The olfactory neurosensory cells are continuously being produced by mitosis and differentiation of basal cells of the olfactory epithelium, and lost by desquamation. Each receptor neuron survives for about two months; observations in animals indicate that the replacement is probably of cells lost by wear and tear rather than of cells that die because of an innately short life span. Consequently, there are always new axons growing along the olfactory nerves and into the olfactory bulbs.

The olfactory system is exquisitely sensitive to minute amounts of excitants in the air. Direct stimulation of the receptors, convergence of many neurosensory cells on neurons of the olfactory bulb, and facilitation by neuronal circuits in the bulb are among the factors responsible for the low threshold. Smell is a chemical sense, as is taste. In order for a substance to be smelled it must enter the nasal cavity as a gas or as an aerosol. An odoriferous substance must also be soluble in water for it to be taken up by the fluid that covers the olfactory epithelium. That a large range of odors and aromas can be appreciated may be due in part to the existence of neurosensory cells with different chemical specificities.

The olfactory system adapts rather quickly to a continuous stimulus, so that the odor becomes unnoticed. Older persons usually have reduced acuity of smell, probably caused by a progressive reduction in the population of neurosensory cells in the olfactory epithelium.

OLFACTORY BULB, TRACT, AND STRIAE

The olfactory tract extends forward from its point of attachment to the brain in front of the anterior perforated substance (see Fig. 17–3). The olfactory bulb appears as a slight terminal expansion of the tract, situated above the cribriform plate of the ethmoid bone.

The olfactory bulb has a characteristic cytoarchitecture in animals that rely heavily on the sense of smell. There are five layers (Fig. 17–2): nerve fiber layer (olfactory axons) on the surface, layer of glomeruli, external plexiform layer, layer of mi-

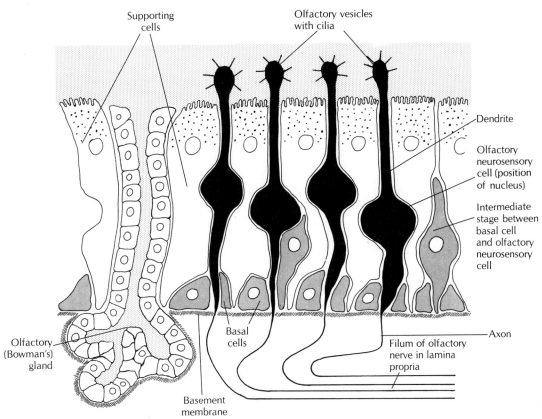

FIGURE 17-1.
The olfactory epithelium.

tral cells, and granule cell layer, which in its deeper parts also contains the myelinated axons that comprise the medullary center of the olfactory bulb. The center contains nests of ependymal cells, which are vestiges of the extension of the lateral ventricle into the bulb in embryonic life. The layers are irregular and indistinct in the olfactory bulb of adult humans, although they are obvious in the fetal stages of development.

The principal cells of the olfactory bulb are the **mitral cells,** whose cell bodies form a single layer. Their dendrites extend into the glomeruli, where they are contacted by axons of neuroepithelial cells, and into the external plexiform layer, where they receive input from centrifugal fibers of the olfactory tract. The axons of the mitral cells

run in the olfactory tract, and constitute the main output of the bulb. **Tufted cells** are similar to the mitral cells, but their somata lie in the external plexiform layer.

The olfactory bulb contains interneurons of two types. **Periglomerular cells** have dendrites within the glomeruli that receive synaptic input from neuroepithelial cells and from centrifugal fibers of the olfactory tract. There are also dendrodendritic synapses with the dendrites of the mitral cells. The axons of the periglomerular cells enter the external plexiform layer to contact the dendrites of mitral cells associated with other glomeruli. The most numerous interneurons are the **granule cells,** which have no axons and are located in the deepest layer of the olfactory bulb. Their dendrites receive axoden-

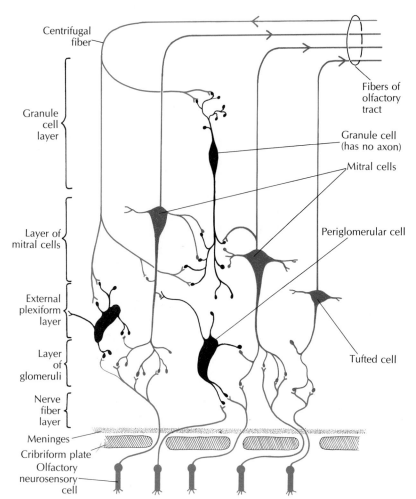

Centrifugal fiber

Granule cell layer

Layer of mitral cells

External plexiform layer

Layer of glomeruli

Nerve fiber layer

Meninges
Cribriform plate
Olfactory neurosensory cell

Fibers of olfactory tract

Granule cell (has no axon)

Mitral cells

Periglomerular cell

Tufted cell

FIGURE 17-2.
Neuronal circuitry of the olfactory bulb.

dritic contacts from mitral cells and from the centrifugal fibers. Other dendrites form dendrodendritic synapses with mitral cell dendrites. Some of these synaptic arrangements are shown in Figure 17–2. The complex circuitry of the olfactory bulb recalls that of the retina and indicates that, as is the case with visual images, sensory data are partially analyzed and edited before reaching the cerebral olfactory areas.

A small group of nerve cells, making up the **anterior olfactory nucleus,** is situated at the transition between the olfactory bulb and olfactory tract. Collateral branches of axons of mitral and tufted cells terminate in this nucleus; fibers originating in the anterior olfactory nucleus pass through the anterior commissure to the contralateral olfactory bulb.

Impulses from the olfactory bulb are conveyed to olfactory areas for subjective appreciation of odors and aromas. These areas also establish connections with other parts of the brain for emotional and visceral responses to olfactory stimuli. The olfactory tract expands into the small **olfactory trigone** at the rostral margin of the anterior perforated substance. Most of the axons of the tract pass into the **lateral olfactory stria** (Fig. 17–3), which goes to the lateral olfactory area. Other axons of the olfactory tract, constituting the **intermediate olfactory stria,** leave the olfactory trigone to enter the anterior perforated sub-

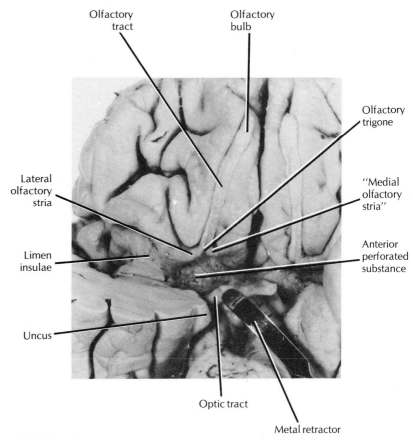

Olfactory tract

Olfactory bulb

Olfactory trigone

Lateral olfactory stria

"Medial olfactory stria"

Limen insulae

Anterior perforated substance

Uncus

Optic tract

Metal retractor

FIGURE 17-3.

A portion of the ventral surface of the brain, showing some of the components of the olfactory system. The anterior portion of the right temporal lobe has been cut away. (× 1)

stance, which is the intermediate olfactory area. The name "medial olfactory stria" is applied to a ridge that was once thought to carry olfactory fibers to the septal area. It is now known, however, that no such connection exists.

OLFACTORY AREAS OF THE CEREBRAL HEMISPHERE

The anatomy of the olfactory areas and the projections from these areas to other parts of the brain are important topics in the discipline of comparative neurology. The details are many and complex, in view of the dominance of smell in the lives of

lower animals. These topics are only briefly discussed here because of the infrequency with which disorders of this system are encountered.

The **lateral olfactory area** receives afferents from the olfactory bulb through the lateral olfactory stria (Figs. 17-3 and 17-4). The area consists of the paleocortex of the **uncus**, cortex of the **entorhinal area** (the anterior part of the parahippocampal gyrus) in the temporal lobe, and cortex in the region of the limen insulae (Fig. 17–3). The uncus, entorhinal area, and limen insulae are collectively known as the **pyriform cortex** (or lobe) because the homologous area has a pear-shaped outline in

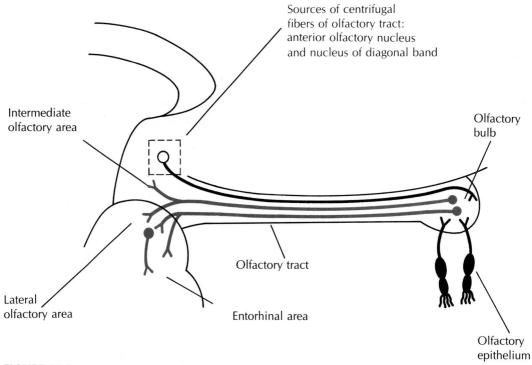

FIGURE 17-4.
Components of the olfactory tract.

macrosmatic animals. Part of the **amygda-loid body** (amygdala) is also included in the lateral olfactory area; this nucleus is situated above the tip of the temporal horn of the lateral ventricle, immediately beneath the lentiform nucleus (see Fig. 18–3). The amygdala is a nuclear complex that consists of a dorsomedial portion continuous with the cortex of the uncus and a larger ventrolateral portion. The dorsomedial portion consists of the **corticomedial group of nuclei;** it receives olfactory fibers, whereas the ventrolateral portion is a component of the limbic system. The lateral olfactory area is the principal region for awareness of olfactory stimuli, and is therefore called the **primary olfactory area.**

The anterior perforated substance, situated between the olfactory trigone and the optic tract (see Fig. 17–3), derives its name from the penetration of many small blood vessels into the brain in this region.

It contains several groups of neurons that receive fibers from the olfactory trigone and together constitute the **intermediate olfactory area.** The **diagonal band of Broca,** immediately in front of the optic tract and beneath the gray matter, connects the ventrolateral portion of the amygdala with the septal area, and is therefore a fiber bundle of the limbic system. However, the adjacent **nucleus of the diagonal band** is a major source of centrifugal fibers to the olfactory bulb, the other source being the contralateral anterior olfactory nucleus. The septal area, on the medial surface of the frontal lobe ventral to the rostrum of the corpus callosum, was formerly also known as the "medial olfactory area," but it does not receive any fibers of the olfactory tract. The septal area is a component of the limbic system of the brain, and can no longer be assigned a role in olfaction as well.

Olfactory stimuli readily produce visceral responses through the autonomic nervous system; examples are salivation when there are pleasing aromas from the preparation of food, and nausea when an odor is very unpleasant. The main projection from the olfactory areas to autonomic nuclei is through the **medial forebrain bundle,** although most of its fibers originate in the septal area. This bundle, which is smaller in humans than in macrosmatic animals, traverses the lateral part of the hypothalamus and gives off fibers to hypothalamic nuclei. Descending fibers from the hypothalamus proceed to autonomic nuclei in the brain stem and spinal cord. Most of the fibers of the medial forebrain bundle that continue beyond the hypothalamus end in raphe reticular nuclei; others end in the dorsal nucleus of the vagus nerve and in the nucleus of the tractus solitarius.

The hippocampal formation in the temporal lobe is a major component of the limbic system, and it receives input from the entorhinal area. Although the functions of the limbic system are poorly understood, they undoubtedly include a role in emotions and subsequent responses that are important for survival. The olfactory areas project as well to the mediodorsal thalamic nucleus, which, with the prefrontal cortex, exerts an influence on mood. The entorhinal area also has direct connections through subcortical association fibers with the neocortex of the temporal lobe and of the orbital surface of the frontal lobe.

Neurological signs caused by dysfunction of the olfactory system may have diagnostic significance. A tumor, usually a meningioma, in the floor of the anterior cranial fossa may interfere with the sense of smell because of pressure on the olfactory bulb or olfactory tract. It is necessary to test each nostril separately because the olfactory loss is likely to be unilateral. A lesion that affects the lateral olfactory area may cause "uncinate fits," characterized by an imaginary disagreeable odor, by movements of the lips and tongue, and often by a "dreamy state."

SUGGESTED READING

Brodal A: Neurological Anatomy in Relation to Clinical Medicine, 3rd ed. New York, Oxford University Press, 1981

Brunjes PC, Frazier LL: Maturation and plasticity in the olfactory system of vertebrates. Brain Res Rev 11:1–45, 1986

Doucette JR, Kiernan JA, Flumerfelt BA: The reinnervation of olfactory glomeruli following transection of primary olfactory axons in the central or peripheral nervous system. J Anat 137:1–19, 1983

Graziadei PPC, Karlan MS, Monti Graziadei GA, Bernstein JJ: Neurogenesis of sensory neurons in the primate olfactory system after section of the fila olfactoria. Brain Res 186:289–300, 1980

Hinds JW, Hinds PL, McNelly NA: An autoradiographic study of the mouse olfactory epithelium: Evidence for long-lived receptors. Anat Rec 210:375–383, 1984

Nakashima T, Kimmelman CP, Snow JB: Structure of human fetal and adult olfactory neuroepithelium. Acta Otolaryngol 110:641–646, 1984

Scalia E, Winans, SS: The differential projections of the olfactory bulb in mammals. J Comp Neurol 161:31–56, 1975

Shepherd GM: The olfactory bulb: A simple system in the mammalian brain. In Kandel ER (ed): Handbook of Physiology, Section 1: The Nervous System, Vol 1: Cellular Biology of Neurons, pp 945–968. Bethesda, American Physiological Society, 1977

EIGHTEEN

Limbic System

Certain components of the cerebral hemispheres and diencephalon are brought together under the heading of the limbic system of the brain. The concept of such a system having special functions developed from comparative neuroanatomical studies and neurophysiological investigations. The terminology is rather vague, however, and is not used consistently by all authors. The **"limbic lobe"** was originally defined by Broca in 1878 as a ring of gray matter on the medial aspect of each hemisphere. The largest components of the "lobe" are the hippocampus, parahippocampal gyrus, and cingulate gyrus. The term **limbic system** is less precise. The broadest interpretation, which is probably the most useful, includes the aforementioned structures together with the dentate gyrus, amygdaloid body, septal area, hypothalamus (especially the mamillary bodies), and anterior and some other nuclei of

the thalamus. Bundles of myelinated axons that interconnect these regions (fornix, mamillothalamic fasciculus, stria terminalis, and stria medullaris thalami) are also parts of the system.

The limbic system is concerned with emotions important to survival, together with visceral and motor responses involved in defense and reproduction, and with processes involved in memory. The limbic system has also been called the **visceral brain** because of its substantial influence on visceral functions through the autonomic nervous system.

HIPPOCAMPAL FORMATION

The hippocampal formation consists of the hippocampus, the dentate gyrus, and most of the parahippocampal gyrus. (The anterior end of the parahippocampal gyrus is occupied by the entorhinal area, which is

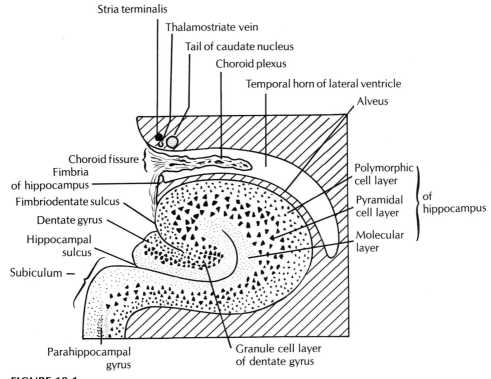

Stria terminalis
Thalamostriate vein
Tail of caudate nucleus
Choroid plexus
Temporal horn of lateral ventricle
Alveus
Choroid fissure
Fimbria
of hippocampus
Fimbriodentate sulcus
Dentate gyrus
Hippocampal
sulcus
Subiculum —
Parahippocampal
gyrus
Polymorphic
cell layer
Pyramidal
cell layer
Molecular
layer
of
hippocampus
Granule cell layer
of dentate gyrus

FIGURE 18-1.
Simplified coronal section through the hippocampal formation (medial surface at the left).

transitional between paleocortex and neocortex histologically and is included in the lateral olfactory area.)

The **hippocampus** develops in the fetal brain by a process of continuing expansion of the medial edge of the temporal lobe in such a way that the hippocampus comes to occupy the floor of the temporal horn of the lateral ventricle (see Figs. 16–10 and 18–1). In the mature brain, therefore, the parahippocampal gyrus on the external surface is continuous with the concealed hippocampus. The hippocampus is C-shaped in coronal section. The outline bears some resemblance to a ram's horn, and the hippocampus is sometimes called Ammon's horn (cornu ammonis), Ammon being the name of an Egyptian deity with a ram's head. The ventricular surface of the hippocampus is made up of a thin layer of white matter called the **alveus**, which

consists of fibers that enter and leave the hippocampal formation. The fibers constitute the **fimbria** of the hippocampus along its medial border, and then continue as the crus of the fornix after the hippocampus terminates beneath the splenium of the corpus callosum.

Continued growth of the cortical tissue composing the hippocampus is responsible for the **dentate gyrus** (Fig. 18–1). This gyrus occupies the interval between the fimbria of the hippocampus and the parahippocampal gyrus; its surface is toothed or beaded—hence the name "dentate" gyrus. The **hippocampal sulcus** is a groove between the parahippocampal and dentate gyri, and the **fimbriodentate sulcus** lies between the dentate gyrus and the fimbria. The **choroid fissure** in this location is dorsal to the fimbria of the hippocampus.

Although the parahippocampal gyrus is

included in the limbic lobe as defined anatomically, most of its cortex is of the six-layered type or nearly so. In the region of the gyrus known as the **subiculum** (see Fig. 18–1), there is a transition between neocortex and the archicortex of the hippocampus, in which there are the following three layers.

1. The **molecular layer,** consisting of delicate nerve fibers and scattered small neurons, is continuous with the outermost layer of neocortex.
2. The prominent **pyramidal cell layer** is composed of large neurons, many of them having a pyramidal outline. Dendrites of cells in this layer extend into the molecular layer, and their axons traverse the alveus on their way to the fornix. This layer is continuous with layer 5 (internal pyramidal) of the neocortex.
3. The **polymorphic cell layer** is similar to the innermost layer (layer 6) of the neocortex. This layer includes neurons that contribute fibers to the fornix. Other neurons are comparable to the cells of Martinotti of neocortex because their axons extend into the molecular layer.

The dentate gyrus also has three layers. The cytoarchitecture differs from that of the hippocampus in that the pyramidal cell layer is replaced by a **granule cell layer** of small neurons. Efferent fibers from the gyrus terminate in the hippocampus; few, if any, enter the fornix. The cytoarchitecture and connections of the dentate gyrus suggest that it is a reinforcing and regulating part of the hippocampal formation.

Knowledge of the connections of the hippocampal formation is derived almost entirely from observations on laboratory animals. The modern tracing methods based on axoplasmic transport have yielded particularly informative results. The organization of the major pathways is evidently the same in all mammalian species that have been studied, so it is reasonable to conclude that equivalent neural circuitry exists also in humans.

Afferent Connections

The hippocampal formation receives a large contingent of fibers from the entorhinal area. There are two populations of such fibers. The axons of the **perforant path** from the entorhinal area pass through the subiculum to end in the dentate gyrus, and the **alvear path** traverses the subcortical white matter and the alveus, to end in the hippocampus. The hippocampal formation receives olfactory information from the entorhinal area, which is part of the lateral olfactory area. The entorhinal area communicates with widespread areas of neocortex through association fibers of the medullary center. Through these connections, as well as through others involving the parahippocampal cortex generally, the hippocampal formation can be informed of the higher activities of the brain.

Afferent fibers for the hippocampal formation are also present in the fornix and fimbria. These come from the anterior thalamic nuclei, the posterior part of the hypothalamus, including the mamillary bodies, the septal area, the substantia innominata, the ventral tegmental area, the raphe nuclei, and the parabrachial nucleus. The fornix also carries commissural fibers, which come from the contralateral entorhinal area and hippocampus. Some of the fibers from the septal area travel in the longitudinal striae, which are embedded in the indusium griseum, an attentuated layer of archicortex on the dorsal surface of the corpus callosum. The medioventral thalamic nucleus also has connections with several components of the limbic system, and therefore participates in its complex circuitry.

Efferent Connections

The connections by means of association fibers through which the hippocampal formation receives information from the neocortex are paralleled by connections that provide for spread of activity from the hippocampal formation to the same cortex.

The fornix is notable as the largest discrete efferent pathway of the hippocampal formation.

The **fornix,** which consists of more than a million fibers in humans, contains myelinated axons that originate in the hippocampus and in the subiculum of the parahippocampal gyrus. As described previously, the axons first traverse the alveus on the ventricular surface of the hippocampus on their way to the fimbria. The fimbria continues as the **crus** of the fornix, which begins at the posterior limit of the hippocampus beneath the splenium of the corpus callosum (Fig. 18–2). The crus curves around the posterior end of the thalamus and joins its partner to form the **body** of the fornix. A small **hippocampal commissure** at the convergence of the crura consists of decussating fibers that proceed from the hippocampus and entorhinal area of one hemisphere to the hippocampal formation of the opposite hemisphere. The body of the fornix separates into **columns,** each of which curves ventrally in front of the interventricular foramen. Here the anterior commissure lies immediately in front of the column of the fornix. Some fibers separate from the column just above the anterior commissure; these constitute the precommissural portion of the fornix and are distributed to the septal area, the anterior part of the hypothalamus, and the substantia innominata. The postcommissural portion of the column of the fornix is much larger. It gives off a bundle of fibers that ends in the anterior and lateral dorsal thalamic nuclei and then continues through the hypothalamus, where it is the landmark for dividing the hypothalamus into medial and lateral areas. Most of the fibers terminate in the mamillary body, and the remainder end in the ventromedial nucleus of the hypothalamus.

There are reciprocal connections between the mamillary body and anterior nuclei of the thalamus through the **mamillothalamic fasciculus** (bundle of Vicq d'Azyr), which is readily demonstrable by

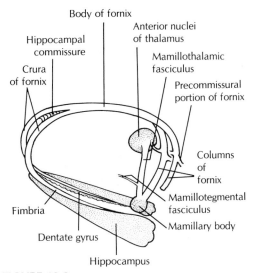

FIGURE 18-2.
The fornix and related pathways of the limbic system.

gross dissection (see Fig. 11–15). The anterior and lateral dorsal thalamic nuclei are in reciprocal communication with the cingulate gyrus through fibers that travel around the lateral side of the lateral ventricle. The cingulate gyrus is also in reciprocal communication with the parahippocampal gyrus through the cingulum, a prominent association fasciculus in the limbic lobe. The structures composing the limbic system are therefore closely integrated, with abundant provision for feedback within the system.

AMYGDALOID BODY (AMYGDALA)

The amygdaloid body consists of several groups of neurons situated between the anterior end of the temporal horn of the lateral ventricle and the ventral surface of the lentiform nucleus (Fig. 18–3). The dorsomedial portion of the amygdaloid body, known as the **corticomedial group** of nuclei, blends with the cortex of the uncus. It received fibers from the olfactory bulb and is part of the lateral olfactory area. The larger ventrolateral portion consists of the **central** and **basolateral groups** of nuclei,

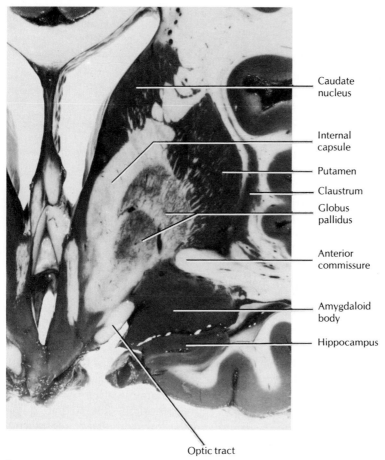

Caudate
nucleus

Internal
capsule

Putamen

Claustrum

Globus
pallidus

Anterior
commissure

Amygdaloid
body

Hippocampus

Optic tract

FIGURE 18-3.
Coronal section through the region of the brain that includes the
amygdaloid body, stained by a method that differentiates gray matter
(dark) and white matter *(light).* This is a portion of the section shown in
Figure 12-3. (× 2)

which have no direct input from the olfactory bulb, although they connect with the dorsomedial portion and with the olfactory cortex in the entorhinal area. The central and basolateral groups are included in the limbic system on the basis of the results of experiments involving stimulation and ablation in laboratory animals and clinical observations in humans. They are in communication with the septal area through the diagonal band of Broca.

The basolateral group has widespread connections, most of which are not in the form of well-defined fiber bundles. Using the shortest routes there are reciprocal connections with cortex of the frontal and temporal lobes, the cingulate gyrus, the thalamus (especially its mediodorsal nucleus), and the catecholamine nuclei and raphe nuclei of the reticular formation. Afferents have also been traced from the substantia nigra, the ventral tegmental area, and the substantia innominata. The most discrete efferent bundle of the amygdala is the **stria terminalis.** The slender fasciculus follows the curvature of the tail of the caudate nucleus, continuing along the groove between the caudate nucleus and thalamus in the floor of the central part of the lateral ventricle. Most of the constituent fibers terminate in the septal area and in the anterior part of the hypothalamus, but some enter the medial forebrain bundle and go to various parts of the brain stem, including the dorsal nucleus of the vagus nerve and the nucleus of the tractus solitarius.

The central nuclei of the amygdala receive afferent fibers from the corticomedial and basolateral nuclei, and have projections similar to those of the basolateral group.

CIRCUITS OF THE LIMBIC SYSTEM

The largest components of the limbic system contain a ring of interconnected neurons. It is often named after Papez (the circuit of Papez), who postulated in 1937 that these parts of the brain "constitute a harmonious mechanism which may elaborate functions of central emotion, as well as participate in emotional expression." Not many of the connections of the system were known at that time. It is now realized that the traffic of nerve impulses proceeds in both directions around the "ring" (Fig. 18–4). The input to the circuit of Papez is from the neocortex, thalamus, septal area, raphe nuclei, ventral tegmental area, and the catecholamine nuclei of the reticular formation. The output is partly to the neocortex, but also to regions of the reticular formation that influence the autonomic nervous system indirectly. The largest descending pathway is the **mamillotegmental fasciculus,** which consists of collateral branches of axons in the mamillothalamic fasciculus. These descending fibers terminate in the raphe nuclei of the reticular formation of the midbrain (Fig. 18–5).

The principal connections of the basolateral and central groups of nuclei of the amygdala are also shown in Figures 18–4 and 18–5. Here again reciprocal connec-

tions with neocortical areas are prominent. The descending output is partly through the **stria terminalis** to the septal area and to the anterior part of the hypothalamus. The septal area sends fibers in the stria medullaris thalami to the **habenular nuclei.** These project through the fasciculus retroflexus to the **interpeduncular nucleus,** and the pathway continues through the reticular formation to autonomic nuclei. Direct hypothalamospinal fibers in the **dorsal longitudinal fasciculus** comprise another pathway whereby the limbic system is able to influence preganglionic autonomic neurons.

The septal area and amygdala are also connected with lower levels of the neuraxis through the **medial forebrain bundle.** This contains both ascending and descending fibers and interconnects the septal area, hypothalamus, and raphe nuclei of the reticular formation. Some of its fibers reach the dorsal nucleus of the vagus and the nucleus of the tractus solitarius.

FUNCTIONAL CONSIDERATIONS

Ablation or stimulation of portions of the limbic system in monkeys and in other experimental animals provides some indication of its function. Bilateral removal of the temporal lobes, which include the hippocampal formations and amygdaloid bodies, is followed by docility and lack of emotional responses such as fear or anger to situations that normally arouse those responses. The animals exhibit increased sexual activity, and the sexual drive may be perverted, being directed toward either sex, a member of another species, or even inanimate objects. Lesions confined to the amygdala produce comparable changes in behavior, although sexual behavior is less affected.

In humans removal of both temporal lobes results in the Klüver–Bucy syndrome (first described in the monkey), characterized by a voracious appetite, increased (sometimes perverse) sexual activ-

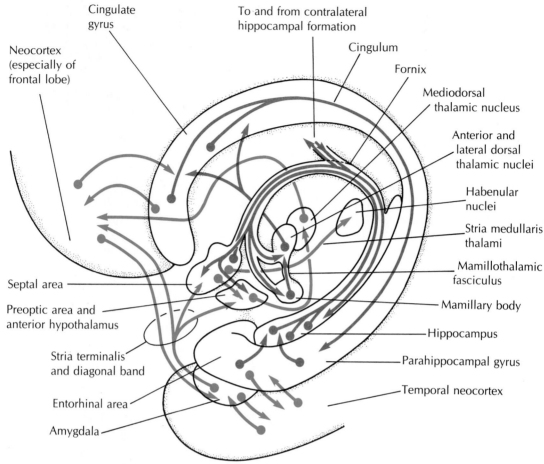

FIGURE 18-4.
Limbic connections in the forebrain and diencephalon.

ity, and docility. Electrical stimulation of the amygdala in humans induces feelings of fear or anger.

Results of studies of this type led to the view that the limbic system represents a phylogenetically old part of the brain and that it is responsible for such strong affective reactions as fear, anger, and emotions associated with sexual behavior. Changes in visceral function accompany these emotions, and electrical stimulation of the hippocampus, amygdala, or cingulate gyrus has been shown to produce a wide range of visceral responses in experimental animals. These include changes in gastrointestinal movements and secretion, pilo-

erection, and pupillary dilation. Respiratory movements are also changed.

The assignment of a role in memory to the limbic system, in particular the hippocampus, is an interesting development of recent years. Impairment of memory is evident following bilateral temporal lobectomy or when arterial occlusion, having caused an infarction in the hippocampal formation of one side, is followed at a later time by a similar infarction in the other hemisphere. Interruption of the major circuit within the limbic system, such as occurs when both mamillary bodies are involved in a lesion, may also result in a memory defect. Those with such lesions

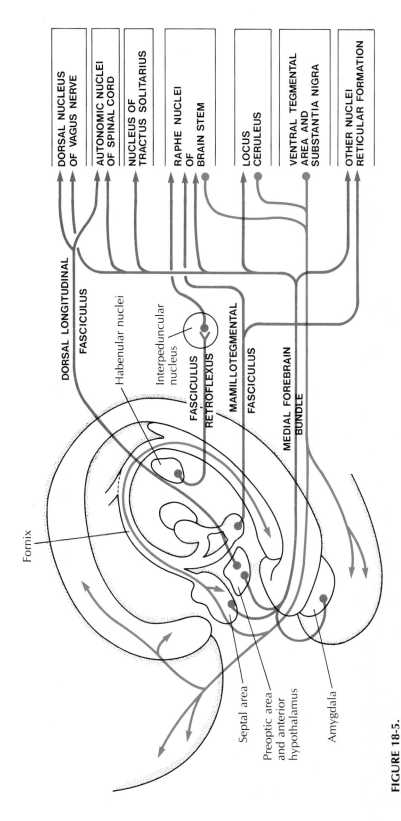

FIGURE 18-5.
Pathways leading into and out of the telencephalic and diencephalic components of the limbic system.

forget information obtained recently and are unable to commit anything to memory. This is not to say that memory traces are stored in the hippocampus. Although there are only hypotheses at this point, one possibility is that long-term memory is a function of the cerebral cortex generally, depending perhaps on macromolecular changes in these neurons superimposed on their other activities. It has been further proposed that there is a tendency for these changes to decay with time; there would therefore be no memory beyond a short interval in the absence of a mechanism that promotes retention of memory. It is envisaged that the hippocampus may provide a bias against "forgetting" through its avenues of communication with the cerebral cortex generally. The consolidation of recent memories may occur during phases of sleep when there are rapid eye movements (REM sleep). At such times, the serotonergic raphe neurons, which project to the hippocampal formation, are active. When the hippocampi are no longer functional, memories of earlier events are retained because these have already been established. However, there is amnesia for events that occurred subsequent to the lesion because the mechanism for retention or consolidation of memory is no longer operating. The probable role of the hippocampus in memory is a subject for continuing research.

Amnesia may also follow bilateral lesions in the mediodorsal nuclei of the thalamus, as in Korsakoff's syndrome. The mediodorsal nuclei are connected with the prefrontal cortices, and these are involved in higher mental functions, although not specifically with memory. Such lesions in the thalamus are likely to interrupt the mamillothalamic fibers as well, which may contribute to the amnesia.

Involvement of the hippocampus in the sleep-waking cycle has also been postulated. In deep sleep, when the electroencephalogram (EEG) recorded over the neocortex shows regular, synchronized rhythms, the hippocampal EEG (recorded with a needle electrode) is desynchronized. In the waking state, however, the neocortical record is desynchronized and the hippocampus generates a slow, regular rhythm.

SUGGESTED READING

Horel JA: The neuroanatomy of amnesia. A critique of the hippocampal memory hypothesis. Brain 101:403–45, 1978

Klüver H, Bucy PC: "Psychic blindness" and other symptoms following bilateral temporal lobectomy in rhesus monkeys. Am J Physiol 119:352–353, 1937

Papez JW: A proposed mechanism for emotion. Arch Neurol Psychiat 38:725–734, 1937

Penfield W, Milner B: Memory deficit produced by bilateral lesions in the hippocampal zone. Arch Neurol Psychiat 79:475–497, 1958

Price JL, Amaral DG: An autoradiographic study of the projections of the central nucleus of the monkey amygdala. J Neurosci 1:1242–1259, 1981

Raisman J, Cowan WM, Powell TPS: The extrinsic efferent, commissural and association fibres of the hippocampus. Brain 88:963–996, 1965

Shepherd GM: Neurobiology. New York, Oxford University Press, 1983

Smith OA, DeVito JL: Central neural integration for the control of autonomic responses associated with emotion. Annu Rev Neurosci 7:43–65, 1984

Stephan H: Evolutionary trends in limbic structures. Neurosci Biobehav Rev 7:367–374, 1983

Swanson LW, Mogenson GJ: Neural mechanisms for the functional coupling of autonomic, endocrine and somatomotor responses in adaptive behavior. Brain Res Rev 3:1–34, 1981

Symonds C: Disorders of memory. Brain 89:625–644, 1966

Terzian H, Dalle Ore G: Syndrome of Klüver and Bucy: Reproduced in man by bilateral removal of the temporal lobes. Neurology 5:373–380, 1955

Victor M: The amnesic syndrome and its anatomical basis. Can Med Assn J 100:1115–1125, 1969

von Cramon DY, Hebel N, Schuri U: A contribution to the anatomical basis of thalamic amnesia. Brain 108:993–1008, 1985

REVIEW
OF THE
MAJOR
SYSTEMS

NINETEEN

General Sensory Systems

Impulses originating in general sensory receptors initiate reflex responses through pathways in the spinal cord and in the brain stem, and impulses from certain of these receptors reach the cerebellum. The circuits are important in neurophysiology, and their interruption by a disease process results in various types of sensory deficit and usually also in some form of motor dysfunction. This chapter deals with the pathways from the general sensory receptors to the thalamus and thence to the cerebral cortex, where the sensations are appreciated subjectively. With an understanding of the anatomy of these pathways, an appraisal of sensory deficits provides information concerning the location of a lesion in the central nervous system.

Sensory fibers that enter the spinal cord in dorsal roots of spinal nerves segregate in such a way that there are two main general sensory systems. The first of these,

generally regarded as the more primitive, includes one or more synaptic relays in the dorsal gray horn. Spinal neurons give rise to axons that cross the midline and ascend in the ventrolateral white matter to the thalamus. This is the **spinothalamic system** for pain and temperature. It is also the main pathway for the less discriminative form of touch usually referred to as light touch, and probably also for some modified forms of touch, notably firm pressure.

The second system includes large numbers of primary afferent fibers that turn rostrally in the ipsilateral dorsal funiculus of the spinal cord and do not end until they reach the medulla. Smaller numbers of fibers in the dorsal funiculus, together with fibers in the dorsal part of the lateral funiculus, arise ipsilaterally from neurons in the dorsal horn. All of these fibers terminate in certain nuclei in the lower medulla, from which axons cross the midline and then ascend as the medial lemniscus to the thalamus. Hence, this second pathway is called the **medial lemniscus system.** It is concerned primarily with discriminative aspects of sensation, especially the awareness of position and movement of parts of the body and the tactile recognition of shapes and textures and of changes in the positions of stimuli that move across the surface of the skin.

The spinoreticulothalamic pathway conducts impulses for cutaneous sensation; it is therefore closely related functionally to the spinothalamic system. The association is seen especially in central conduction for pain. In fact, the spinothalamic pathway and the less direct spinoreticulothalamic pathway, with their projections to the cerebral cortex, may be combined under the term **ventrolateral** (or anterolateral) **system.** The comparable term **dorsomedial system** is then used for the medial lemniscus system.

The general sensory pathways are said to consist of primary, secondary, and tertiary neurons, the cell bodies of which are in sensory ganglia, the spinal cord or brain stem, and the thalamus, respectively. However, the concept of a simple relay of three neurons is not accurate because interneurons are commonly interposed between the major neurons of a pathway. In addition, the activity of the secondary neurons is influenced by descending fibers that originate in the cerebral cortex and in the brain stem.

SPINOTHALAMIC SYSTEM

The spinothalamic system is also known as the "pathway for pain and temperature" because these modalities of sensation are transmitted to the brain in the spinothalamic tract. However, it is also concerned with tactile sensation, as has already been noted.

Receptors

The receptors for pain (nociceptors) consist of nonencapsulated endings of periph-
eral nerve fibers; these fibers are the smaller components of group A, with thin myelin sheaths, and unmyelinated group C fibers. These simple endings are phylogenetically old receptors; although not exclusively concerned with pain they appear to be the only type of receptor that responds to painful stimuli. Pain may be felt as two waves, separated by an interval of a few tenths of a second. The first wave is sharp and localized, with conduction by group A fibers. The second wave, which is rather diffuse and still more disagreeable, depends on group C fibers, with a slow conduction speed. The two waves are most easily noticed in the feet (as when treading on something sharp) because of the greater lengths of the conducting axons in the nerves of the lower limb.

The mechanism of perception of pain is inseparable from that of the initiation of inflammation, which is the response of living tissue to any kind of injury. Injured cells release several substances known as mediators, which act upon venules and nerve endings. The venules dilate, causing redness of the affected area, and become permeable to blood plasma, which leaks out to cause swelling of the tissue. Simultaneous stimulation of the nociceptive endings results in perception of pain. However, nerve impulses do not pass solely to the central nervous system: they are also propagated antidromically along other peripheral branches of the afferent fiber. In the case of cutaneous group C fibers, the impulses cause a peptide neurotransmitter known as substance P to be released into the interstitial tissues of the dermis. This results in degranulation of mast cells (which thereby release more mediators), dilation of arterioles, and sometimes edema in the area surrounding the injury. In the skin, the total result constitutes the **triple response** (of Lewis): a red mark and a wheal, surrounded by a flare of neurogenic arteriolar vasodilation. A neurally mediated phenomenon such as this, which does not involve any synapses, is called an **axon reflex.** Other examples are known experimentally, but the axon reflex just described is the only one of clinical interest.

The question of identity of receptors for temperature has not yet been resolved. They are probably morphologically nondescript free nerve endings, similar to those for pain. The nerve fibers are of similar caliber to those conducting impulses for pain. The receptors for light touch are nonencapsulated nerve endings, Merkel and peritrichial endings, and Meissner's corpuscles. Ruffini endings and pacinian corpuscles respond to firm pressure on the skin, a modified form of touch. Conduction for light touch and pressure in peripheral nerves is by myelinated group A fibers of medium diameter.

Ascending Central Pathway

Cell bodies of small and intermediate size in the dorsal root ganglia have central processes that constitute the lateral division of the dorsal rootlets. These fibers conduct impulses from pain and temperature receptors (Fig. 19-1). (Afferents for light touch and pressure enter the dorsal gray horn through the medial division of the dorsal rootlets.) The pain and temperature fibers enter the **dorsolateral tract** (of Lissauer) of the spinal cord, in which ascending and descending branches travel in most instances for lengths that correspond to one segment. A few of the axons travel as far as four segments rostral or caudal to their levels of entry.

The terminals and the collateral branches of the fibers in the dorsolateral tract enter the dorsal horn, where they arborize profusely and end mainly in laminae I, II, and V (see Fig. 5-6). Lamina II (the **substantia gelatinosa** of Rolando) is an important region in which patterns of incoming sensory impulses are modified. The greatly branched dendrites of the gelatinosa cells are contacted not only by primary afferent axons but also by reticulospinal fibers, notably those derived from the raphe nuclei of the medulla. (Descend-

ing pathways that modulate transmission in the ascending sensory pathways are discussed later in the chapter). The axons of the cells in the substantia gelatinosa ascend and descend in the dorsolateral tract and in adjacent white matter, mostly for a distance no greater than the length of one segment, but occasionally for as many as four segments. Throughout its length the axon of a gelatinosa cell gives off branches that end by synapsing on neurons of laminae I through IV. Most of the **tract cells** whose axons constitute the spinothalamic tract are situated in lamina V. The dendrites of these tract cells extend into laminae II, III, and IV, where they are contacted by primary afferent fibers for pain and temperature, by axons of the gelatinosa cells, and by primary afferents for light touch and pressure in the medial division of the dorsal rootlets. These connections are shown diagrammatically in Figure 5-7.

From the foregoing description it will be noted that the tract cells receive synaptic input from primary afferent fibers and from other neurons of the dorsal horn. The most prominent members of the latter group of neurons are those of the substantia gelatinosa that are, in their turn, contacted by primary afferents and by descending reticulospinal fibers.

Axons of the tract cells in lamina V, together with a few in laminae I, VII, and VIII, cross the midline in the ventral white commissure. Continuing through the ventral horn of gray matter, the fibers ascend in the **spinothalamic tract,** situated in the ventral part of the lateral funiculus and in the adjoining region of the ventral funiculus. Proceeding in a cephalad direction, fibers are continually being added to the internal aspect of the tract. At upper cervical levels, therefore, fibers from sacral segments are most superficial, followed by fibers from lumbar and thoracic segments, and those from cervical segments are closest to the gray matter.

The ascending tracts of the spinal cord continue into the medulla without appre-

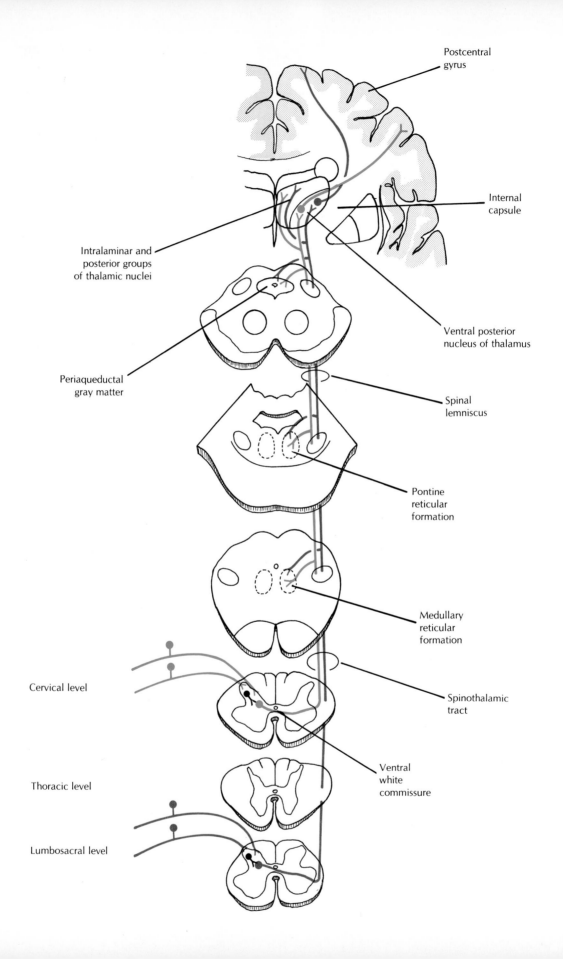

Postcentral
gyrus

Internal
capsule

Intralaminar and
posterior groups
of thalamic nuclei

Ventral posterior
nucleus of thalamus

Periaqueductal
gray matter

Spinal
lemniscus

Pontine
reticular
formation

Medullary
reticular
formation

Cervical level

Spinothalamic
tract

Ventral
white
commissure

Thoracic level

Lumbosacral level

ciable change of position initially. At the level of the inferior olivary nucleus the spinothalamic tract traverses the lateral medullary zone (Monakow's area) between the inferior olivary nucleus and the nucleus of the spinal tract of the trigeminal nerve, where it is close to the lateral surface of the medulla. At this level, and throughout the remainder of the brain stem, the spinothalamic fibers constitute most of the **spinal lemniscus,** which also includes fibers of the spinotectal tract destined for the superior colliculus. The spinal lemniscus continues through the ventrolateral region of the dorsal pons and close to the surface of the tegmentum in the midbrain, running along the lateral edge of the medial lemniscus. In their passage through the brain stem, the spinothalamic fibers give off collateral branches that terminate in the medullary and pontine reticular formation and in the periaqueductal gray matter of the midbrain.

Most of the spinothalamic fibers end in the ventral posterior nucleus of the thalamus. This nucleus consists of two parts: the ventral posterolateral division (VPl), in which spinothalamic fibers and the medial lemniscus terminate, and the ventral posteromedial division (VPm), which receives trigeminothalamic fibers. The somatotopic representation is such that the contralateral lower limb is represented dorsolaterally and the contralateral upper limb ventromedially in the VPl; the opposite side of the head is represented in the VPm.

The cortical projection consists of neurons in the ventral posterior nucleus whose axons traverse the posterior limb of the internal capsule and corona radiata to reach the somesthetic area in the parietal lobe. The contralateral half of the body, exclusive of the head, is represented as inverted in the dorsal two thirds of the somesthetic area. Beginning ventrally the sequence is therefore hand, arm, trunk, and thigh, followed by representation of the remainder of the lower limb and the perineum on the medial surface of the hemisphere. The cortical area for the hand is disproportionately large, providing for maximal sensory discrimination. The somatotopic arrangement at various levels of the sensory pathways forms the basis for recognition of the site of stimulation.

Some fibers of the spinal lemniscus end in other thalamic nuclei, notably those of the posterior and intralaminar groups. The posterior group projects to the insula, and also to adjacent cortex, including that of the second general sensory area, which is at the lower end of the postcentral gyrus. The intralaminar nuclei project diffusely to the frontal and parietal lobes of the cerebral cortex. The latter projections form part of the ascending reticular activating system, which is thought to be involved in the maintenance of a conscious, alert state.

Pain

Pain is a common complaint, and it is therefore necessary to become conversant with the anatomy, physiology, and pharmacology of this symptom. The mechanisms whereby peripheral nerve endings respond to injurious stimuli have already been reviewed. The central pathways concerned with pain will now be discussed in further detail.

Spinal Mechanisms

Perception of pain is thought to be modified by neural mechanisms in the dorsal horn. In addition to the influence of reticulospinal and corticospinal fibers, to be discussed further on, the transmission of

---

FIGURE 19-1.

The spinothalamic system for pain, temperature, light touch, and pressure. The pathway from the lower limb is shown in red and from the upper limb in blue.

impulses for pain to the brain appears to be altered by dorsal root afferents for sensory modalities other than pain. Afferent fibers of larger diameter, especially those for touch and deep pressure, end in laminae III and IV. These same laminae receive axons of gelatinosa cells, on which a large proportion of the pain afferents of smaller diameter end; they are also abundantly penetrated by dendrites of the spinothalamic tract cells, most of which have their cell bodies in lamina V. The trains of impulses coming through the larger fibers are thought to cause synaptic inhibition of the tract cells concerned with nociception. This mechanism probably operates when pain arising in deep structures such as muscles and joints is relieved by counterirritation (*i.e.*, by rubbing the overlying skin or by applying a mild irritant, such as a liniment).

The simplest defensive reflex initiated by pain is the **flexor reflex,** which involves at least two synapses in the spinal cord and causes withdrawal of a limb from the source of a sudden painful stimulus. In quadrupeds there is also a **crossed extensor reflex** in which the withdrawal is assisted by extension of the contralateral limb. In normal humans the crossed extensor reflex is largely suppressed as a result of activity in descending tracts of the spinal cord, but both it and the flexor reflex are conspicuous and, because of a lowered threshold, troublesome in paraplegic patients.

Ascending Pathways

Impulses that signal pain are transmitted rostrally in the spinothalamic and spinoreticular tracts (Fig. 19-2); some fibers with this function appear to be present in the dorsolateral funiculus as well. Tractotomy or surgical transection of the ventro-lateral region of the spinal cord, which contains the spinothalamic and spinoreticular tracts, results in almost complete loss of the ability to experience pain on the opposite side of the body below the level of the lesion. However, the sensibility usually returns gradually over several weeks. The recovery is probably a consequence of synaptic reorganization and increased usage of intact alternative pathways. A surgical cut in the midline of the spinal cord (commissural myelotomy) causes prolonged analgesia in the segments affected by the lesion.

Pain is still felt, although poorly localized, after destruction of an area of cortex that includes the primary somesthetic area. This clinical observation led to the assumption that painful sensations reached the level of consciousness within the thalamus. It is more likely, however, that spinothalamic and reticulothalamic afferents to the posterior and intralaminar groups of thalamic nuclei, and their connections with the second somesthetic and other areas of cortex, are responsible for the persistence of sensibility to pain in patients with a destructive lesion that involves the primary somesthetic area. The ventral posterior nucleus of the thalamus and the primary somesthetic area are undoubtedly necessary for the accurate localization of the site of the painful stimulus.

Descending Pathways

As noted below, descending pathways modify the activity of all ascending systems of fibers; they are prominent in controlling the conscious and reflex responses to noxious stimuli. Both the subjective awareness of pain and the occurrence of defensive reflexes may be suppressed under circumstances of intense emotional

FIGURE 19-2.

Ascending pathways for the appreciation of pain. The spinothalamic system is shown in red and the spinoreticular and reticulothalamocortical pathways in blue.

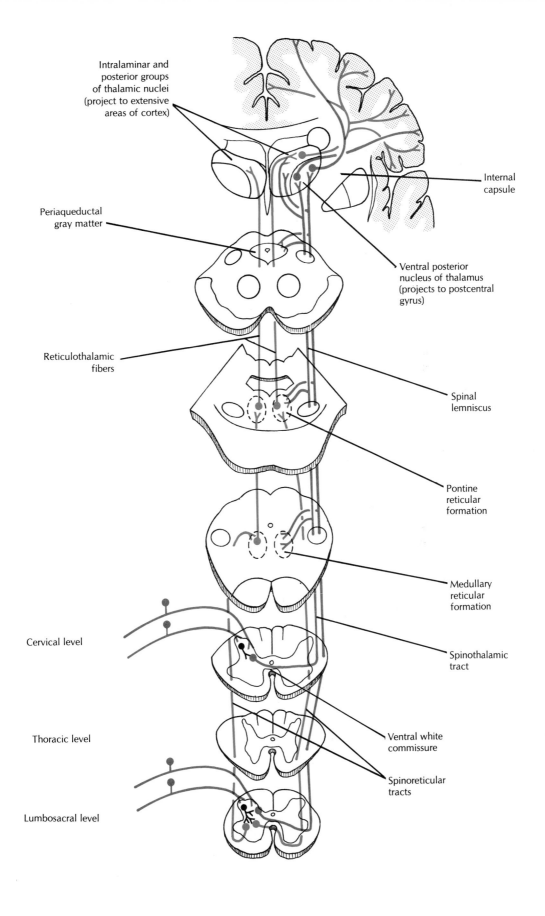

Intralaminar and posterior groups of thalamic nuclei (project to extensive areas of cortex)

Internal capsule

Periaqueductal gray matter

Ventral posterior nucleus of thalamus (projects to postcentral gyrus)

Reticulothalamic fibers

Spinal lemniscus

Pontine reticular formation

Medullary reticular formation

Cervical level

Spinothalamic tract

Thoracic level

Ventral white commissure

Spinoreticular tracts

Lumbosacral level

stress. This effect is probably mediated by **corticospinal fibers** that originate in the parietal lobe and terminate in laminae IV and V of the dorsal horn. It will be recalled that lamina V is the site of most of the cells of origin of the spinothalamic tract, and that dendrites of these cells extend into lamina IV.

Control of a more subtle kind is exerted by certain reticulospinal pathways. The best understood of these is the **raphespinal tract,** which arises from neurons in the raphe nuclei of the medullary reticular formation, mainly those of the nucleus raphe magnus. The unmyelinated axons of this tract traverse the dorsolateral funiculus of the spinal cord, and are believed to use serotonin as a neurotransmitter. The highest density of serotonin-containing boutons (observable by a histochemical method for the amine) is seen in lamina II (the substantia gelatinosa). The nucleus raphe magnus is itself influenced by descending fibers from the periaqueductal gray matter of the midbrain. Electrical stimulation of the nucleus raphe magnus or the periaqueductal gray matter causes profound analgesia. This is reversed either by transection of the dorsolateral funiculus or by administration of naloxone or similar drugs that antagonize the actions of morphine and related alkaloids of opium. Furthermore, the analgesic action of opiates is suppressed by transection of the dorsolateral funiculus.

The actions of the opiates and their antagonists are attributable to selective binding molecules (**opiate receptors**) on the surfaces of neurons in several parts of the brain. The normal function of the opiate receptor is to bind naturally occurring pentapeptides, known as **enkephalins.** These serve either as neurotransmitters or as neuromodulators. Neurons that contain enkephalins have been identified immunohistochemically, and include some of the gelatinosa cells of lamina II and some of the large tract cells (Waldeyer cells) of lamina I. Enkephalins also occur in the periaqueductal gray matter and in the nu-

cleus raphe magnus. These same regions also have high concentrations of opiate receptors. The analgesic action of morphine and of related opiates can be attributed to simulation of the effects of endogenously secreted enkephalins upon neurons bearing opiate receptors on their surfaces. The major anatomical sites of action are evidently the periaqueductal gray matter, the nucleus raphe magnus, and laminae I and II of the dorsal horn. Many other parts of the central nervous system contain enkephalins, mainly in local circuit neurons. These regions may be the sites of other pharmacological actions of the opiates, such as nausea, suppression of coughing, euphoria, and the development of addiction.

Information about the descending pathways that modulate pain has led not only to increased understanding of the sites of action of the opium alkaloids but also to a technique for the relief of chronic pain. An electrode stereotaxically implanted into the periaqueductal gray matter enables a patient to relieve pain instantly by switching on an electrical stimulator. The analgesia often lasts for several hours after cessation of stimulation.

MEDIAL LEMNISCUS SYSTEM

The set of sensory pathways known as the medial lemniscus system is for proprioception, fine touch, and vibration. In contrast to the spinothalamic system, in which ascending fibers cross the midline at spinal segmental levels, the pathways that constitute the medial lemniscus system ascend ipsilaterally in the cord and cross the midline in the caudal half of the medulla.

Receptors

The medial lemniscus system is especially important in humans because of the discriminative quality of the sensations as perceived subjectively and their value in the learning process. The characteristics of fine or discriminative touch are that the subject can recognize the location of the stimulated points with precision and is aware that two points are touched simultaneously even though they are close together (two-point discrimination). These qualities accentuate recognition of textures and of moving patterns of tactile stimuli. Of the receptors responding to touch, Meissner's corpuscles, which have been found only in primates, have a special significance in discriminative touch. They are most abundant in the ridged hairless skin of the palmar surface of the hand; preferential sites for Meissner's corpuscles correspond to those areas in which two-point discrimination is best developed. Several additional touch receptors noted in connection with the spinothalamic system also produce sensations through the medial lemniscus system. Pacinian corpuscles are the principal receptors for the sense of vibration, although this modality, once believed to be served exclusively by the dorsal funiculi, is now known to be carried also in the lateral white matter of the spinal cord.

With respect to proprioception, the dorsomedial pathway provides information concerning the precise position of parts of the body, the shape, size, and weight of an object held in the hand, and the range and direction of movement. The proprioceptors are neuromuscular spindles, neurotendinous spindles or Golgi tendon organs, and endings in and near to the capsules and ligaments of joints. All of them function in pathways through various parts of the nervous system that affect muscle action. Conscious proprioception (kinesthesia) was once thought to depend mainly on receptors in joints, but it is now realized that the input from muscle spindles is probably of greater significance than the input from other proprioceptors.

Ascending Central Pathways

The pathways for discriminative touch and for proprioception are now known to differ with respect to conduction from the lower limbs. The pathways for the two main sensory modalities of the medial lemniscus system are therefore described separately.

Discriminative Touch

The primary sensory neurons for discriminative touch (and for proprioception) are the largest cells in the dorsal root ganglia; their processes are large group A fibers with thick myelin sheaths (Fig. 19-3). The central processes are in the medial group of fibers of each rootlet, and they bifurcate on entering the **dorsal funiculus.** The short descending branches are described further on. Most of the ascending branches proceed ipsilaterally to the medulla. Above the midthoracic level the dorsal funiculus consists of a medial **fasciculus gracilis** and a lateral **fasciculus cuneatus.** The fibers of the fasciculus gracilis, which enter the spinal cord below the midthoracic level, terminate in the **nucleus gracilis;** fibers of the fasciculus cuneatus, coming from the upper thoracic and cervical spinal nerves, end in the **nucleus cuneatus.** More precisely, there is a lamination of the dorsal funiculus according to segments. Fibers that enter the spinal cord in lower sacral segments are most medial, and fibers from successively higher segments ascend in an orderly manner along the lateral side of those already present.

Axons of neurons in the nuclei gracilis and cuneatus curve ventrally as **internal arcuate fibers,** cross the midline of the medulla in the decussation of the medial lemnisci, and continue to the thalamus as the **medial lemniscus.** This substantial tract is situated between the midline and the inferior olivary nucleus in the medulla, in the most ventral portion of the tegmentum of the pons, and lateral to the red nucleus in the tegmentum of the midbrain. The medial lemniscus and spinothalamic tract intermingle in the dorsal region of the subthalamus before entering the ventral posterior nucleus of the thalamus. The fibers of the medial lemniscus, in contrast to

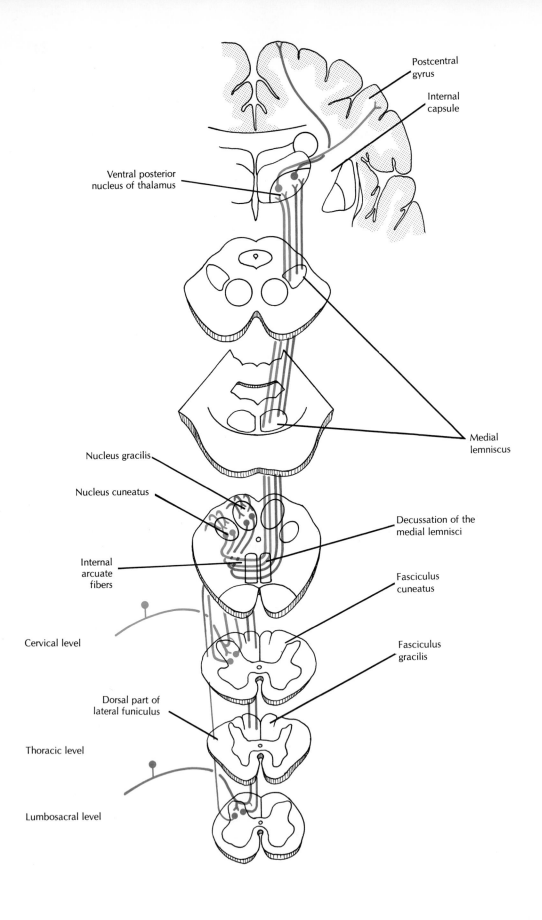

Postcentral gyrus

Internal capsule

Ventral posterior nucleus of thalamus

Medial lemniscus

Nucleus gracilis

Nucleus cuneatus

Decussation of the medial lemnisci

Internal arcuate fibers

Fasciculus cuneatus

Cervical level

Fasciculus gracilis

Dorsal part of lateral funiculus

Thoracic level

Lumbosacral level

those of the spinothalamic tract, all terminate in the ventral posterior nucleus.

A topographic arrangement of fibers is maintained throughout the medial lemniscus. In the medulla the larger dimension of the lemniscus is vertical as seen in cross section; fibers for the lower limb are most ventral (adjacent to the pyramid), and fibers for the upper part of the body are most dorsal. On entering the pons the medial lemniscus "rotates" through 90 degrees; from here to the thalamus fibers for the lower limb are in the lateral part of the lemniscus, and those for the upper part of the body are in its medial portion. This pattern conforms with the representation of the body in the ventral posterior nucleus of the thalamus (VPl). The pathway is completed by a projection from this nucleus to the primary somesthetic cortex of the parietal lobe.

Proprioception

The central pathway for conscious awareness of position and movement differs for sensory data from the lower and upper limbs (Fig. 19-4). The simpler pathway is that for the **upper limb,** which corresponds with the one just described. That is, the ascending branches of primary afferent fibers terminate in the nucleus cuneatus, from which the impulses are relayed through the medial lemniscus to the ventral posterior nucleus of the thalamus and thence to the first general sensory area of the cerebral cortex. The pathway for the **lower limb** is a series of four neurons. The primary afferent fibers enter the cord from the lumbar and sacral dorsal roots; they bifurcate into ascending and descending branches in the dorsal funiculus, but the former only go part of the way up the spinal cord. They terminate in the **nucleus dorsalis** (nucleus thoracicus), which is a column of cells within lamina VII, on the medial side of the dorsal horn in segments C8 through L3. The neurons in the nucleus dorsalis give rise to axons that ascend ipsilaterally as the **dorsal spinocerebellar tract** in the dorsolateral funiculus. Before entering the inferior cerebellar peduncle, some of the constituent axons give off collateral branches, which remain in the medulla. These collaterals from the dorsal spinocerebellar tract are concerned with conscious proprioception from the lower limb. They end in the **nucleus Z** of Brodal and Pompeiano. This is rostral to the nucleus gracilis, of which it may be functionally an outlying part. The cells of nucleus Z give rise to internal arcuate fibers that cross the midline and join the medial lemniscus. The remainder of the pathway is the same as for the upper limb, with a synapse in the ventral posterior thalamic nucleus (VPl) and thalamocortical fibers projecting to the leg area of the sensory cortex.

The different neuroanatomical substrates of proprioception from the upper and lower limbs have functional consequences. Thus, the dorsal funiculi do not conduct impulses concerned with proprioception in the lower limbs further rostrally than the thoracic segmental levels. The nucleus gracilis, unlike the nucleus cuneatus, is not concerned with proprioception at all, and the neural pathway to the cortex for the lower limb consists of four principal neurons, whereas that for the upper limb consists of only three. It is also noteworthy that the same axons (those of the dorsal spinocerebellar tract) not only convey information that eventually reaches consciousness in the cerebral cortex but also participate in the entirely unconscious workings of the cerebellum.

FIGURE 19-3.
The medial lemniscus system for discriminative tactile sensation. The pathway from the lower limb is shown in red and from the upper limb in blue. (The spinomedullary fibers, as opposed to the axons of primary sensory neurons, convey some information for most modalities of general sensation.)

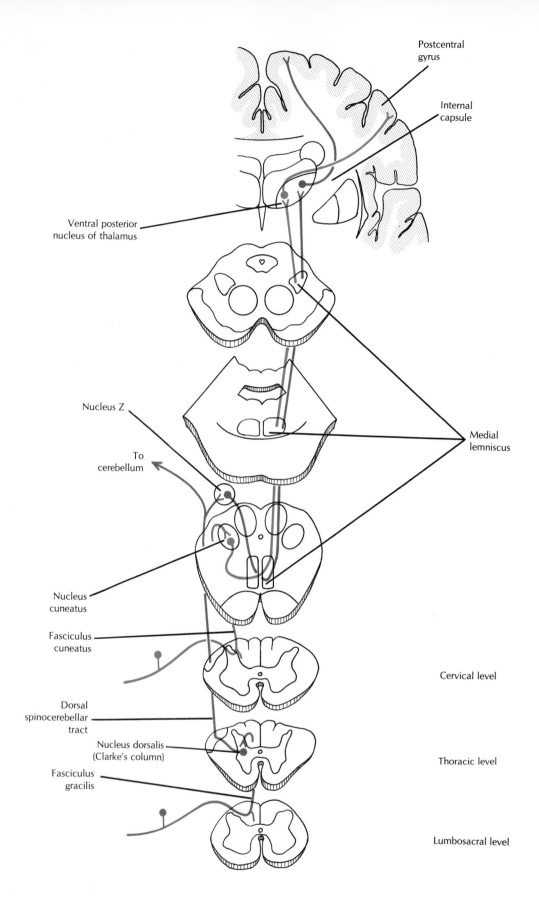

Postcentral
gyrus

Internal
capsule

Ventral posterior
nucleus of thalamus

Nucleus Z

To
cerebellum

Medial
lemniscus

Nucleus
cuneatus

Fasciculus
cuneatus

Cervical level

Dorsal
spinocerebellar
tract

Nucleus dorsalis
(Clarke's column)

Thoracic level

Fasciculus
gracilis

Lumbosacral level

Spinomedullary Neurons

The short descending branches of the primary neurons in the dorsal funiculus accumulate in the fasciculus septomarginalis in the lower half of the spinal cord and in the fasciculus interfascicularis in the upper half of the cord. They terminate in the spinal gray matter, as do some ascending branches that do not travel as far as the medulla. In addition, many of the ascending and descending branches give off collaterals to the spinal gray matter. Some of the fibers entering the gray matter, especially those concerned with proprioception, establish connections for spinal reflexes, and the remainder terminate on tract cells. Axons of the tract cells ascend ipsilaterally, not only in the dorsal funiculus, but in the dorsolateral funiculus as well (see Fig. 19–3). All of these fibers terminate in the nuclei gracilis and cuneatus alongside the primary ascending fibers. However, these tract cells, especially those sending axons into the dorsolateral funiculus, convey some information for most modalities of cutaneous and deep sensation. This relatively small population of afferents to the nuclei gracilis and cuneatus therefore broadens the role of the medial lemniscus system to some extent, beyond that of a pathway for discriminative touch and proprioception.

Spinocervicothalamic Pathway

Axons of tract cells in the dorsal horn ascend ipsilaterally in the dorsolateral funiculus to the **lateral cervical nucleus.** This nucleus is embedded in the white matter, just lateral to the tip of the dorsal horn in spinal segments C1 and C2, and extends into the lower medulla. It projects to the contralateral thalamus by means of fibers that are included in the medial lemniscus. In some animals this is a significant pathway for all types of cutaneous sensation. In humans, however, the lateral cervical nucleus is inconspicuous; in many instances the nucleus cannot be identified, although it may be merged with the apex of the dorsal horn. The spinocervicothalamic pathway has to be considered as a possible supplementary pathway in humans, but its significance as a component of the medial lemniscus system has yet to be determined.

SENSORY PATHWAYS FOR THE HEAD

The back of the head and much of the external ear are supplied by branches of the second and third cervical nerves, whose central connections are with the spinothalamic and medial lemniscus systems. General sensations arising elsewhere in the head are mediated almost entirely by the trigeminal nerve. Small areas of the skin and larger areas of mucous membrane are supplied by the facial, glossopharyngeal, and vagus nerves, but the central connections of the general sensory components of these nerves are the same as for the trigeminal nerve.

The cell bodies of primary sensory neurons of the trigeminal nerve, with the exception of those in the mesencephalic nucleus, are in the trigeminal ganglion (see Fig. 8–8). The peripheral processes have a wide distribution through the ophthalmic, maxillary, and mandibular divisions of the nerve. The central processes enter the pons in the sensory root. Some of these fibers terminate in the pontine trigeminal nucleus, many descend in the spinal trigeminal tract and end in the associated nucleus, and still others bifurcate, with a branch ending in each nucleus.

There is a spatial arrangement of fibers in the sensory root and the spinal tract that corresponds to the divisions of the trigem-

FIGURE 19-4.
Pathways for conscious proprioception. The pathway from the lower limb is shown in red and from the upper limb in blue.

inal nerve. In the sensory root ophthalmic fibers are dorsal, mandibular fibers ventral, and maxillary fibers in between. Because of a rotation of the fibers as they enter the pons, the mandibular fibers are dorsal and the ophthalmic fibers ventral in the spinal trigeminal tract. The most dorsal part of this tract includes a bundle of fibers from the facial, glossopharyngeal, and vagus nerves. The cell bodies of the primary sensory neurons are in the geniculate ganglion of the facial nerve and in the superior ganglia of the glossopharyngeal and vagus nerves. Fibers in the facial and vagus nerves supply parts of the external ear, acoustic canal, and tympanic membrane. The glossopharyngeal and vagus nerves supply the mucosa of the back of the tongue, pharynx, esophagus, larynx, auditory (eustachian) tube, and middle ear.

Pain and Temperature

The fibers for pain and temperature terminate in the pars caudalis of the **nucleus of the spinal trigeminal tract;** the pars caudalis is in the lower medulla and upper three cervical segments of the spinal cord. (There is some evidence that the pars interpolaris receives pain afferents from the teeth.) The portion of the pars caudalis in the cervical cord receives sensory data from areas of distribution of the trigeminal nerve and upper cervical spinal nerves. The cellular characteristics of the pars caudalis are similar to those of laminae I through IV of the dorsal gray horn of the spinal cord. The continuity of the substantia gelatinosa (lamina II) with a layer of small cells in the pars caudalis is particularly conspicuous.

Neurons in the reticular formation immediately medial to the pars caudalis of the nucleus of the spinal trigeminal tract correspond to lamina V of the spinal gray matter. The tract cells whose axons project to the thalamus are in both the nucleus of the spinal tract and in the adjacent reticular formation. These axons of the second

order neurons cross to the opposite side of the medulla and continue rostrally in the **ventral trigeminothalamic tract.** The tract terminates mainly in the ventral posterior nucleus of the thalamus (VPm), and thalamocortical fibers complete the pathway to the ventral one third of the somesthetic area of cortex. The axons of the tract cells associated with the pars caudalis, similar to those of the spinothalamic tract, also have branches that end in the intralaminar and posterior nuclear groups of the thalamus, thus providing for distribution of the sensory information to areas of cortex beyond the confines of the first sensory area. From the foregoing description it is evident that the pathway for pain and temperature from the head corresponds quite closely to that of the spinothalamic system.

Touch

The central pathway for tactile sensation from the head is similar to the one just described for pain and temperature, differing mainly in the sensory trigeminal nuclei involved. For light touch the second order neurons are in the pars interpolaris and pars oralis of the **nucleus of the spinal trigeminal tract** and in the **pontine trigeminal nucleus.** For discriminative touch they are in the pontine trigeminal nucleus and the pars oralis of the nucleus of the spinal trigeminal tract. The second order neurons project to the contralateral ventral posterior nucleus of the thalamus (VPm) through the **ventral trigeminothalamic tract.** In addition, smaller numbers of fibers, crossed and uncrossed, proceed from the pontine trigeminal nucleus to the same thalamic nucleus in the **dorsal trigeminothalamic tract.**

Proprioception

The primary sensory neurons for proprioception in the head are unique in that most of their cell bodies are in a nucleus in the brain stem instead of in a sensory ganglion. Comprising the **mesencephalic trigeminal nucleus,** they are unipolar neurons similar to most primary sensory neurons elsewhere. The peripheral branch of the single process proceeds through the trigeminal nerve without interruption; these fibers supply proprioceptors in the trigeminal area of distribution, such as those related to the muscles of mastication. The other branch of the single process synapses with cells in the adjacent reticular formation, the axons of which join the **dorsal trigeminothalamic tract,** or terminate in the trigeminal motor nucleus for reflex action. The innervation of proprioceptors in muscles receiving their motor supply from cranial nerves other than the trigeminal is discussed in Chapter 8.

The neurons of the mesencephalic trigeminal nucleus also send peripheral branches to receptors in the sockets of the teeth. These receptors detect pressure on the teeth and participate in the reflex control of the force of biting. The only other type of sensation perceived by a tooth is pain, which may originate within the dentin, the pulp, or from the periodontal tissues.

DESCENDING PATHWAYS INVOLVED IN SENSATION

The conscious perception of any sensation involves a sequence of neurons that form a pathway from the receptors to the cerebral cortex. For each of the ascending pathways described in this chapter there are two or three levels at which synapses occur; these are sites such as the dorsal horn, nuclei gracilis and cuneatus, and ventral posterior nucleus of the thalamus. The synapses exist, not to delay the passage of nerve impulses, but rather to accommodate convergence in some of the pathways. They also allow the upward traffic in neurally coded information to be modified by activity in other parts of the central nervous system through descending pathways (Fig. 19-5).

The first general sensory area of the **cerebral cortex** sends fibers to all the regions in which ascending somesthetic pathways are interrupted by synapses. Thus, there are projections from this part of the cortex to the ventral posterior thalamic nucleus, to the nuclei gracilis and cuneatus, to the sensory nuclei of the trigeminal nerve, and to the dorsal horn of the spinal cord. The corticofugal fibers destined for the medulla and spinal cord travel in the corticobulbar and corticospinal tracts, which were once thought of as being entirely motor in function. It is of interest that most of the corticospinal fibers from the first sensory area terminate in laminae IV and V of the dorsal horn, whereas fibers from the premotor and motor areas end in the ventral horn, especially in lamina VII. The corticospinal fibers of sensory significance are augmented by a few descending fibers in the dorsal funiculus that originate in the nuclei gracilis and cuneatus.

The other major source of descending fibers associated with the somesthetic pathways is the **reticular formation.** The inhibitory projection to the dorsal horn from the nucleus raphe magnus of the medulla has already been discussed in connection with the neuroanatomy of pain. Other reticulospinal fibers arise in the oral and caudal pontine reticular nuclei and in the gigantocellular reticular nucleus of the medulla. The reticulospinal tracts terminate mostly in lamina VII of the spinal gray matter, next to the sites of termination of corticospinal and vestibulospinal fibers, and they are concerned with the control of the motor neurons in lamina IX. Some reticulospinal axons, however, end in lamina VI at the base of the dorsal horn, and these probably synapse with dendrites of the tract cells in the adjacent lamina V. As was seen in Chapter 9, the cells of origin of the pontine and medullary reticulospinal tracts receive synaptic input from spinoreticular fibers, from other neurons in the reticular formation, and from the cerebral cortex. The corticoreticular projection

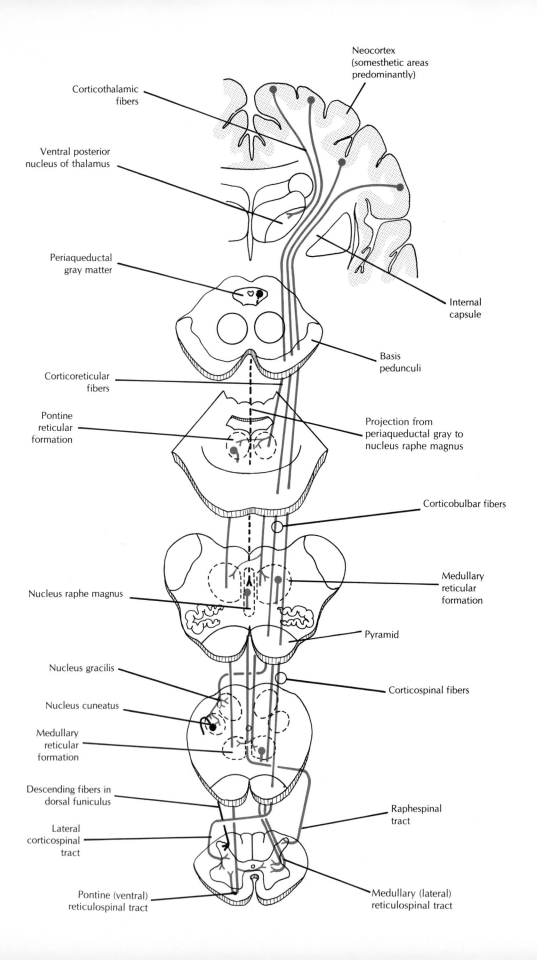

Neocortex
(somesthetic areas
predominantly)

Corticothalamic
fibers

Ventral posterior
nucleus of thalamus

Periaqueductal
gray matter

Internal
capsule

Basis
pedunculi

Corticoreticular
fibers

Projection from
periaqueductal gray to
nucleus raphe magnus

Pontine
reticular
formation

Corticobulbar fibers

Medullary
reticular
formation

Nucleus raphe magnus

Pyramid

Nucleus gracilis

Corticospinal fibers

Nucleus cuneatus

Medullary
reticular
formation

Descending fibers in
dorsal funiculus

Raphespinal
tract

Lateral
corticospinal
tract

Medullary (lateral)
reticulospinal tract

Pontine (ventral)
reticulospinal tract

comes from many parts of the cortex, but most abundantly from the motor and sensory areas of the frontal and parietal lobes.

The functions of these descending pathways are not known with certainty. It is probable that they promote attentiveness to particular stimuli. Connections are present that would enable the cerebral cortex and other parts of the brain to lower the threshold of conscious perception for a modality of sensation in any part of the body. Similarly, it would be possible to increase the thresholds for stimuli to which attention is not being paid, thereby protecting the higher levels of the ascending systems from a deluge of irrelevant information. As noted previously, corticospinal fibers are probably involved in the suppression of pain when there is intense emotional stress.

CLINICAL CONSIDERATIONS

Spinothalamic System

Inflammatory reactions in dorsal roots of spinal nerves or in peripheral nerves and pressure on spinal nerve roots by a herniated intervertebral disk stimulate pain and temperature fibers, causing painful and burning sensations in the area supplied by the affected roots or nerves. An effect opposite to that of irritation is produced by local anesthetic drugs. These are most effective in blocking the conduction of impulses along group C fibers, so that low doses may reduce pain perception while having little or no effect on tactile sensibility. Ischemia of a nerve, such as that resulting from a tight tourniquet, preferentially blocks conduction in group A fibers. Pain, with a burning character, is the only sensation that can be perceived

before the failure of conduction in an ischemic nerve becomes complete.

Degenerative changes in the region of the central canal of the spinal cord interrupt pain and temperature fibers as they decussate in the ventral white commissure. The best example is syringomyelia, which is characterized by central cavitation of the spinal cord. When the disease process is most marked in the cervical enlargement, as is frequently the case, the area of anesthesia includes the hands, arms, and shoulders (yokelike anesthesia).

A lesion that includes the ventrolateral part of the spinal cord on one side results in loss of pain and temperature sensibility below the level of the lesion and on the opposite side of the body. If, for example, the spinothalamic and spinoreticular tracts are interrupted on the right side at the level of the first thoracic segment, the area of anesthesia includes the left leg and the left side of the trunk. Careful testing of the upper margin of sensory impairment will show that cutaneous areas supplied by the first and second thoracic nerves are spared. Some impulses from these areas reach the contralateral pathways above their interruption because of the short ascending branches of dorsal root fibers in the dorsolateral tract. Surgical section of the pathway for pain (tractotomy or chordotomy) may be required for relief of intractable pain. Tractotomy is most likely to be considered in later stages of malignant disease of a pelvic viscus; interruption of the pain pathway may be unilateral or bilateral, depending on circumstances prevailing in the particular patient. An alternative procedure is commissural myelotomy, in which decussating spinothalamic and spinoreticular fibers are cut by a median incision at and a few segments above the level of the source of the pain.

FIGURE 19-5.

Descending pathways that modulate the transmission of sensory information from the spinal cord to the cerebral cortex.

The spinal lemniscus may be included in an area of infarction in the brain stem. An example is provided by Wallenberg's lateral medullary syndrome; the area of infarction usually includes the spinal lemniscus and the spinal tract of the trigeminal nerve and its associated nucleus. The principal sensory deficit is for pain and temperature sensibility on the side of the body opposite the lesion, but on the same side for the face.

The standard method of testing for integrity of the pain and temperature pathway is to stimulate the skin with a pin and to ask whether it feels sharp or dull. Temperature perception usually need not be tested separately; if such testing is required, the method used is to touch the skin with test tubes containing warm or cold water. Light touch is tested with a wisp of cotton.

Medial Lemniscus System

Sensory deficits involving proprioception and discriminative touch result from interruption of the medial lemniscus system anywhere along its course. For example, the dorsal and dorsolateral funiculi are sites of symmetrical demyelination in subacute combined degeneration of the spinal cord, and conduction may be interrupted at any level by trauma, by infarction, or by the plaques of multiple sclerosis. The usual test for proprioception is to move the patient's finger or toe, asking him to state when the movement begins and to state the direction of movement. In the Romberg test any abnormal unsteadiness is noted when the patient stands with the feet together and the eyes closed, thereby evaluating proprioception in the lower limbs. Another useful test is to ask the patient to identify an object held in the hand with the eyes closed. Proprioception is especially helpful in recognizing the object on the basis of shape and size (stereognosis) as well as its weight. This is a sensitive test that the patient may perform unsuccessfully when there is a lesion in the

parietal association cortex, even though the pathway to the somesthetic area is intact.

For testing of two-point touch discrimination, two pointed objects are applied lightly to the skin simultaneously. A suitable test object can be devised from a paper clip. Normally, simultaneous stimuli may be detected in a fingertip when the stimuli are 3 mm to 4 mm apart, or even less. Thorough testing of two-point discrimination is a tedious procedure. A simpler test is for the examiner to ask the subject to identify simple figures "drawn" on the skin with the finger or with some other blunt object. This test relies on the ability to recognize the distance and direction of movement of the stimulus across the surface of the skin. It is highly specific for the dorsal funiculi of the spinal cord provided that there is no lesion in the cerebral cortex that is causing aphasia or agnosia.

Another sensory test is to ask the patient whether vibration as well as touch or pressure is felt when a tuning fork, preferably with a frequency of 128 Hz, is placed against a bony prominence such as an ankle or a knuckle. The sense of vibration is often reduced in the elderly, but even slight vibration should be felt in the young. For identifying the site of a lesion in the central nervous system, this test is less valuable than the examination of proprioception and discriminative touch. However, diminished perception of vibration is often the first sign of disease affecting a peripheral nerve.

Sensation from the Head

The most common sensory abnormality affecting the face and scalp is herpes zoster. This disease is caused by a virus (the same one that causes chickenpox) that infects the neurons in sensory ganglia. Burning pain and itching, commonly in the field of distribution of one of the three divisions of the trigeminal nerve, is accompanied by a skin eruption. This is not usually a serious condition except when corneal ulceration results from infection of the ganglion cells concerned with the ophthalmic division of the trigeminal nerve. However, the disability is occasionally prolonged by postherpetic neuralgia, which may be particularly painful and recalcitrant to treatment. Herpes zoster may also affect the geniculate ganglion or the superior vagal ganglion, causing an eruption on the tympanic membrane and parts of the external auditory canal and concha of the auricle; this is classical clinical evidence for the anatomy of the dual cutaneous innervation of this region.

A less common condition causing pain in the fields of distribution of one or more divisions of the trigeminal nerve is trigeminal neuralgia, described in Chapter 8.

Thalamic Lesions

Surgically or pathologically produced lesions in the ventral posterior nucleus of the thalamus cause profound loss of all sensations other than pain on the opposite side of the body. The intralaminar and posterior groups of nuclei in the thalamus are probably almost as important as the ventral posterior nucleus in the central pathway for pain.

A lesion involving the thalamus may result in the thalamic syndrome, characterized by exaggerated and exceptionally disagreeable responses to cutaneous stimulation. The syndrome may also include spontaneous pain and evidence of emotional instability, such as unprovoked laughing and crying.

SUGGESTED READING

Albe-Fessard D, Berkley KJ, Kruger L, Ralston HJ, Willis WD: Diencephalic mechanisms of pain sensation. Brain Res Rev 9:217–296, 1985

Basbaum AI, Fields HL: Endogenous pain control systems: Brainstem spinal pathways and endorphin circuitry. Annu Rev Neurosci 7:309–338, 1984

Beers RF, Bassett EG (eds): Mechanisms of Pain and Analgesic Compounds. Miles International Symposium Series, No 11. New York, Raven Press, 1979

Brodal A: Neurological Anatomy in Relation to Clinical Medicine, 3rd ed. New York, Oxford University Press, 1981

Cook AW, Nathan PW, Smith MC: Sensory consequences of commissural myelotomy. A challenge to traditional anatomical concepts. Brain 107:547–568, 1984

Darian-Smith I: Touch in primates. Annu Rev Neurosci 5:155–194, 1982

Hensel H: Thermoreception and Temperature Regulation. Monographs of the Physiological Society, No 38. London, Academic Press, 1981

McLean A: C.N.S. Neurological Examination. Toronto, Collier-Macmillan, 1980

Wall PD: The sensory and motor role of impulses travelling in the dorsal columns toward cerebral cortex. Brain 93:505–524, 1970

Wall D, Noordenbos W: Sensory functions which remain after complete transection of dorsal columns. Brain 100:505–524, 1977

Walton J: Essentials of Neurology, 5th ed. London, Pitman, 1982

Webster KE: Somaesthetic pathways. Br Med Bull 33:113–120, 1977

Willis WD: Nociceptive pathways: Anatomy and physiology of nociceptive ascending pathways. Phil Trans R Soc Lond [Biol] 308:253–268, 1985

TWENTY

Visual System

The visual pathway begins with photoreceptors in the retina from which nerve impulses reach the visual cortex in the occipital lobe through a series of neurons. There are two types of photoreceptor cell; rods have a special role in peripheral vision and vision under conditions of low illumination, whereas cones, which function in bright light, are responsible for central discriminative vision and for the detection of colors. The responses of the photoreceptors are transmitted by bipolar cells to ganglion cells within the retina, and axons of ganglion cells reach the lateral geniculate nucleus of the thalamus through the optic nerve and optic tract. The final relay is from the lateral geniculate nucleus to the visual cortex by way of the geniculocalcarine tract. In addition, some fibers from the retina terminate in various parts of the midbrain, in the pulvinar of the thalamus, and in the hypothalamus.

The following account of the visual system is restricted to a discussion of the nervous elements and presupposes a general understanding of the structure of the eye.

RETINA

Optic vesicles evaginate from the prosencephalon at an early stage of embryonic development. Each optic vesicle "caves in" to form the optic cup, which consists of two layers and is connected to the developing brain by the optic stalk. The outer layer of the optic cup becomes the pigment epithelium of the retina, and the inner layer differentiates into the complex neural layer of the retina. The optic stalk becomes the optic nerve.

In addition to photoreceptors, bipolar cells, and ganglion cells, the neural layer contains association neurons and neuroglial cells. The complex neuronal pattern of the retina resembles that of the gray matter of the brain. Similarly, the optic nerve corresponds histologically to the white matter of the brain rather than to a peripheral nerve. The retina and the optic nerve are, therefore, outgrowths of the brain that are specialized for sensitivity to light, for some modification of sensory data, and for transmission of the resulting information to the thalamus and cerebral cortex.

Retinal Landmarks

Certain specialized regions serve as landmarks that need to be identified before the cellular components of the retina are described.

The basic cell layers of the retina, listed from the choroid to the vitreous body, are the pigment epithelium, rods and cones, bipolar cells, and ganglion cells (Fig. 20-1). Axons of ganglion cells run toward the posterior pole of the eye and enter the optic nerve at the **optic papilla** or **optic disk.** The papilla is slightly medial to the posterior pole, about 1.5 mm in diameter, and pale pink in color. The nerve fibers are heaped up as they converge at the margin of the optic papilla, and then pass through the fibrous tunic (sclera) of the eyeball into the optic nerve. The optic papilla is a blind spot because it contains only nerve fibers.

The **macula lutea,** the central area of the retina in line with the visual axis, is a specialized region about 5 mm in diameter that abuts on the lateral edge of the optic papilla. The name macula lutea (yellow spot) is derived from the presence of a diffuse yellow pigment (xanthophyll) among the neural elements in this location. However, the yellow color is apparent only when the retina is examined with red-free light, and the macula is therefore not ordinarily seen when the ocular fundus is inspected with an ophthalmoscope. The macula is specialized for acuity of vision; the function of the yellow pigment is probably to screen out some of the blue part of the visible spectrum, thereby protecting the photoreceptors from the dazzling effect of strong light.

The **fovea** (or fovea centralis) is a depression in the center of the macula; the fovea is about 1.5 mm in diameter and is separated from the edge of the optic disk by a distance of about 2 mm. Visual acuity is greatest at the fovea, the center of which contains only cone receptors. The capillary network present elsewhere in the retina is absent from the center of the fovea. When the retina is viewed with an ophthalmoscope the fovea appears darker than the reddish hue of the retina generally because the black melanin pigment in the choroid and the pigment epithelium is not screened by capillary blood. The visible fovea is frequently referred to as the "macula" in an ophthalmoscopic examination of the retina.

The functional retina terminates anteriorly along an irregular border, the **ora serrata.** Forward of this line the ciliary portion of the retina consists of a double layer of columnar epithelium, with the outer layer being pigmented.

Pigment Epithelium

The pigment epithelium, consisting of a single layer of cells, reinforces the light-absorbing property of the choroid in reducing the scattering of light within the eye (see Fig. 20-1). Each pigment cell has a flat hexagonal base that adheres to Bruch's glassy membrane of the choroid. The basal portion of the cell contains the nucleus and a few pigment granules. Processes extending from the free surface of the cell interdigitate with the outer photosensitive regions of rods and cones. The processes, which are filled with granules of melanin pigment, isolate individual photoreceptors and enhance visual acuity. In lower vertebrates there is a movement of pigment granules toward the tips of the

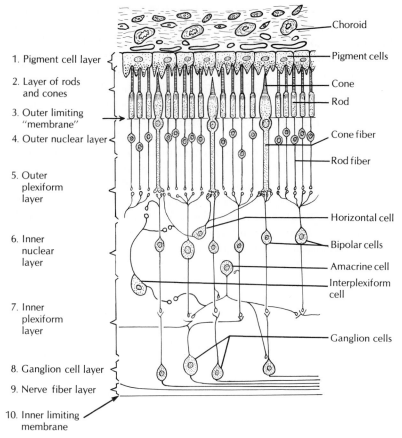

FIGURE 20-1.
Schematic representation of the cellular components of the retina.

processes, which also change in length and shape, in response to bright light. Such a response has not been described in mammals.

The pigment epithelium is fixed to the choroid but is not as firmly attached to the neural part of the retina. Detachment of the retina, such as may follow a blow to the eye or occur spontaneously, consists of separation of the neural layers from the pigment epithelium. Fluid accumulates in the space thus created between the parts of the retina derived from the two layers of the optic cup. Retinal detachment is a serious condition that can lead to complete blindness of the eye if untreated.

Photoreceptors

The light-sensitive part of the photoreceptor is the outer portion adjacent to the pigment epithelium. The incident light therefore has to pass through almost all of the retina before being detected. This arrangement, known as the inverted retina, is present in all vertebrates. It does not introduce a significant barrier to light because the retina is transparent and at no point is more than 0.4 mm thick. When they consist of layers of cells, the photoreceptive parts of the eyes of invertebrate animals are called retinas, but their cellular organization is always quite different from that of the vertebrate retina. The neural connections are on the opposite side to that from which the light approaches; hence, invertebrate retinas are not inverted.

Rods

The number of rods (also known as rod cells or bacilliform cells) in the human retina is of the order of 130 million, outnumbering cones by nearly twenty to one. Rods are lacking in the central part of the fovea and become progressively more numerous from that point to the ora serrata. The distribution is such that rods are important for peripheral vision. Each rod consists of three portions: the outer segment, inner segment, and rod fiber. The outer and inner segments are about 2 μm thick and their combined lengths vary from 60 μm near the fovea to 40 μm at the periphery of the retina. The **rod fiber** consists of a slender filament that includes the nucleus in an expanded region and terminates as an end bulb in synaptic contact with bipolar and association neurons.

In electron micrographs most of the light-sensitive **outer segment** is occupied by about 700 double-layered membranous disks or flattened saccules (Figs. 20-2 and 20-3). The membranous disks contain the pigment **rhodopsin** (visual purple), which gives the retina a purplish red color when removed from the eye and viewed under dim light. Rhodopsin consists of a protein, opsin, in loose chemical combination with retinal, a derivative of vitamin A. A quantum of light absorbed by a rhodosin molecule changes its configuration. A subsequent series of reactions results in hyperpolarization of the surface membrane of the inner segment and rod fiber, with consequent inhibition of the release of the neurotransmitter, which is secreted continuously in darkness.

The photochemical properties of rhodopsin and the summation of excitation in the visual pathway through the retina are responsible for the sensitivity of the rod system to low illumination (twilight or night vision). The rod-free area of the fovea is night blind, and a faint point of light such as a dim star is best detected by looking slightly away from it.

The **inner segment** of a rod contains the organelles generally found in cells. A region adjacent to the outer segment, known as the **ellipsoid,** contains numerous elongated mitochondria. A cilium extends into the outer segment from one of two centrioles situated at the junction of the outer and inner segments (Fig. 20-3). The remainder of the inner segment contains neurofibrils, vesicles, and granular endoplasmic reticulum. This region is known as the **myoid** because in lower vertebrates it is contractile in response to changes in light intensity. A contractile property has not been established for the corresponding region in higher vertebrates, including humans.

Cones

The cone photoreceptors, although less numerous than rod photoreceptors, are especially important because of their role in visual acuity and in color vision. Similar to the rod, the cone consists of an outer and inner segment and a cone fiber.

The tapering **outer segment** of a cone consists principally of double-layered disks, varying in number from 1000 in cones at the fovea to several hundred at the periphery of the retina (Fig. 20-2). There are differences in detail between the disks of cones and rods, including somewhat closer stacking of the disks in cones. The disks undoubtedly carry visual pigment molecules but the photosensitive compounds of cones have not yet been chemically identified, despite intensive research. To account for the sensitivity of cones to colors, one theory has proposed that there are three cone types, each con-

(Text continues on p. 302)

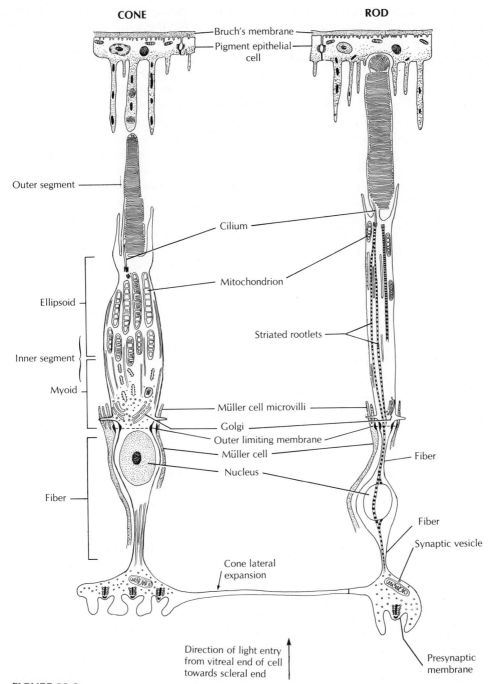

CONE **ROD**

Bruch's membrane
Pigment epithelial cell

Outer segment

Cilium

Mitochondrion

Ellipsoid

Striated rootlets

Inner segment

Myoid

Müller cell microvilli
Golgi
Outer limiting membrane
Müller cell
Nucleus

Fiber

Fiber

Fiber

Synaptic vesicle

Cone lateral expansion

Direction of light entry
from vitreal end of cell
towards scleral end

Presynaptic membrane

FIGURE 20-2.

Ultrastructural components of rods and cones. The striated rootlets are prominent structures in the cytoplasm of rods whose function is obscure. (Modified by permission from Enoch JM, Tobey FL [eds]: Springer Series in Optical Sciences, Vol 23. Heidelberg, Springer-Verlag, 1981. Courtesy of Dr. B. Borwein)

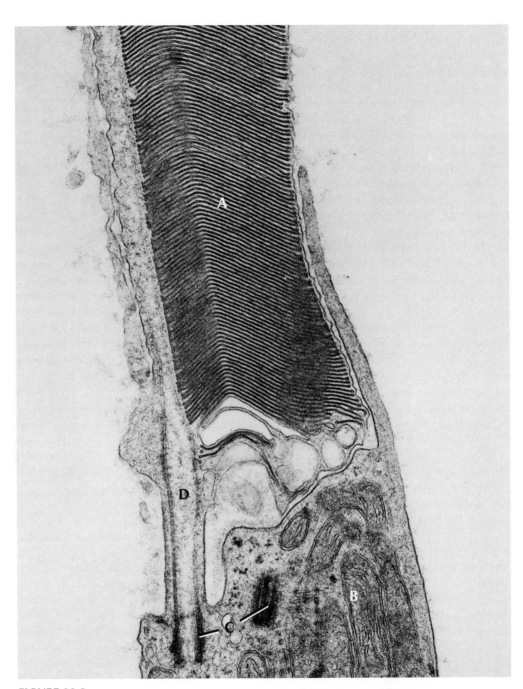

FIGURE 20-3.
Electron micrograph of a rod from the human retina, showing a portion of the outer segment and the adjoining region of the inner segment. **(A)** Membranous disks. **(B)** Mitochondria in the ellipsoid. **(C)** Centrioles. **(D)** Cilium. (× 36,000; Courtesy of Dr. M. Hogan)

taining one of three photosensitive substances that provide differential sensitivity to red, green, and blue light. The **inner segment** of a cone is thicker than the inner segment of a rod, and it contains a larger ellipsoid and a larger amount of granular endoplasmic reticulum. Cones contain a cilium similar to that of rods.

The **cone fiber** is thicker than a rod fiber, and the nucleus is in an expansion adjacent to the inner segment. The fiber expands again terminally, establishing synaptic contact with bipolar and association neurons.

The human retina contains about 7 million cones. The central part of the fovea, the foveola, contains about 35,000 cones and no rods; there are some 100,000 cones in the whole of the fovea. The proportion of cones to rods remains high throughout the macular area for central vision, but it steadily decreases from the macula to the periphery of the retina. The fovea is specialized in other ways for visual acuity. In this region the cones are longer and more slender than elsewhere (75 μm × 1.0 μm at the fovea and 40 μm × 6 μm at the periphery). The cone fibers and bipolar cells diverge from the center of the fovea, producing a slight concavity and reducing any slight impediment to light passing through the retina. Such scattering of light as may be caused by capillary blood flow is eliminated by the absence of a retinal capillary network at the center of the fovea.

Figure 20-4 illustrates cone photoreceptors as they appear in a scanning electron micrograph.

Bipolar Cells

There are several types of bipolar cell according to morphological and physiological properties. These are true neurons interposed between photoreceptor cells and ganglion cells (see Fig. 20-1). One bipolar cell is contacted by numerous rods (ranging from 10 near the macula to 100 at the periphery); the summation of excitation is

an important factor in the sensitivity of the rod system to small amounts of light. Although there is some convergence of cones on bipolar cells in the peripheral parts of the retina there is none at the fovea, at which point visual acuity is greatest. There each cone fiber synapses with the dendrites of several bipolar cells. The synaptic terminals of cone fibers also have lateral expansions that contact the presynaptic parts of nearby rod fibers.

Ganglion Cells

Ganglion cells are rather large neurons with clumps of Nissl material, forming the last retinal link in the visual pathway (see Fig. 20-1). The bipolar cells contact both dendrites and somata of ganglion cells. The axons of ganglion cells form a layer of nerve fibers adjacent to the vitreous body. The fibers converge on the optic papilla from all directions, with those from the lateral part of the retina curving above or below the macula. On reaching the papilla bundles of fibers pass through foramina in the sclera, which at this point is called the **lamina cribosa,** and then constitute the optic nerve. The axons acquire myelin sheaths only after traversing the sclera, although in a few people bundles of myelinated axons are present in the retina, where they appear ophthalmoscopically as white streaks.

Excitation and inhibition of ganglion cells depend on properties of photoreceptors and bipolar cells that are atypical of most neurons elsewhere. The presynaptic part of a photoreceptor leaks its transmitter continuously in darkness. The release of transmitter is suppressed by illumination. Thus, the activity of the receptor cell is suppressed by light. This inhibition of sensory receptors by their specific stimulus, which is unique to the retina, is probably a consequence of the fact that a dark image on an illuminated background is as important biologically as an isolated source of light in an otherwise dark visual field. With respect to bipolar cells, there

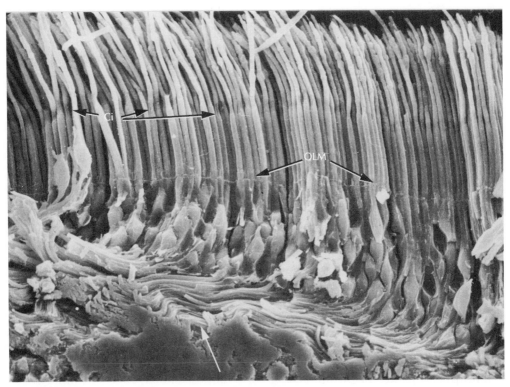

FIGURE 20-4.
Scanning electron micrograph of foveal cones in a monkey. There is a constriction of each photoreceptor at the base of its cilium **(Ci)**. The outer limiting membrane **(OLM)** appears as a thin line. The inner cone fibers *(arrow)* turn sharply back at an angle to the photoreceptors and their nuclei. (By permission from Enoch JM, Tobey FL [eds]: Springer Series in Optical Sciences, Vol 23. Heidelberg, Springer-Verlag, 1981. Courtesy of Dr. B. Borwein)

is no impulse conduction along these neurons, and their processes or neurites (and those of other retinal interneurons) are all called dendrites. Some bipolars respond to the transmitter from the photoreceptors with hyperpolarization of the cell membrane. Others respond to the same transmitter with partial depolarization. The quantity of transmitter released by the presynaptic neurites of a bipolar neuron varies with the magnitude of the partial depolarization of the cell.

Association Neurons

Synaptic transmission in the retina is subject to modification by interneurons known as association neurons (Fig. 20-1).

Horizontal cells are in the outer part of the zone occupied by the cell bodies of the bipolar cells. Their dendrites make synaptic contact with the synaptic terminals of the photoreceptors and with the dendrites of bipolar cells, which they inhibit. **Amacrine cells** are in the inner part of the zone occupied by the cell bodies of the bipolar cells. The dendrites of an amacrine cell all emerge from the same side of the cell, to ramify and then terminate in the synaptic complexes between bipolar and ganglion cells, and upon cells of the type to be described next. Amacrine cells contain many putative transmitters, and there are probably inhibitory and excitatory types. The **interplexiform cells** are interspersed among the cell bodies of the bipolars. They are postsynaptic to amacrine cells and presynaptic to horizontal and bipolar cells, thus providing a feedback loop through which neural information is passed back from the inner to the outer of the two layers of retinal synapses.

Neuroglial Cells

The innermost layers of the retina contain astrocytes similar to those present in the gray matter of the brain. There are also large numbers of radial neuroglial cells, called **cells of Müller.** These extend from the interface between the nerve fiber layer of the retina and the vitreous body to the junction of the inner segments of rods and cones and the rod and cone fibers. Microvilli project from the outer end of a Müller's cell, which is connected to photoreceptor cells by zonulae adherentes. Müller's cells therefore extend throughout almost the whole thickness of the retina; lateral processes are given off that intervene between the neuronal elements of the retina and give these neuroglial cells a supporting role, among other possible functions.

Histological Layers

When studied in sections stained with hematoxylin and eosin, the retina is described as consisting of ten layers (Fig. 20-5). These layers can now be defined in relation to the cells that constitute the retina (see Fig. 20-1). Layer 1 is the **pigment epithelium,** and layer 2 consists of the outer and inner segments of **rods** and **cones.** Layer 3 is called the **outer limiting membrane** because it appears as a delicate line in histological sections. In fact, it is not a membrane but rather the row of zonulae adherentes where the outer ends of Müller's cells make contact with photoreceptor cells. Layer 4, the **outer nuclear layer,** consists of nuclei of rods and cones. Layer 5, the **outer plexiform layer,** includes principally rod and cone fibers and

dendrites of bipolar cells. Layer 6 is called the **inner nuclear layer;** it is comprised of nuclei of bipolar cells, horizontal cells, amacrine cells, interplexiform cells, and cells of Müller. Layer 7, the **inner plexiform layer,** consists mainly of presynaptic dendrites of bipolar cells and postsynaptic dendrites of ganglion cells. The cell bodies of **ganglion cells** are in layer 8, and the axons of these cells constitute layer 9, the **nerve fiber layer.** Layer 10 is the **inner limiting membrane** formed by the expanded inner ends of Müller's cells.

Blood Supply

The retina receives nourishment from two sources. The central artery of the retina enters the eye through the optic disk and its branches spread out over the inner surface of the retina. Fine branches penetrate the retina and form a capillary network that extends to the outer border of the inner nuclear layer. The capillary bed drains into retinal veins that converge on the optic papilla to form the central vein of the retina. The other source of nourishment is from the capillary layer of the choroid, which is separated from the retina by Bruch's glassy membrane. This is a composite structure that consists of the basement membrane of the pigment epithelium and the innermost layer of the choroid, which is an orderly array of elastic and collagen fibrils, 1 to 2 μm thick. Soluble nutrients and metabolites of small molecular size can diffuse through Bruch's membrane, but macromolecules such as plasma proteins cannot. The outer part of the retina, extending from the pigment epithelium to the outer border of the inner nuclear layer, is devoid of capillaries.

PATHWAY TO THE VISUAL CORTEX

There is a point-to-point projection from the retina to the lateral geniculate nucleus of the thalamus and from this nucleus to the visual cortex of the occipital lobe.

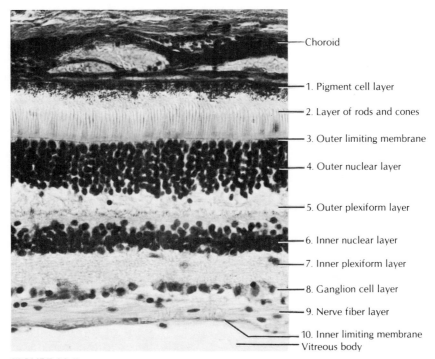

Choroid

1. Pigment cell layer

2. Layer of rods and cones

3. Outer limiting membrane

4. Outer nuclear layer

5. Outer plexiform layer

6. Inner nuclear layer

7. Inner plexiform layer

8. Ganglion cell layer

9. Nerve fiber layer

10. Inner limiting membrane
Vitreous body

FIGURE 20-5.
Section of human retina showing histological layers. (Stained with alum-hematoxylin and eosin, × 350)

There is therefore a spatial pattern of cortical excitation according to the retinal image of the visual field. Before discussing the components of the visual pathway, it may be useful to establish certain general rules concerning the projection from the retina to the cortex.

For the purpose of describing the retinal projection, each retina is divided into nasal and temporal halves by a vertical line that passes through the fovea. A horizontal line, also passing through the fovea, divides each half of the retina into upper and lower quadrants. The macular area for central vision is represented separately from the remainder of the retina. Figure 20-6 illustrates the following rules with respect to the central projection of retinal areas.

1. Fibers from the right halves of the two retinae terminate in the right lateral ge-

niculate nucleus, and the visual information is then relayed to the visual cortex of the right hemisphere. The converse holds true, of course, for the contralateral projection.

2. Fibers from the upper quadrants peripheral to the macula end in the medial part of the lateral geniculate nucleus, and impulses are relayed to the anterior two thirds of the visual cortex above the calcarine sulcus.

3. Fibers from the lower quadrants peripheral to the macula end in the lateral portion of the geniculate nucleus, with a relay to the anterior two thirds of the visual cortex below the calcarine sulcus.

4. The macula projects to a relatively large posterior region of the lateral geniculate nucleus, which in turn sends fibers to the posterior one third of the visual cortex in the region of the occipital

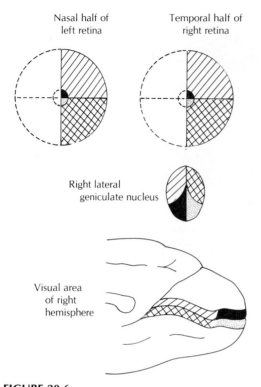

Nasal half of
left retina

Temporal half of
right retina

Right lateral
geniculate nucleus

Visual area
of right
hemisphere

FIGURE 20-6.
Projection of the retina on the lateral geniculate
nucleus and visual cortex.

pole. The portions of the lateral geniculate nucleus and the visual cortex that receive fibers from the macula, which is only 5 mm in diameter, are disproportionately large because of the role of the macula in central vision with maximal discrimination.

Visual defects that result from interruption of the pathway at any point from the retina itself to the visual cortex are described in terms of the visual field rather than the retina. *The retinal image of an object in the visual field is inverted and reversed from right to left,* just as an image on the film in a camera is inverted and reversed. The following rules therefore apply to the nuclear and cortical representation of regions of the visual field.

1. The left visual field is represented in the right lateral geniculate nucleus and in the visual cortex of the right hemisphere, and vice versa.
2. The upper half of the visual field is represented in the lateral portion of the lateral geniculate nucleus and in the visual cortex below the calcarine sulcus.
3. The lower half of the visual field is projected on the medial portion of the lateral geniculate nucleus and on the visual cortex above the calcarine sulcus.

Optic Nerve, Optic Chiasma, and Optic Tract

Each optic nerve in humans contains about 1 million fibers, all of them myelinated; the large number of fibers is indicative of the importance of human vision. The optic nerve is surrounded by extensions of the meninges; the pia mater adheres to the nerve and is separated from the arachnoid by an extension of the subarachnoid space. The dura mater forms an outer sheath, and the meningeal extensions around the nerve fuse with the fibrous scleral coat of the eyeball. The nerve fibers are arranged in fasciculi that are separated by connective tissue septa continuous with the sheath of pia mater. Each fasciculus is further divided into small bundles by the cytoplasmic processes of fibrous astrocytes. Intimate ensheathment of the optic axons is by oligodendrocytes, whose processes penetrate between individual fibers. The myelin sheaths are formed by these oligodendrocytes rather than by Schwann cells because the optic nerve is in effect a tract of the central nervous system.

The central artery and central vein of the retina traverse the meningeal sheaths and are included in the anterior part of the optic nerve. An increase in pressure of cerebrospinal fluid around the nerve impedes the return of venous blood. Edema or swelling of the optic disk (papilledema) results; this is a valuable indication of an increase in intracranial pressure.

The partial crossing of optic nerve fibers in the optic chiasma is a requirement for binocular vision. Fibers from the nasal or medial half of each retina decussate in the chiasma and join uncrossed fibers from the temporal or lateral half of the retina to form the optic tract. Impulses conducted to the right cerebral hemisphere by the right optic tract therefore represent the left half of the field of vision, whereas the right visual field is represented in the left hemisphere. Immediately after crossing in the chiasma fibers from the nasal half of the retina loop forward for a short distance in the optic nerve. A lesion affecting the optic nerve adjacent to the chiasma may therefore cause a temporal field defect with respect to the opposite eye, in addition to blindness in the eye whose optic nerve has been interrupted. The optic tract curves around the rostral end of the midbrain and ends in the lateral geniculate nucleus of the thalamus.

Some of the fibers from the retina leave the optic chiasma and tract to proceed to sites other than the lateral geniculate nucleus. These will be described after the pathway for conscious visual sensation has been discussed.

Lateral Geniculate Nucleus, Geniculocalcarine Tract, and Visual Cortex

The lateral geniculate nucleus is responsible for a small swelling, the lateral geniculate body, beneath the posterior projection of the pulvinar of the thalamus. The nucleus, in which the great majority of the fibers of the optic tract terminate, consists of six layers of cells, numbered consecutively from ventral to dorsal. Within the general pattern shown in Figure 20-6 and described previously, crossed fibers of the optic tract terminate in layers 1, 4, and 6, whereas uncrossed fibers end in layers 2, 3, and 5.

The geniculocalcarine tract originating in the lateral geniculate nucleus first traverses the retrolentiform and sublenti-

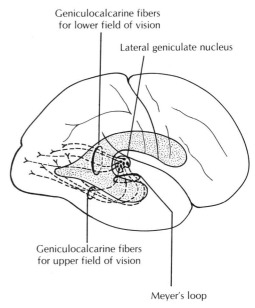

FIGURE 20-7.
The geniculocalcarine projection.

form parts of the internal capsule. Its fibers then pass around the lateral ventricle, curving posteriorly toward their termination in the visual cortex (Fig. 20-7). Some of the geniculocalcarine fibers travel far forward over the temporal horn of the lateral ventricle. These fibers, which constitute the **temporal** or **Meyer's loop** of the geniculocalcarine tract, terminate in the visual cortex below the calcarine sulcus. It is evident from the retinal projection shown in Figure 20-6 that a temporal lobe lesion involving Meyer's loop causes a defect in the upper visual field on the side opposite the lesion. A lesion in the parietal lobe, on the other hand, may involve geniculocarine fibers that proceed to the visual cortex above the calcarine sulcus; the result is then a defect in the lower visual field on the side opposite the lesion.

The **visual cortex** occupies the upper and lower lips of the calcarine sulcus on the medial surface of the cerebral hemisphere. The area is much larger than suggested by cortical maps because of the depth of the calcarine sulcus. The visual cortex is thin heterotypical cortex of the granular type (area 17 of Brodmann); it is marked by the line of Gennari and is known alternatively as the **striate area.** There is a detailed point-to-point projection of the retina on the lateral geniculate nucleus and on the visual cortex. The size of the retinal point is reduced to the diameter of a single cone for most acute vision in the central part of the fovea. Precise coordination of movements of the eyes ensures that the retinal patterns of excitation correspond with one another, as required for binocular vision. The **visual association cortex,** corresponding to areas 18 and 19 of Brodmann, is involved in recognition of objects, perception of color and depth, and other complex aspects of vision.

VISUAL DEFECTS CAUSED BY INTERRUPTION OF THE PATHWAY

Certain general rules governing defects in the visual field as a result of a lesion involving the visual pathway are indicated in Figure 20-8. The first example is an obvious one; severe degenerative disease or trauma involving an optic nerve results in blindness in the corresponding eye. Example 2 refers to interruption of decussating fibers in the optic chiasma, which causes bitemporal hemianopsia if the full thickness of the chiasma is interrupted. The most common lesion affecting the optic chiasma is a pituitary tumor pressing on it from below, which first interrupts fibers from the inferior nasal quadrants of both retinae. The visual defect begins as a scotoma in each upper temporal quadrant of the visual field, and spreads throughout the temporal fields as the chiasma is increasingly affected. Pressure on the lateral edge of the optic chiasma (example 3) happens rarely, but may occur when there is an aneurysm of the internal carotid artery in this location. The field defect, in the case of pressure on the right edge of the chiasma, is nasal hemianopsia for the right eye. Interruption of the right optic tract

(example 4) causes left homonymous hemianopsia.

Example 5 refers to a lesion involving the geniculocalcarine tract or the visual cortex. An extensive right-sided lesion results in left homonymous hemianopsia, except that central vision may remain intact (macular sparing). Decussating fibers that would provide bilateral cortical representation of the macula are lacking, and it is likely that a slight shifting of the patient's fixation or gaze during examination of the visual fields is responsible for the phenomenon known as macular sparing. Lesions affecting only a portion of the geniculocalcarine tract or the visual cortex cause field defects of lesser proportions than hemianopsia. An example is provided by the upper quadrantic defect in the opposite visual field following interruption of fibers comprising Meyer's loop in the white matter of the temporal lobe.

It is important to remember that defects in the visual field can result from lesions of the eye as well as of the central pathways or cortex. For example, chronic glaucoma and senile degeneration of the macula result in areas of blindness in the center of the field, often bilaterally.

VISUAL REFLEXES

A small bundle of fibers from the optic tract bypasses the lateral geniculate nucleus and enters the superior brachium. These fibers, which constitute the afferent limb of reflex arcs, terminate in the pretectal area and in the superior colliculus.

The **pupillary light reflex** is tested in the routine neurological examination; the response consists of constriction of the pupil when light, as from a pen flashlight, is directed into the eye. Impulses from the retina impinge on the pretectal area, which is immediately rostral to the superior colliculus. Impulses are relayed to the Edinger–Westphal nucleus of the oculomotor complex, then to the ciliary ganglion in the orbit, and finally to the sphincter

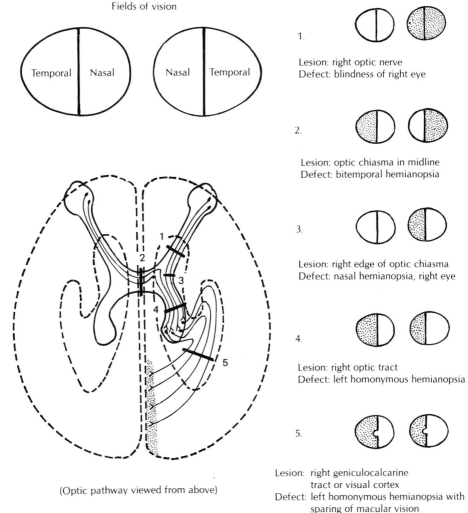

Fields of vision

(Optic pathway viewed from above)

1.
Lesion: right optic nerve
Defect: blindness of right eye

2.
Lesion: optic chiasma in midline
Defect: bitemporal hemianopsia

3.
Lesion: right edge of optic chiasma
Defect: nasal hemianopsia, right eye

4.
Lesion: right optic tract
Defect: left homonymous hemianopsia

5.
Lesion: right geniculocalcarine
tract or visual cortex
Defect: left homonymous hemianopsia with
sparing of macular vision

FIGURE 20-8.
Visual field defects caused by lesions affecting different parts of the visual pathway.

pupillae muscle in the iris. Both pupils constrict in response to light entering one eye because the pretectal area sends some fibers across the midline in the posterior commissure to the contralateral Edinger–Westphal nucleus.

Visual impulses from the retina that reach the superior colliculus collaborate with impulses from the occipital cortex, frontal eye field, and spinal cord, which are the sources of most of the afferent fibers to the colliculus. The layered cytoar-chitecture of the superior colliculus, to-gether with its diverse sources of afferent fibers, indicates that considerable integra-tive activity occurs in the region. Efferent fibers go to the accessory oculomotor nu-clei, paramedian pontine reticular forma-tion, pretectal area, and cervical segments of the spinal cord. This last pathway is known as the tectospinal tract.

The functions of the retinal afferents of the superior colliculus cannot be easily separated from the functions of the other afferents. The efferent fibers to the accessory oculomotor nuclei and to the paramedian pontine reticular formation are part of the pathway for control of both voluntary and involuntary movement of the eyes, as is described in Chapter 8. An indirect connection to the Edinger–Westphal nucleus, by way of the pretectal area, controls the contractions of the ciliary and sphincter pupillae muscles in accommodation (see below). The importance of the tectospinal tract in humans is not definitely known, but this pathway is thought to function in movements of the head as required for fixation of gaze.

Accommodation, or the **accommodation–convergence reaction,** consists of ocular convergence, pupillary constriction, and thickening of the lens when attention is directed to a near object. The reflex is tested in the routine neurological examination by asking the subject to examine an object held about a foot from the eyes after looking into the distance, and noting whether or not there is pupillary constriction. When attention is directed to a near object the medial recti muscles contract for convergence of the eyes. At the same time contraction of the ciliary muscle allows the lens to thicken, increasing its refractive power, and pupillary constriction sharpens the image on the retina.

For accommodation to near objects, impulses from the visual association cortex reach the midbrain through fibers traversing the superior brachium, and terminate in the superior colliculus. The subsequent connections to the nuclei of those cranial nerves that supply the extraocular muscles, and to the Edinger–Westphal nucleus, have already been described. The frontal eye field, which is necessary for voluntary conjugate movements of the eyes, is not involved in convergence. The pathways for constriction of the pupil in the light and accommodation reflexes are known to be different because they may be dissociated by disease. This occurs, for example, in central nervous system syph-

ilis, in which there is loss of pupillary constriction in response to light but not to accommodation (the Argyll Robertson pupil). The precise site of the lesion causing dissociation of the responses is not known. The small size and slight irregularity of the Argyll Robertson pupil are probably caused by local disease of the iris.

There is dilation of the pupils in response to severe pain or strong emotional states. The pathway begins with fibers from the thalamus and hippocampal formation to the hypothalamus, from which impulses reach the intermediolateral cell column of the spinal cord both directly and through a relay in the reticular formation. The pathway continues to the superior cervical ganglion of the sympathetic trunk, and it is completed by postganglionic fibers in the carotid plexus to the dilator pupillae muscle in the iris. At the same time the parasympathetic supply to the sphincter pupillae muscle is inhibited.

OTHER OPTIC CONNECTIONS

Results of experimental investigations in animals have revealed that the axons of retinal ganglion cells end in several parts of the brain in addition to the lateral geniculate nucleus, pretectal area, and superior colliculus.

The **retinohypothalamic tract** is formed by collateral branches of optic axons that leave the dorsal surface of the optic chiasma and terminate in the suprachiasmatic nucleus of the hypothalamus. The visual input synchronizes the circadian rhythm of the firing pattern of the neurons of the suprachiasmatic nucleus with the changes in ambient illumination. This is responsible for the influence of different levels of illumination on the antigonadotrophic activity of the pineal gland; in some animals, the retinohypothalamic tract regulates seasonal changes in the secretion of pituitary gonadotrophins.

The **accessory optic tract** consists of small fascicles that pass from the optic tract into the cerebral peduncle. They end in various small nuclei in the tegmentum of the midbrain. These nuclei project, both directly and through a synaptic relay in the inferior olivary complex, to the flocculonodular lobe of the cerebellum. (The principal input to this part of the cerebellum is from the vestibular system.) The connections indicate that the accessory optic tract may be involved in coordination of movements of the eyes and head.

Other optic axons end in thalamic nuclei other than the lateral geniculate nucleus. The main area of termination of such fibers is the **pulvinar,** which projects to the cortex of the occipital lobe, including the visual areas. The function of this alternative pathway from the retina to the cerebral cortex is not yet understood, but there is evidence in animals that it may permit some residue of conscious vision after destruction of the lateral geniculate body.

As is the case with other sensory systems, there are fibers that pass in directions opposite to those of the main flow of incoming visual information. Thus, the primary and associational visual cortices project upon the lateral geniculate nucleus and pulvinar. There is now convincing evidence for the existence of centrifugal fibers in the optic nerve in some mammals. They come from the pretectal area and from the ventral part of the hypothalamus. Equivalent fibers are well known in birds and fishes, in which they terminate among the amacrine cells of the retina.

SUGGESTED READING

Borwein B: The retinal receptor. A description. In Enoch JM (ed): Optics of Vertebrate Retinal Receptors, Chap 2. Berlin, Springer-Verlag, 1982

Boycott BB, Dowling JE: Organization of the primate retina: Light microscopy. Phil Trans R Soc Lond [Biol] 255:109–184, 1969

Hubel DH, Wiesel TN: Brain mechanisms of vision. Sci Am 241:150–162, 1979

Itaya SK: Retinal efferents from the pretectal area in the rat. Brain Res 201:436–441, 1980

Kanako A: Retinal bipolar cells: Their function and morphology. Trends Neurosci 5:219–222, 1983

Mariani AP: Biplexiform cells: Ganglion cells of the primate retina that contact photoreceptors. Science 216:1134–1136, 1982

Missoten L: Estimation of the ratio of cones to neurons in the fovea of the human retina. Invest Ophthalmol 13:1045–1049, 1974

Rodieck RW: Visual pathways. Annu Rev Neurosci 2:193–225, 1975

Stone J, Dreher B: Parallel processing of information in the visual pathways. Trends Neurosci 5:441–446, 1982

Terubayashi H, Fujisawa H, Itoi M, Ibata Y: Hypothalamoretinal centrifugal projection in the dog. Neurosci Lett 40:1–6, 1983

Van Essen DC: Visual areas of the mammalian cerebral cortex. Annu Rev Neurosci 2:227–263, 1979

Wurtz RH, Albano JE: Visual-motor function of the mammalian superior colliculus. Annu Rev Neurosci 3:189–226, 1980

TWENTY-ONE

Auditory System

Hearing is second in importance among the special senses of humans, yielding first place only to sight. Their role in language accounts to a large extent for the reliance placed on these special senses.

The auditory system consists of the external ear, middle ear, cochlea of the internal ear, cochlear nerve, and pathways in the central nervous system. The external ear consists of the auricle or pinna and the external acoustic meatus, with the latter being separated from the middle ear by the tympanic membrane. The function of the external ear is to collect sound waves, which cause a resonant vibration of the tympanic membrane. The vibration is transmitted across the middle ear cavity by a chain of three ossicles, the malleus, incus, and stapes. The malleus is attached to the tympanic membrane and articulates with the incus, which articulates in turn with the stirrup-shaped stapes. The foot plate of the stapes occupies the fenestra vestibuli in the wall between the middle and internal ears; the rim of the foot plate is attached to the margin of the fenestra vestibuli by the annular ligament, composed of elastic connective tissue. The ossicles constitute a bent lever with the longer of the two arms attached to the tympanic membrane, and the area of the foot plate of the stapes is considerably less than the area of the tympanic membrane. The vibratory force of the tympanic membrane is therefore magnified about 15 times at the fenestra vestibuli; the substantial increase in force is important because the sound waves are transferred from air to a fluid medium. Protection against the effect of sudden, excessive noise is provided by reflex contraction of the tensor tympani and stapedius muscles, which are inserted on the malleus and stapes, respectively.

The internal ear, which has a dual function, consists of the **membranous labyrinth** encased in the **bony labyrinth.** Certain parts of the internal ear contain sensory areas for the vestibular system, which is discussed in Chapter 22. The cochlear portion of the internal ear contains the organ of Corti (spiral organ), from which nerve impulses arise as a result of the sound waves produced in the fluid in the cochlea by vibration of the stapes. The nerve impulses are conducted to the brain stem by the cochlear division of the vestibulo-cochlear nerve, reaching the auditory area of the cerebral cortex through several synaptic relays or causing reflex responses through connections in the brain stem. Although the present chapter is concerned primarily with the organ of Corti and the central pathways, the main features of the bony and membranous labyrinths are reviewed as an aid in understanding how vibration of the stapes results in stimulation of sensory cells in the organ of Corti

and initiation of nerve impulses traveling to the brain.

BONY AND MEMBRANOUS LABYRINTHS

The bony labyrinth (Fig. 21-1) is in the petrous portion of the temporal bone, which forms a prominent oblique ridge between the middle and posterior cranial fossae. The labyrinth is a system of tunnels within the bone. A preparation such as that represented in Figure 21-1 is made by chipping away the surrounding cancellous bone until only the walls of the tunnels (which are of compact bone) remain. The **fenestra vestibuli** (oval window) in which the foot plate of the stapes fits is in the wall of the **vestibule,** the middle part of the bony labyrinth. The **fenestra cochleae** (round window) is situated below the fenestra vestibuli; it is closed by a thin membrane that makes pressure waves possible

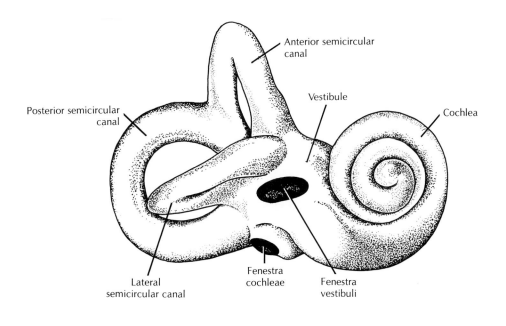

FIGURE 21-1.
Anterolateral view of the right bony labyrinth.

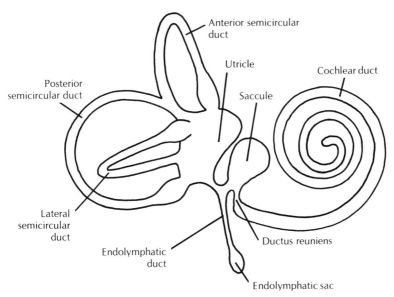

FIGURE 21-2.
Anterolateral view of the right membranous labyrinth.

in the fluid in the internal ear. The fluid would otherwise be enclosed completely in a rigid "box," except for the source of the waves at the fenestra vestibuli. Three **semicircular canals** extend posterolaterally from the vestibule, and the **cochlea** constitutes the anteromedial portion of the bony labyrinth. The cochlea has the shape of a snail shell; its base abuts against the deep end of the internal acoustic meatus, which opens into the posterior cranial fossa. Nerve fibers emerging from the base of the cochlea constitute the cochlear nerve, whereas fibers concerned with the vestibular portion of the internal ear constitute the vestibular nerve. The two divisions of the vestibulocochlear nerve leave the internal acoustic meatus and are attached to the brain stem at the junction of the medulla and pons.

The delicate membranous labyrinth conforms, for the most part, to the contours of the bony labyrinth (Fig. 21-2). However, there are two dilations, the **utricle** and the **saccule,** in the vestibule of the bony labyrinth. Three **semicircular ducts** arise from the utricle. There is a patch of sensory epithelium supplied by the vestibular

nerve on the inner surface of the utricle, the saccule, and each semicircular duct. The saccule is continuous with the **cochlear duct** through a narrow channel known as the ductus reuniens. The cochlear duct contains a highly specialized strip of sensory epithelium along its entire length; this is the organ of Corti (spiral organ), the end organ for hearing.

The lumen of the membranous labyrinth is continuous throughout and filled with **endolymph,** whereas the interval between the membranous and bony labyrinths is filled with **perilymph.** The vestibular portion of the membranous labyrinth is suspended within the bony labyrinth by trabeculae of connective tissue. However, the cochlear duct is firmly attached along two sides to the wall of the cochlear canal.

COCHLEA

The **cochlear canal** makes two and a half turns around a bony pillar or core, the **modiolus,** in which there are channels for nerve fibers and blood vessels. The cochlea is most conveniently described as if it were resting on its base (Fig. 21-3), although its base in fact faces posteromedially.

The cochlear canal, the cavity of this portion of the bony labyrinth, is divided by two partitions into three spiral spaces. The middle of these is the **cochlear duct** (scala media)—that is, the portion of the membranous labyrinth within the cochlea, which contains endolymph. The cochlear duct is firmly fixed to the inner and outer walls of the cochlear canal. The remaining spiral spaces are the **scala vestibuli** and the **scala tympani,** which contain perilymph. The unspecialized wall of the cochlear duct apposing the scala vestibuli is called the **vestibular** or **Reissner's membrane,** whereas the wall apposing the scala tympani constitutes the specialized **basilar membrane,** on which the organ of Corti rests.

The basilar membrane is of special importance in the physiology of hearing because it responds to vibration of the stapes in the following manner. As shown in Figure 21-4, vibration of the foot plate of the stapes produces corresponding waves in the perilymph, beginning with that of the vestibule. The vestibule opens into the scala vestibuli, which communicates with the scala tympani through a small aperture, the **helicotrema,** at the apex of the cochlea. The sound waves may be thought of as passing along the scala vestibuli and into the scala tympani through the helicotrema, causing vibration of the basilar membrane from the scala tympani. However, the helicotrema is a minute orifice, and it is more likely that the basilar membrane vibrates in response to sound waves transmitted through the endolymph in the cochlear duct from the scala vestibuli to the scala tympani. These same waves create a vibration of the membrane closing the fenestra cochleae at the base of the scala tympani; this is essential in order to eliminate the damping of pressure waves in bone-encased fluid that would otherwise occur.

The scala vestibuli and scala tympani are lined by a single layer of squamous cells of mesenchymal origin, with this layer resting on periosteum where the scalae are bounded by the bony labyrinth. The perilymph filling the scala vestibuli and scala tympani is a watery fluid, similar in composition to cerebrospinal fluid. In fact there is a communication between the perilymph-filled spaces of the bony labyrinth and the subarachnoid space. It consists of a narrow channel in the petrous portion of the temporal bone, extending from the scala tympani in the basal turn of the cochlea to an extension of the subarachnoid space around the ninth, tenth, and eleventh cranial nerves as they traverse the jugular foramen.

The **cochlear** or **spiral ganglion** consists of cells in a spiral configuration at the periphery of the modiolus (see Fig. 21-3). The primary sensory neurons of both divisions of the vestibulocochlear nerve are bipolar rather than unipolar as in other cerebrospinal nerves, retaining this embryonic characteristic of primary sensory neurons. The peripheral processes are dendrites in the sense of conduction toward the cell bodies, but in all other characteristics they are axons. These processes reach the organ of Corti by traversing openings in the osseous spiral lamina projecting from the modiolus, where myelin sheaths terminate. The central processes (axons) traverse channels in the modiolus, enter the internal acoustic meatus from the base of the cochlea, and continue in the cochlear division of the vestibulocochlear nerve. There is a small anastomotic connection between the vestibular and cochlear nerves within the external acoustic meatus. As will be seen, this carries efferent nerve fibers to the cochlea.

Cochlear Duct

Certain specialized regions in the wall of the cochlear duct need to be described (Fig. 21-5). The organ of Corti is considered separately because of its complex structure and importance as the receptor of acoustic stimuli.

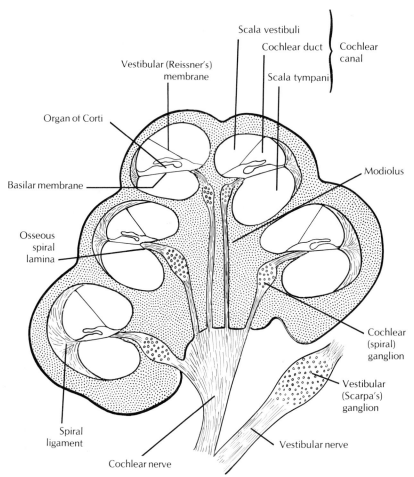

FIGURE 21-3.
Section through the cochlea.

Vibration of the **basilar membrane** is essential in the transduction of a mechanical stimulus (sound waves) to the electrical potential of a nerve impulse in the organ of Corti. The inner edge of the basilar membrane is attached to the **osseous spiral lamina,** which projects from the modiolus like the thread on a screw. The outer edge of the membrane is attached to the **spiral ligament,** consisting of a thickening of the periosteum along the outer wall of the cochlear canal. The basilar membrane consists of collagen fibers and sparse elastic fibers embedded in a ground substance, with most of the fibers being directed across the membrane. The surface presenting to the scala tympani is covered by a thin layer of vascular connective tissue and a single layer of squamous cells. The width of the basilar membrane increases steadily from the beginning of the basal turn of the cochlea to the apex; this is made possible by a progressive narrowing of the osseous spiral lamina and spiral ligament in the same direction. The width of the membrane at any point determines the pitch of sound to which it responds maximally. High tones therefore cause maximal vibration in the basal turn of the cochlea and low tones near the apex. The range of

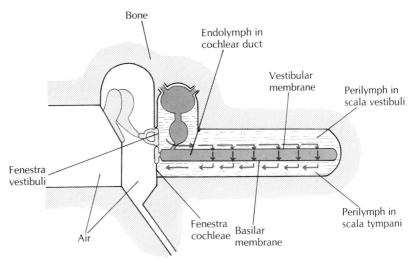

FIGURE 21-4.
Schematic representation of the manner in which sound waves in the perilymph and endolymph cause vibration of the basilar membrane.

audible frequencies in the human ear is from 20 to 20,000 Hz. (With advancing age there is a gradual decrease in perception of high frequencies.) The range extends over 11 octaves, of which 7 are used in musical instruments such as the piano. Ordinary conversation falls within the range of 300 to 3000 Hz.

The **vestibular** or **Reissner's membrane** consists of two layers of simple squamous epithelium separated by a trace of connective tissue. The outer wall of the cochlear duct is specialized as the **stria vascularis**, which consists of cuboidal epithelium overlying vascular connective tissue, and which produces endolymph. This is similar to intracellular fluid in respect to its high concentration of potassium ions and low concentration of sodium ions. Endolymph fills the membranous labyrinth; absorption takes place into venules surrounding the endolymphatic sac in the dura mater on the posterior surface of the petrous portion of the temporal bone. This sac is an expansion of the endolymphatic duct arising from the communication between the saccule and the utricle (see Fig. 21-2).

The epithelial lining of the membranous labyrinth, including the specialized sensory areas for the auditory and vestibular systems, is ectodermal in origin. The epithelium differentiates from the cells lining the **otic vesicle.** This is formed by an invagination of ectoderm at the level of the hindbrain of the early embryo.

Organ of Corti

The **organ of Corti** or **spiral organ** (Fig. 21-5) consists of supporting cells and sensory cells. The latter are specialized for conversion of a mechanical stimulus into the ionic and electrical events that constitute a nerve impulse.

Supporting cells containing bundles of tonofibrils are of two types, pillar cells and phalangeal cells. There are two rows of **pillar cells,** inner and outer, on each side of the **tunnel of Corti.** The number in each row is of the order of 5000. Each cell consists mainly of a compact bundle of tonofibrils (the pillar), extending from the basilar membrane to the surface of the organ of Corti. The tonofibrils appear in electron micrographs as compact arrays of

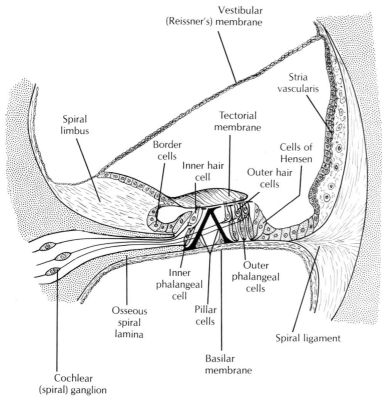

FIGURE 21-5.
Structure of the cochlear duct and spiral organ (organ of Corti).

microtubules. The inner and outer pillars converge, and each pillar ends in a flange directed outward. The nucleus of the pillar cell is in a cytoplasmic region in the acute angle between the pillar and the basilar membrane.

The **phalangeal cells** afford intimate support for the sensory cells; they are arranged as a single row of inner phalangeal cells and three to five rows of outer phalangeal cells, with the number of rows increasing from the base to the apex of the cochlea. The base of the slender flask-shaped phalangeal cell rests on the basilar membrane, and a bundle of tonofibrils extends the length of the cell. Some of the tonofibrils form a supporting shelf for the base of a sensory cell, and the remainder continue alongside a sensory cell. At the surface of the organ of Corti, the tonofibrils of phalangeal and pillar cells form a thin

reticular plate in which holes accommodate the ends of sensory cells. The organ of Corti is completed on the inner side by **border cells** and on the outer side by **cells of Hensen.** The fluid in the tunnel of Corti and the interstitial fluid in much of the organ of Corti have a chemical composition similar to that of perilymph rather than endolymph. The high concentration of potassium ions in endolymph would prevent impulse conduction by the nerve fibers crossing the tunnel of Corti to reach the outer hair cells.

The sensory cells are called **hair cells** because of the hairlike projections from their free ends. There is a single row of inner hair cells, numbering about 7000; the outer hair cells, of which there are some 25,000, are arranged in three rows in the basal turn of the cochlea, increasing to five rows at the apex. The hairs project from the cell along a V- or W-shaped line, with their tips embedded in the tectorial membrane. The number of hairs per cell ranges from 50 to 150, with the largest number on hair cells at the base of the cochlea and the smallest number on cells at the apex. The hairs are microvilli of an unusual type; there is also a single cilium, but this disappears in the adult. The inner and outer hair cells differ in certain details of ultrastructure and innervation. The roles of the inner and outer hair cells are probably different in some respects, although their separate contributions to acoustic input to the brain have yet to be fully determined.

Processes of sensory neurons are in synaptic contact with the hair cells. From 90% to 95% of the sensory neurons in the spiral ganglion have myelinated processes that end upon inner hair cells. Each inner hair cell is contacted by approximately ten such neurons, but each neuron contacts only one inner hair cell. The remaining 5% to 10% of sensory neurons have unmyelinated processes that branch in the organ of Corti. Each outer hair cell is contacted by one such branch.

The cochlear nerve contains efferent fibers originating in the superior olivary nuclei in the pons. These axons terminate on the outer hair cells (where their synaptic terminals outnumber those of the afferent fibers) and upon the preterminal parts of the sensory neurites that innervate the inner hair cells. The efferent axons are inhibitory to both the receptor cells and the sensory fibers.

The **tectorial membrane** is a ribbonlike structure of gelatinous consistency; it is attached to the **spiral limbus,** a thickening of the periosteum on the osseous spiral lamina. The tectorial membrane extends over the organ of Corti, and the tips of the hairs of the sensory cells are embedded in the membrane.

It is basic to the physiology of the cochlea that a particular region of the basilar membrane, depending on the pitch of sound, responds by maximal vibration. Bending of the hairs reduces the membrane potential of the hair cells, causing release of their chemical transmitter and initiation of action potentials in the sensory nerve endings. Regardless of the pitch of sound, vibration of the basilar membrane begins at the base of the cochlea and travels along the membrane with increasing magnitude to a point determined by the pitch. At this point the vibration suddenly dies away, and impulses reaching the brain from the place of maximal stimulation of the organ of Corti are interpreted as a particular pitch of sound. Tonotopic localization is sharpened by the inhibitory effect of efferent fibers in the cochlear nerve and feedback circuits in the central pathway to the auditory cortex. Increase in intensity of sound causes maximal vibration in a larger region of the basilar membrane, thereby activating more hair cells and neurons. Persistent exposure to excessively loud sounds causes degenerative changes in the organ of Corti at the base of the cochlea. This results in high tone deafness, which is prone to occur in workers who are exposed to the sound of compression engines or jet engines and in those who work for long hours on farm tractors. High tone deafness was formerly encountered most frequently among workmen in boiler factories and is still sometimes known as "boiler-makers' disease."

AUDITORY PATHWAYS

The **cochlear nerve** consists principally of axons or central processes of cells in the spiral ganglion, most of which are myelinated. It traverses the internal acoustic meatus in the petrous portion of the temporal bone as a component of the vestibulocochlear nerve. The internal acoustic meatus also contains the labyrinthine artery (a branch of the basilar artery) and the facial nerve. On emerging from the meatus, the cochlear nerve continues to the junction of the medulla and pons. The afferent fibers

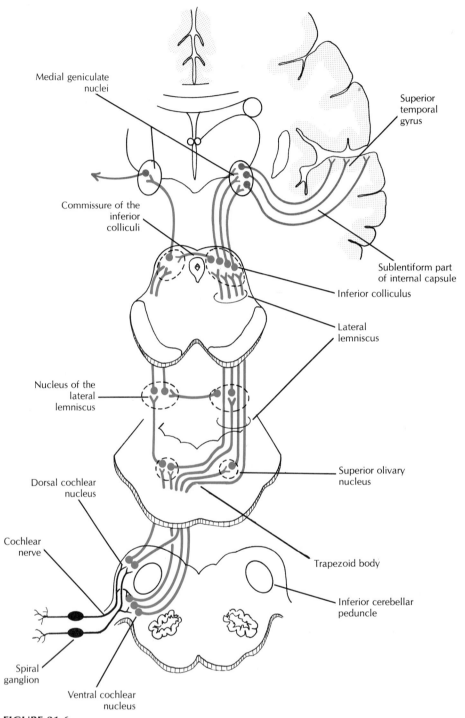

FIGURE 21-6.
The ascending auditory pathway.

then bifurcate, one branch ending in the **dorsal cochlear nucleus** and the other branch in the **ventral cochlear nucleus** (Fig. 21–6). The cochlear nuclei are situated superficially in the rostral end of the medulla adjacent to the base of the inferior cerebellar peduncle. A tonotopic pattern of axonal endings has been demonstrated in both nuclei in experimental animals and probably exists in humans. The dorsal and ventral cochlear nuclei differ in cellular organization, and the pattern of axonal endings in the ventral nucleus is more precise than in the dorsal nucleus. It is therefore probable that the nuclei also differ in their contribution to the central pathways and to the overall functioning of the auditory system.

Pathway to the Auditory Cortex

The pathway to the cerebral cortex is characterized by one or more synaptic relays between the cochlear nuclei and the specific thalamic nucleus for hearing, the medial geniculate nucleus (Fig. 21-6). There is a relay in the inferior colliculus, and additional synaptic interruptions may occur in the superior olivary nucleus and in the nucleus of the lateral lemniscus. The pathway is also characterized by a significant ipsilateral projection to the cortex. In view of the complicated nature of the pathway the transmission of acoustic data to the cortex can best be described after certain components of the pathway in the brain stem have been identified.

The **superior olivary nucleus** is situated in the ventrolateral corner of the dorsal portion or tegmentum of the pons at the level of the motor nucleus of the facial nerve (see Fig. 7-9). (Although considered here as a unit, the nucleus is a complex of four nuclei, whose connections differ in detail.) Auditory fibers that cross the pons in the ventral part of the tegmentum constitute the **trapezoid body;** these fibers pass ventral to the ascending fibers of the medial lemniscus or intersect them. Nerve

cells situated among the transverse fibers on each side constitute the nucleus of the trapezoid body, which is the most medially situated nucleus of the superior olivary complex. The **lateral lemniscus,** the ascending auditory tract, extends from the region of the superior olivary nucleus, through the lateral part of the pontine tegmentum, and close to the surface of the brain stem in the isthmus region between the pons and midbrain. The **nucleus of the lateral lemniscus** consist of cells situated among the fibers of the tract in the pons.*

The projection from the cochlear nuclei to the inferior colliculus and then to the medial geniculate nucleus, through the components of the pathway just identified, is as follows. Fibers from the **ventral cochlear nucleus** proceed to the region of the ipsilateral superior olivary nucleus, in which some of the fibers terminate. The majority continue across the pons, with a slight forward slope; these fibers, together with others contributed by the superior olivary nucleus, constitute the trapezoid body. On reaching the region of the superior olivary nucleus on the other side of the brain stem the fibers either continue into the lateral lemniscus or terminate in the superior olivary nucleus, from which fibers are added to the lateral lemniscus. Fibers from the **dorsal cochlear nucleus** pass over the base of the inferior cerebellar peduncle and continue obliquely to the region of the contralateral superior olivary nucleus. Most of the fibers join the lateral lemniscus; the remainder end in the superior olivary nucleus, from which axons are contributed to the lateral lemniscus. In addition to these, some efferents of the dorsal cochlear nucleus terminate in the ipsilateral superior olivary nucleus.

Impulses conveyed by the lateral lem-

---

* As noted in the appropriate chapters, the cerebellum receives impulses of both acoustic and optic origin, as does the reticular formation of the brain stem in connection with the ascending reticular activating system.

niscus reach the **inferior colliculus** in the midbrain with or without a synaptic relay in the nucleus of the lateral lemniscus. The complexity of neuronal organization in the inferior colliculus indicates that, far from being a simple relay station, it is capable of complex integrative activity. Fibers from the inferior colliculus traverse the inferior brachium and end in all parts of the **medial geniculate nucleus.** (A few fibers of the lateral lemniscus have been described as bypassing the inferior colliculus and proceeding directly through the inferior brachium to the medial geniculate nucleus.) The termination of axons in the ventral part of the medial geniculate nucleus of experimental animals produces a spiral tonotopic pattern corresponding to the spiral of the cochlea, and a similar pattern is probably present in humans.

The last link in the auditory pathway consists of the **auditory radiation** in the sublentiform part of the internal capsule, through which the medial geniculate nucleus projects on the **auditory cortex** of the temporal lobe. This auditory area, corresponding to areas 41 and 42 of Brodmann, is in the floor of the lateral sulcus, extending only slightly on the lateral surface of the hemisphere. A landmark is provided by the two most anterior of the transverse temporal gyri (Heschl's convolutions) on the dorsal surface of the superior temporal gyrus (see Fig. 15–3). The area receives afferent fibers from the tonotopically organized ventral part of the medial geniculate nucleus. The tonotopic pattern in the auditory area is such that fibers for sounds of low frequency end in the anterolateral part of the area, whereas fibers for sounds of high frequency terminate in its posteromedial part. Analysis of acoustic stimuli at a higher neural level, notably the recognition and interpretation of sounds on the basis of past experience, occurs in the auditory association cortex of the temporal lobe (Wernicke's area). In addition to its afferents from the auditory area, the association cortex also receives projections from regions of the medial geniculate nucleus other than from its tonotopically organized ventral part. Wernicke's area, it will be recalled, makes an important contribution to sensory aspects of language as well as functioning as auditory association cortex.

Above the level of the cochlear nuclei the auditory pathway is both crossed and uncrossed, because a significant number of axons from the cochlear nuclei ascend in the lateral lemniscus of the same side. In addition, the nuclei of the lateral lemnisci and the inferior colliculi of the two sides are connected by commissural fibers. Consequently, any loss of hearing that follows a unilateral cortical lesion is so slight as to make detection difficult in audiometric testing. Most lesions in the vicinity of the auditory cortex also involve Wernicke's area and cause receptive aphasia when the dominant hemisphere for language is involved. The latter disability obscures any slight auditory deficiency.

The directions and distances of sources of sound are determined from the discrepancy in time of arrival of the stimulus in the left and right ears. Results obtained from investigations with animals indicate that the different inputs to the brain from the two cochleae are compared and analyzed in the superior olivary nuclei, although the auditory cortex is necessary if the coded information transmitted rostrally from the medulla is to have any meaning. The most severe loss of ability to judge the sources of sounds is that caused by unilateral deafness resulting from disease of the ear. The condition is equivalent to the loss of binocular vision that results from blindness in one eye.

Descending Fibers in the Auditory Pathway

Parallel with the neurons conducting information from the organ of Corti to the auditory cortex, there are descending and efferent neurons that conduct impulses in the reverse direction. The descending connections consist of the following: corticogeniculate fibers, which originate in the auditory and adjoining cortical areas and terminate in all parts of the medial geniculate nucleus; corticocollicular fibers, from the same cortical areas to the inferior colliculi of both sides; colliculoolivary fibers, from the inferior colliculus to the superior olivary nucleus; and colliculocochleonuclear fibers, from the inferior colliculus to the dorsal and ventral cochlear nuclei. Except for the corticocollicular projection, which includes both crossed and uncrossed fibers, these descending pathways are ipsilateral.

As indicated earlier, control is also exerted by the central nervous system over the initiation of nerve impulses in the organ of Corti. Olivocochlear fibers, constituting the **olivocochlear bundle** (of Rasmussen), originate in the superior olivary nuclei. The axons leave the brain stem in the vestibular division of the vestibulocochlear nerve and then cross over into the cochlear division by forming an anastomotic branch, located in the internal acoustic meatus. The endings of these inhibitory fibers, which contain synaptic vesicles, are applied to the outer hair cells and to the terminal parts of the afferent neurites that supply the inner hair cells. The efferent fibers for the outer hair cells originate in both superior olivary nuclei, whereas those for neurites supplying inner hair cells come from the ipsilateral nucleus only.

The central transmission of data from the sensory hair cells is therefore far more than just a relay to the cortex. In the various cell stations of the pathway there is a complex processing of acoustic data that provides for refinement of such qualities as pitch, timbre, and volume of sound perception. In particular, feedback inhibition sharpens the perception of pitch, especially through the olivocochlear bundle. This is accomplished by inhibition in the organ of Corti except for the region in which the basilar membrane is responding by maximal vibration to a particular frequency of sound waves (auditory sharpening). Central inhibition probably suppresses background noise when attention is being concentrated on a particular acoustic stimulus.

Reflexes

A few acoustic fibers from the inferior colliculus pass forward to the superior colliculus, which influences motor neurons of the cervical region of the spinal cord through the tectospinal tract. The superior colliculus also influences neurons of the oculomotor, trochlear, and abducens nuclei through indirect connections in the brain stem. These pathways provide for reflex turning of the head and eyes toward the source of a sudden loud sound.

Fibers from the superior olivary nucleus, and probably from the nucleus of the lateral lemniscus, terminate in the motor nuclei of the trigeminal and facial nerves for reflex contraction of the tensor tympani and stapedius muscles, respectively. Contraction of these muscles in response to loud sounds reduces the vibration of the tympanic membrane and the stapes.

SUGGESTED READING

Békésy G von: Experiments in Hearing. Wever EG (trans). New York, McGraw-Hill, 1960

Brodal A: Neurological Anatomy in Relation to Clinical Medicine, 3rd ed, pp 602–639. New York, Oxford University Press, 1981

Celesia GG: Organization of auditory cortical areas in man. Brain 99:403–414, 1976

Clopton BM, Winfield JA, Flammino FJ: Tonotopic organization: Review and analysis. Brain Res 76:1–20, 1974

Dallos P, Billone MC, Durrant JD, Wong C-y, Raynor S: Cochlear inner and outer hair cells: Functional differences. Science 177:356–358, 1972

Fitzpatrick KA: Cellular architecture and topographic organization of the inferior colliculus of the squirrel monkey. J Comp Neurol 164:185–207, 1975

Kelly JP: Auditory System. Chap 23 in Kandel ER, Schwartz JH (eds): Principles of Neural Science, pp 258–268. New York, Elsevier-North Holland, 1981

Klinke R, Galley N: Efferent innervation of vestibular and auditory pathways. Physiol Rev 54:316–357, 1974

Masterson RB: Neural mechanisms for sound localization. Annu Rev Physiol 46:275–287, 1984

Moskowitz N: Comparative aspects of some features of the central auditory system of primates. Ann NY Acad Sci 167:357–369, 1969

Smith CA, Rasmussen GL: Recent observations on the olivocochlear bundle. Ann Otol Rhinol Laryngol 72:489–506, 1963

Somjen GG: Neurophysiology—The Essentials. Baltimore, Williams & Wilkins, 1983

Spoendlin H: Anatomy and physiology of cochlear innervation. Am J Otolaryngol 6:453–467, 1985

TWENTY-TWO

Vestibular System

Three sources of sensory information are used by the nervous system in the maintenance of equilibrium. These are the eyes, proprioceptive endings throughout the body, and the vestibular portion of the internal ear. The role of the vestibular system, especially in relation to visual information, is illustrated by the individual who has congenital atresia of the vestibular apparatus, usually accompanied by cochlear atresia and deaf–mutism. Such a person can orient himself satisfactorily by visual guidance but becomes disoriented in the dark or if submerged while swimming. In addition, vestibular impulses caused by motion of the head contribute to appropriate movements of the eyes to maintain fixation on an object in the visual field. These functions require the distribution of nerve impulses from the vestibular labyrinth to motor neurons through pathways in the spinal cord, brain stem,

and cerebellum, and there is also a projection to the cerebral cortex.

The static labyrinth represented by the utricle and saccule detects the position of the head with respect to gravity, whereas the kinetic labyrinth represented by the semicircular ducts detects movement of the head. Both parts of the membranous labyrinth function in the maintenance of equilibrium, and the kinetic labyrinth has a special role in coordination of eye movement with movement of the head.

STATIC LABYRINTH

The **utricle** and **saccule** are endolymph-containing dilations of the membranous labyrinth, enclosed by the vestibule of the bony labyrinth (see Figs. 21-1 and 21-2). Except at the maculae or specialized sensory areas, the utricle and saccule are lined by simple cuboidal epithelium derived

325

from the otic vesicle of the embryo and supported by a thin layer of connective tissue. The utricle and saccule are suspended from the wall of the vestibule by connective tissue trabeculae, and they are surrounded by a perilymphatic space lined by a single layer of squamous cells of mesenchymal origin.

Each dilation includes a specialized area of sensory epithelium, the macula, about 2 mm by 3 mm in size. The **macula utriculi** is in the floor of the utricle and parallel with the base of the skull, whereas the **macula sacculi** is vertically disposed on the medial wall of the saccule. The two maculae are histologically identical (Fig. 22-1).

The columnar supporting cells of the maculae are continuous with the cuboidal epithelium lining the utricle and saccule elsewhere. The sensory **hair cells,** of which two types have been identified in electron micrographs, are basically similar to hair cells in the organ of Corti. Type 1 hair cells are flask-shaped, whereas type 2

hair cells are cylindrical. From 40 to 80 hairs project from each cell, together with a cilium (kinocilium) that arises from a centriole (Fig. 22-2*A*). The hairs are microvilli of an unusual type, similar to those of hair cells in the organ of Corti except for their greater length, which may be as much as 100 μm. Bundles of the hairs are the "stereocilia" of light microscopy. The tips of the hairs and cilium are embedded in the gelatinous **otolithic membrane,** in which there are irregularly shaped concretions composed of protein and calcium carbonate. These are variously known as otoliths, otoconia, statoliths, and statoconia.

The cell bodies of the primary sensory neurons are in the **vestibular ganglion** (Scarpa's ganglion), situated at the bottom of the internal acoustic meatus. The peripheral processes, which are dendrites in the sense of conduction toward the cell body but are otherwise like axons, enter the maculae with loss of myelin sheaths and end on the hair cells. The nerve terminals on type 1 hair cells take the form

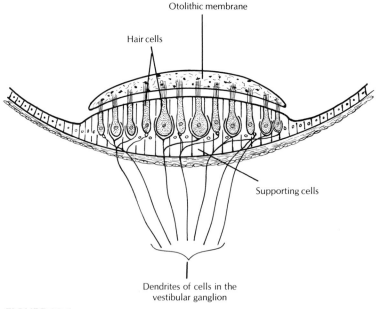

FIGURE 22-1.
Structure of the macula utriculi.

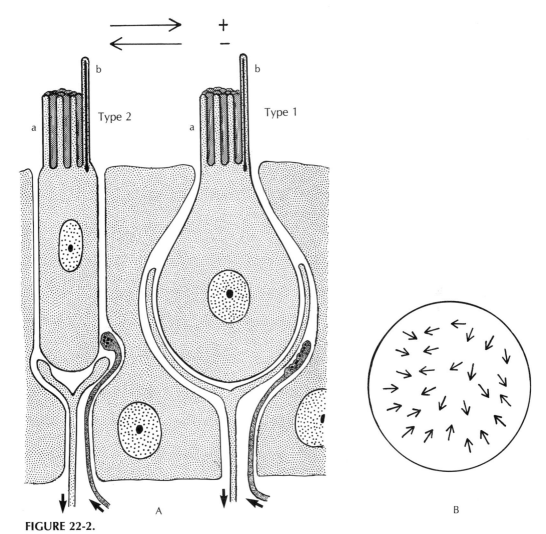

FIGURE 22-2.
(A) Simplified sketch of the two types of hair cell in the macula. Excitation occurs when the hairs or microvilli *(a)* bend in the direction of the cilium *(b)*, whereas inhibition of the hair cells occurs when the hairs bend in the opposite direction.   **(B)** Surface of the macula, showing that hair cells in different regions are stimulated and different nerve fibers activated according to the direction of gravitational pull on the otolithic membrane. This pattern is caused by variations in the position of the cilium relative to the tuft of hairs from one region of the macula to another. Each arrow indicates the direction of gravitational pull for stimulation of hair cells in that location.

of chalicelike branches surrounding the cells, whereas minute terminal swellings make the synaptic contact with type 2 hair cells. In addition, efferent fibers in the vestibular nerve terminate as presynaptic boutons on the type 2 hair cells and on the sensory nerve endings that contact the type 1 cells. These inhibitory fibers originate in the superior and medial vestibular nuclei of the brain stem and possibly also in the fastigial nucleus of the cerebellum.

The otoliths give the otolithic membrane a higher specific gravity than the endolymph, thereby causing bending of the hairs in one direction or another except when the macula is in a strictly horizontal plane. The detailed sensory output of the macula is, however, quite complicated. In each hair cell the cilium is situated at one side of the tuft of hairs, and the position of the cilium at the periphery of the hairs differs from one region of the macula to another. The hair cells are excited when the hairs and the cilium are bent in the direction of the cilium, and they are inhibited when the deflection is in the opposite direction (see Fig. 22-2A). The pattern of afferent impulses conducted by the fibers of the vestibular nerve to the vestibular nuclei and the cerebellum differs, therefore, according to the orientation of the macula to the direction of gravitational pull (Fig. 22-2B). The appropriate changes in muscle tonus follow, as required to maintain equilibrium.

Although the macula is predominantly a static organ, the higher specific gravity of the otolithic membrane with respect to the endolymph allows the macula to respond to quick tilting movements of the head and to rapid linear acceleration and deceleration. Motion sickness is caused predominantly by prolonged, fluctuating stimulation of the maculae. The utricle and saccule are not as efficient sensors of orientation in humans as they are in some lower animals. This is illustrated by the pilot flying a small aircraft without the aid of instruments, whose intended level flight through clouds may be altered considerably without the pilot's being aware of it.

KINETIC LABYRINTH

The three semicircular ducts are attached to the utricle and are enclosed in the semicircular canals of the bony labyrinth (see Figs. 21-1 and 21-2). The **anterior** and **posterior semicircular ducts** are in vertical planes, with the former being transverse to and the latter parallel with the long axis of the petrous portion of the temporal bone. The **lateral semicircular duct** slopes downward and backward at an angle of 30 degrees to the horizontal plane. The semicircular ducts of the two sides form spatial pairs; the lateral ducts are in the same plane, and the anterior vertical duct of one side and the posterior vertical duct of the opposite side are in the same plane. The sensory areas of the semicircular ducts respond only to movement; the response is maximal when movement is in the plane of the duct.

Each semicircular duct has an expansion or **ampulla** at one end, in which the **crista ampullaris** or sensory epithelium is supported by a transverse septum of connective tissue (Fig. 22-3). Situated among the columnar supporting cells are the sensory **hair cells,** whose structural details and mode of innervation conform to those already described for hair cells of the static labyrinth. The hairs and cilium of each hair cell are embedded in gelatinous material that forms the **cupula,** in which otoliths are lacking.

The cristae are sensors of movement of the head, as has been indicated. More specifically they respond to rotary movement, sometimes called angular movement, especially when accompanied by acceleration or deceleration. At the beginning of movement in or near the plane of a semicircular duct the endolymph lags because of inertia, and the cupula swings like a door in a direction opposite to that of the movement of the head. The momentum of the endolymph causes the cupula to swing momentarily in the opposite direction when the movement ceases. The hairs and cilium of the sensory cells bend accordingly. Depending on the direction of movement, this may reduce the membrane potentials of the hair cells, causing release of their chemical transmitter and the initiation of action potentials in the sensory nerve endings.

The cilium is consistently on the side

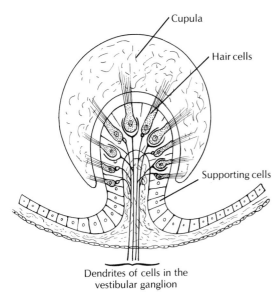

Cupula

Hair cells

Supporting cells

Dendrites of cells in the
vestibular ganglion

FIGURE 22-3.
Structure of the crista ampullaris.

of the tuft of hairs nearest the opening of the ampulla into the utricle. The excitation of hair cells noted above therefore occurs when the flow of endolymph is from the ampulla into the adjacent utricle, whereas there is inhibition of the hair cells when the flow is in the opposite direction. (There is a slight tonic discharge from the hair cells of both the maculae and cristae, even in the absence of bending of the hairs.) The hair cells of the cristae, similar to those of the maculae, are supplied by primary sensory neurons whose bipolar cell bodies are in the **vestibular ganglion.** The pattern of nerve conduction—that is, the particular fibers of the vestibular nerve that are conducting impulses to the vestibular nuclei and cerebellum at any given moment—varies according to the plane in which the head is moving.

VESTIBULAR PATHWAYS

On entering the brain stem at the junction of the medulla and pons, most of the vestibular nerve fibers bifurcate in the usual manner of afferent fibers and end in the vestibular nuclear complex. The remaining fibers enter the cerebellum through the inferior cerebellar peduncle.

Vestibular Nuclei

The vestibular nuclei are situated in the rostral part of the medulla, partly beneath the area vestibuli or lateral area of the floor of the fourth ventricle and extending slightly into the pons (Fig. 22-4). Four vestibular nuclei are recognized on the basis of cytoarchitecture and the details of afferent and efferent connections. The **lateral vestibular nucleus,** also known as **Deiters' nucleus,** consists mainly of large multipolar neurons that resemble typical motor neurons; they have widely branching dendrites, long axons, and prominent Nissl bodies. The **superior, medial,** and **inferior vestibular nuclei** consist of small and medium-sized cells.

Connections with the Cerebellum

The vestibular portion of the cerebellum consists of the flocculonodular lobe, adjacent region of the inferior vermis, and fastigial nuclei. The **vestibulocerebellum** receives fibers from the superior, medial, and inferior vestibular nuclei in addition to receiving a modest number of fibers directly from the vestibular nerve. In the reverse direction fibers from the vestibulocerebellum terminate throughout the vestibular nuclear complex. These afferent and efferent fibers of the vestibulocerebellum occupy the medial portion of the inferior cerebellar peduncle. The role of the cerebellum in maintaining equilibrium is exerted mainly through pathways from the vestibular nuclei to the spinal cord.

Connections with the Spinal Cord

The connection between the vestibular nuclei and the spinal cord is through de-

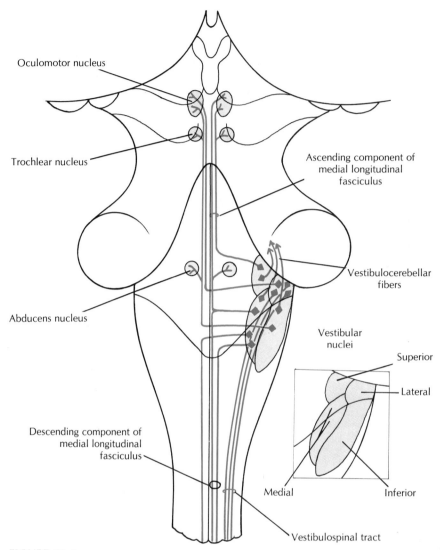

FIGURE 22-4.
Vestibular pathways to the spinal cord and to the nuclei of the abducens, trochlear, and oculomotor nerves.

scending fibers in the vestibulospinal tract and the medial longitudinal fasciculus. (These tracts are sometimes referred to as the lateral and medial vestibulospinal tracts, respectively.)

The **vestibulospinal tract,** which is uncrossed, originates in the lateral vestibular or Deiters' nucleus exclusively. The fibers descend in the medulla dorsal to the in-

ferior olivary nucleus and continue into the ventral funiculus of the spinal cord. Vestibulospinal fibers terminate for the most part in laminae VII and VIII at all levels of the spinal cord, but most abundantly in the cervical and lumbosacral enlargements. A few vestibulospinal fibers synapse with motor neurons in the medial part of the ventral horn (lamina IX) that supply the axial musculature. This tract is of prime importance in regulating muscle tonus so that balance is maintained.

Fibers from the medial vestibular nucleus project toward the midline and turn caudally in the **medial longitudinal fasciculi** of both sides. This fasciculus is adjacent to the midline, close to the floor of the fourth ventricle, and ventral to the central canal of the medulla more caudally. The fibers continue into the medial part of the ventral funiculus of the spinal cord; they influence cervical motor neurons so that the head moves in such a way as to assist in maintaining equilibrium.

Connections within the Brain Stem

The ascending portion of the **medial longitudinal fasciculus** is situated adjacent to the midline in the pons and midbrain, ventral to the floor of the fourth ventricle and the periaqueductal gray matter. The constituent fibers connect the vestibular nuclei with the nuclei of the abducens, trochlear, and oculomotor nerves, and with the accessory oculomotor nuclei of the midbrain. Some of the ascending fibers are uncrossed; others cross the midline at the level of the vestibular nuclei. This portion of the medial longitudinal fasciculus provides for conjugate movement of the eyes, coordinated with movement of the head, to maintain visual fixation. Impulses received by the vestibular nuclei from the cristae ampullares of the kinetic labyrinth are responsible for the ocular adjustments to movement of the head.

The medial longitudinal fasciculus also contains fibers interconnecting the nuclei of the third, fourth, and sixth cranial nerves, and fibers that originate in the paramedian pontine reticular formation (PPRF). These connections, and the effects of lesions of the medial longitudinal fasciculus, are described in Chapter 8.

Excessive or prolonged stimulation of the vestibular system may cause nausea and vomiting. The connections responsible for these effects appear to be collateral branches of efferent fibers from vestibular nuclei, with the branches ending in visceral "centers" and in parasympathetic nuclei in the brain stem. Excessive input from the labyrinth to the vestibular nuclei is probably reduced to some extent by a feedback through the efferent inhibitory fibers in the vestibular nerve. The neural mechanisms governing visceral responses to vestibular stimulation are in fact quite complicated because of the frequent involvement of psychological and emotional factors.

Cortical Representation

Although the vestibular system functions mainly at the levels of the brain stem, cerebellum, and spinal cord, there is a significant pathway from the vestibular nuclei to the cerebral cortex. However, the experimental and clinical evidence concerning the location of the cortical area is conflicting.

Evoked potentials have been recorded in the parietal lobe of the monkey during electrical stimulation of the vestibular nerve. The area thus identified as receiving vestibular information is adjacent to the general sensory area for the head. Sensations of turning or body displacement have been elicited in humans by stimulation of the corresponding area of cortex. It has been stated also that a vestibular area is present in the superior temporal gyrus, anterior to the auditory area. This was based on occasional reports of vertigo or a feeling of dizziness on electrical stimulation of this part of the gyrus in conscious patients, and the occurrence of the same sensation in temporal lobe epilepsy. However, caloric stimulation of the kinetic labyrinth causes a regional increase in blood flow in the superior temporal gyrus posterior to the auditory area, with no such change being recorded from either of the areas to which vestibular function has previously been ascribed.

The ascending pathway from the vestibular nuclei is predominantly crossed, and runs close to the medial lemniscus. The thalamic relay for the cortical projection, wherever that area may be, is thought to be in or near the portion of the ventral posterior nucleus that receives somatosensory fibers for the head (VPm). A vestibular cortical field would contribute information for use in higher motor regulation, and for conscious spatial orientation.

TESTS APPLIED TO THE VESTIBULAR SYSTEM

The vestibular projections to nuclei that supply extraocular muscles and motor neurons in the spinal cord can be demonstrated by strong stimulation of the labyrinth. This may be done by rotating a subject around a vertical axis about ten times in 20 sec, and then stopping the rotation abruptly. The responses are most pronounced if the head is bent forward 30 degrees to bring the lateral semicircular ducts in a horizontal plane. On stopping rotation, momentum acquired by the endolymph causes it to flow past (and deflect) the cupulae of the lateral semicircular ducts more suddenly and rapidly than for most movements.

The responses of the hair cells in the cristae ampullares produce the following signs immediately after rotation ceases. Impulses conveyed by the ascending fibers of the medial longitudinal fasciculus cause nystagmus—that is, a slight oscillatory movement of the eyes consisting of fast and slow components. The direction of nystagmus, right or left, is designated by that of the fast component, which is opposite to the direction of rotation. The subject deviates in the direction of rotation if asked to walk in a straight line, and the finger deviates in the same direction on pointing to an object. These responses are

caused by the effect of vestibulospinal projections on muscle tonus. There is a subjective feeling of turning in a direction opposite to that of rotation, for which both the cortical projection and the nystagmus are presumably responsible. The spread of impulses to visceral centers may produce sweating and pallor, and even nausea in those who are more susceptible.

The **caloric test** is used when there is a reason to suspect a tumor of the vestibulocochlear nerve or a lesion interrupting the vestibular pathway in the brain stem. This procedure has the distinct advantage of testing the pathway from each internal ear separately. The head is positioned so that the lateral semicircular duct is in a vertical plane, and the external acoustic meatus is irrigated with warm or cold water, usually the latter. The ampulla of the duct is near the bone that is undergoing a change of temperature, and the endolymph "rises" or "falls," depending on whether it is warmed or cooled. The procedure causes nystagmus if the vestibular pathway for the side tested is intact.

Labyrinthine irritation or disease may cause vertigo, sometimes accompanied by nausea and vomiting, pallor, a cold sweat, and nystagmus. Paroxysms of labyrinthine irritation constitute Ménière's disease, the cause of which is usually obscure.

SUGGESTED READING

Bender MB: Brain control of conjugate horizontal and vertical eye movements. A survey of the structural and functional correlates. Brain 103:23–69, 1980

Dechesne C, Raymond J, Sans A: The efferent vestibular system in the cat: A horseradish peroxidase and fluorescent retrograde tracers study. Neuroscience 11:893–901, 1984

Deeke L, Schwarz DWF, Fredrickson JM: Nucleus ventroposterior inferior (VPI) as the vestibular thalamic relay in the Rhesus monkey. I. Field potential investigation. Exp Brain Res 200:80–100, 1974

Friberg L, Olsen IS, Roland PE, Paulson OB, Lassen NA: Focal increase of blood flow in the cerebral cortex of man during vestibular stimulation. Brain 108:609–623, 1985

Friedland RP (ed): Selected Papers of Morris B. Bender. Memorial Volume. New York, Raven Press, 1983

Hudspeth AJ: Mechanoelectric transduction by hair cells in the acousticolateralis sensory system. Annu Rev Neurosci 6:187–215, 1983

Penfield W: Vestibular sensation and the cerebral cortex. Ann Otol Rhinol Laryngol 66:691–698, 1957

TWENTY-THREE

Motor Systems

Except for some aspects of visceral function, overt expression of activity in the central nervous system depends on the somatic or skeletal musculature. The muscles are supplied by the motor neurons in the ventral horns of the spinal cord and in the motor nuclei of cranial nerves, with these neurons constituting the final common pathway (Sherrington) for determining muscle action. They are collectively known as the **lower motor neuron,** especially in clinical medicine. Another clinical expression is **upper motor neuron,** which embraces all the descending pathways of the brain and spinal cord involved in the volitional control of the musculature.

Components of the brain responsible for the execution of properly coordinated movements include the cerebral cortex, corpus striatum, thalamus, subthalamic nucleus, red nucleus, substantia nigra, reticular formation, vestibular nuclei, inferior olivary complex, and cerebellum. The connections of these structures have been described elsewhere in this book, but here they are reviewed with particular attention to their influence upon the lower motor neuron.

LOWER MOTOR NEURON AND MUSCLES

Skeletal muscles are supplied by motor neurons of two types, named **alpha** and **gamma** after the diameters of their axons. The large alpha motor neurons innervate the extrafusal fibers that constitute the main mass of the muscle, in which the axon of each neuron branches to supply the muscle fibers. The number supplied by a single neuron varies from only a few for small muscles whose contractions are precisely controlled to several hundred for large muscles that carry out strong but crude movements. An alpha motor neuron and the muscle fibers it supplies constitute a **motor unit.**

Three different types of **extrafusal muscle fiber** are recognized on the basis of physiological and histochemical studies. The type I fibers contract slowly, are resistant to fatigue, and contain little stainable myofibrillar adenosine triphosphatase. Type II fibers have faster contractions, are more rapidly fatigued than those of type I, and have high concentrations of adenosine triphosphatase in their myofibrils. Using other histochemical criteria, the type II muscle fibers are further divided into types IIA and IIB. All the muscle fibers in a motor unit are of the same type, and experimental evidence indicates that the type of fiber is determined by trophic influence of the innervating neuron. In addition to secreting acetylcholine to make the muscle fibers it supplies contract, a motor neuron provides trophic factors, which direct the differentiation of the muscle fibers and are necessary for their continued health. Proteins with myotrophic properties have been isolated from extracts of peripheral nerves.

The different types of muscle fiber respond differently to denervation: type IIB fibers atrophy most rapidly and type I fibers most slowly.

Intrafusal muscle fibers supplied by gamma motor neurons control the length and tension of the neuromuscular spindles. The gamma motor neurons are much less numerous than the alpha motor neurons but are nevertheless important because their patterns of firing determine the thresholds of the sensory nerve endings in the spindles. These endings are the receptors for the spinal stretch reflex, which is ordinarily suppressed as a result of activity in the descending tracts of the spinal cord. The muscle spindles are also receptors for the conscious awareness of position and movement.

LOWER MOTOR NEURON LESIONS

The syndrome of a lower motor neuron lesion occurs when a muscle is paralyzed or weakened as a result of disease or injury affecting the cell bodies or axons of the innervating neurons. Typical causes include poliomyelitis, in which a virus selectively attacks ventral horn cells or equivalent neurons in the brain stem, and injuries to peripheral nerves that transect some or all of the axons. The following clinical features are observed.

1. The muscle tonus is reduced or absent (flaccid paresis or paralysis), owing to interruption of the efferent limb of the tonic stretch reflex.
2. The tendon-jerk reflexes are weak or absent. The cause is the same as that of the flaccidity.
3. The muscles supplied by the affected neurons atrophy progressively. The atrophy is due partly to loss of specific trophic factors normally provided by the motor nerve, and partly to disuse.
4. Fibrillation potentials, caused by random contractions of isolated denervated muscle fibers, can be detected by electromyography. Fibrillation should not be confused with fasciculation, which is visible twitching that occurs at irregular intervals within a muscle. Fasciculation is a rather unreliable diagnostic sign, being quite common in normal muscles.
5. In a partially denervated muscle, the intact nerve fibers sprout at nodes of Ranvier and at motor end plates, with some of the new axonal branches innervating denervated muscle fibers. These changes can be seen in a suitably stained biopsy specimen.

Signs similar to those of a lower motor neuron lesion occur in diseases of muscle in which synaptic transmission at the motor end plate is impaired (myasthenia gravis) or in which the contractile elements function inadequately (various forms of dystrophy, myopathy, and myositis). Biopsy and neurophysiological testing are used when a differential diagnosis cannot be made using clinical criteria.

DESCENDING PATHWAYS TO THE SPINAL CORD

Motor neurons in the spinal cord are influenced by descending fibers from the cerebral cortex, central nuclei of the reticular formation, and the lateral vestibular nucleus. Large tracts of fibers from these sites descend in the lateral and ventral funiculi of the spinal cord. Smaller contingents of descending fibers come from the superior colliculus, medial vestibular nucleus, and certain nuclei in the midbrain.

Corticospinal Tracts

The corticospinal tracts (Figs. 23-1 and 23-2) consist of the axons of cells in the primary motor and premotor areas of the frontal lobe and in the parietal lobe, including the first sensory area. The corticospinal fibers pass through the medullary center, converging as they enter the posterior limb of the internal capsule—that is, the band of white matter between the lentiform nucleus and thalamus. It also contains fibers descending from the cortex to the red nucleus, reticular formation, pontine nuclei, and inferior olivary complex, together with many thalamocortical, corticothalamic, and corticostriate fibers. As will be seen, all these populations of fibers are involved in the control of movement. The corticospinal fibers give off collateral branches to the neostriatum and the thalamus within the internal capsule.

The internal capsule continues into the basis pedunculi of the midbrain. At this level some of the corticospinal axons give off branches that terminate in the red nu-

cleus. The corticospinal fibers occupy the middle three fifths of the basis pedunculi, flanked on each side by and partially intermingled with corticopontine fibers. On reaching the ventral (basal) portion of the pons, the corticospinal tract breaks up into fasciculi that pass caudally with the bundles of corticopontine fibers. At this level some of the corticospinal fibers have collateral branches that synapse with neurons of the pontine nuclei. Such collaterals are greatly outnumbered, however, by direct corticopontine fibers. Other branches from the corticospinal fibers end in the reticular formation of the pons and medulla.

At the caudal limit of the pons the corticospinal axons reassemble to form, on the ventral surface of the medulla, the eminence known as the pyramid. The corticospinal fibers are therefore said to constitute the **pyramidal tract.** The term **pyramidal system** is applied to the corticospinal tracts and the functionally equivalent **corticobulbar (corticonuclear) fibers,** which end in and near the motor nuclei of cranial nerves. At the caudal end of the medulla, about 85% of the corticospinal fibers cross the midline in the decussation of the pyramids and enter the dorsolateral funiculus of the spinal cord, where they form the **lateral corticospinal tract.** The remaining 15% of the pyramidal fibers constitute the **ventral corticospinal tract,** which descends ipsilaterally in the medial part of the ventral funiculus. However, the relative sizes of the two corticospinal tracts are variable. In a small percentage of the population a much larger than usual proportion of the fibers descend ipsilaterally in the ventral tract. Most of them cross the midline at segmental levels and terminate in the gray matter contralateral to their hemisphere of origin.

Within the gray matter, corticospinal axons terminate in the dorsal horn (laminae IV, V, and VI) and in the base of the ventral horn (lamina VII). A few of the fibers pass into the columns of cells that constitute lamina IX and synapse directly with the

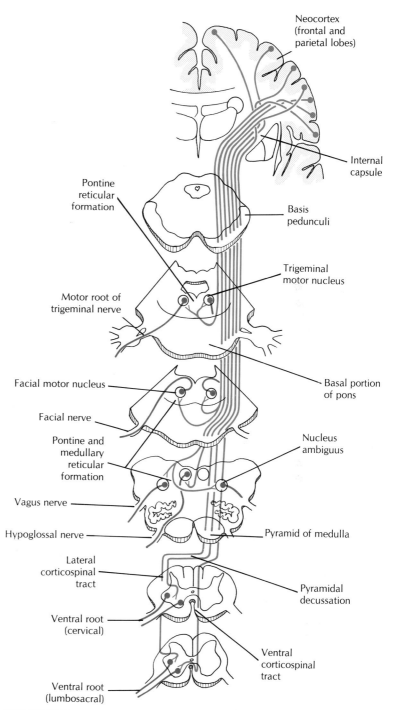

FIGURE 23-1.

The pyramidal system. The corticobulbar and corticospinal neurons are shown in blue and the motor neurons ("lower motor neuron") in red.

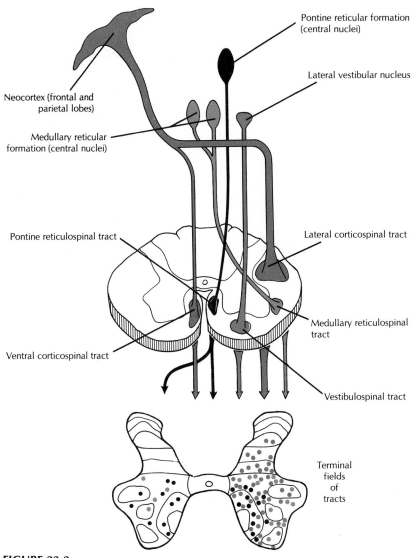

FIGURE 23-2.
Origins, courses, and sites of termination of the major descending pathways concerned with the control of movement.

cell bodies of motor neurons. However, the great majority of corticospinal fibers are able to influence motor neurons only through the mediation of interneurons in the spinal gray matter. Some corticospinal fibers originate in the first somesthetic area of the parietal lobe. These are not motor in function, but instead modulate the transmission of data through general sensory pathways. These fibers end mainly in laminae IV and V. (The positions of the laminae of Rexed are shown in Figure 5–6.)

Selective transection of the monkey's pyramidal tract, which can be best accomplished in the medulla, results in reduced tone in the contralateral musculature and clumsiness in the use of the hands and feet for actions requiring discrete movements of individual fingers and toes. Recovery occurs over the course of a few months but is never complete. The hypotonia is evidently caused by a decreased rate of tonic discharge of gamma motor neurons, with consequent reduction of the sensory input to the cord from the neuromuscular spindles. The stretch reflexes, however, are not abnormal. Neurosurgeons have cut through the middle part of the basis pedunculi in attempts to relieve certain dyskinesias. The effects of this surgical lesion are similar to those of transection of the pyramid in monkeys. These observations indicate that the most important function of the pyramidal tract is to control the precision and speed of skilled movements.

Reticulospinal Tracts

Each half of the spinal cord contains two reticulospinal tracts (Fig. 23-2). Both consist of the axons of cells in the central group of nuclei of the reticular formation. The **pontine reticulospinal tract** arises ipsilaterally in the oral and caudal pontine reticular nuclei. It travels in the ventral funiculus, and its fibers terminate bilaterally in lamina VIII and in the adjacent part of lamina VII. The **medullary reticulospinal tract** originates in the gigantocellular reticular nuclei on both sides of the medulla. The tract descends in the ventral half of the lateral funiculus. Its fibers nearly all end bilaterally in lamina VII; a few of them enter lamina IX, which contains the cell bodies of the motor neurons.

The central nuclei of the reticular formation have several known afferent connections. Fibers from the motor and general sensory regions of the cerebral cortex descend in the internal capsule and cerebral peduncle and are then distributed bilaterally to the reticular formation. Spinoreticular fibers, which are both crossed and uncrossed, and afferents from the ipsilateral cerebellum and lateral group of

reticular nuclei may also be presumed to influence the cells of origin of the reticulospinal tracts.

Within the brain stem the reticulospinal axons have many branches. The short ones synapse with other neurons of the reticular formation; the long branches ascend, often as far as the intralaminar thalamic nuclei. Branching has also been demonstrated in the spinal cord, so that a single axon may have terminations in cervical, thoracic, and lumbar segments. This observation has led to the suggestion that the reticulospinal tracts control coordinated movements of muscles supplied from different segmental levels of the spinal cord, such as those of the upper and lower limbs in walking, running, and swimming. Long propriospinal (spinospinalis) fibers may also be important for synchronization of the movements of the limbs. Electrical stimulation of the regions containing the cell bodies of origin of the reticulospinal tracts results in either excitation or inhibition of either alpha or gamma motor neurons, depending on the exact site of stimulation.

Information about the reticulospinal tracts is derived almost entirely from research with animals. The anatomy of the tracts is constant over a wide phylogenetic range of mammals, so it is likely to hold true also for humans. In view of what is known of other major descending pathways, it seems probable that the reticulospinal tracts mediate control over most movements that do not require dexterity or the maintenance of balance.

Vestibulospinal Tract

This tract (Fig. 23-2), which arises ipsilaterally from the large cells of the lateral vestibular nucleus (Deiters' nucleus), is also known as the lateral vestibulospinal tract. It is composed of myelinated axons of large caliber descending in the ventral funiculus of the spinal white matter. The fibers terminate in the ventral part of lamina VII and in lamina VIII of the gray matter. Some vestibulospinal fibers synapse with the dendrites of both gamma and alpha motor neurons. These dendrites extend outside the territory of lamina IX, which contains their cell bodies, into the adjacent parts of laminae VII and VIII.

Electrical stimulation of the lateral vestibular nucleus in animals causes contraction of ipsilateral extensor muscles of the limbs and spinal column, with relaxation of the flexors. These effects occur to a lesser extent contralaterally as well—a consequence, no doubt, of the fact that many of the neurons in lamina VIII have axons that cross the midline of the spinal cord. Transection of the brain stem above the vestibular nuclei causes a condition known as **decerebrate rigidity,** in which the extensor musculature of the whole body is in a continuous state of contraction. This condition is easily produced in experimental animals and occasionally occurs in patients who have large destructive lesions of the midbrain or upper pons. The extensor spasm is abolished by destruction of the lateral vestibular nucleus, indicating that it is caused by the unopposed excessive activity of vestibulospinal neurons. The principal sources of afferent fibers to the lateral vestibular nucleus are the vestibular nerve, fastigial nucleus of the cerebellum, and vestibulocerebellar cortex. There are no afferents from the cerebral cortex.

The physiological, pathological, and neuroanatomical data summarized above all support the view that the vestibulospinal tract is concerned with the maintenance of upright posture, which results mainly from the action of the extensor muscles in opposing gravity. Orderly functioning of the "antigravity" musculature is essential for balance, both at rest and during locomotion. Although the vestibulospinal tract does not mediate "voluntary" movements dictated by the cerebral cortex, it is essential for such highly skilled

accomplishments of motor coordination as the feats of a gymnast or an acrobat. The learning of those aspects of skilled movement that involve posture and balance, and which are effected through the vestibulospinal tract, probably occur in neuronal circuits that include the inferior olivary complex of nuclei and the cerebellum.

Other Descending Tracts

Two tracts in the medial part of the ventral funiculus terminate throughout the cervical segments of the spinal cord. These are the **tectospinal tract,** from the contralateral superior colliculus, and the descending component of the **medial longitudinal fasciculus.** The latter, which is sometimes called the medial vestibulospinal tract, arises from the medial vestibular nuclei of both sides, but is mainly ipsilateral. Both tracts influence the activity of neurons innervating the muscles of the neck, including those supplied by the accessory nerve. The tectospinal tract and the descending portion of the medial longitudinal fasciculus function in effecting movements of the head as required for fixation of gaze and maintaining equilibrium, respectively. The small **interstitiospinal tract,** from the interstitial nucleus of Cajal and the Edinger–Westphal nucleus in the midbrain, extends along the whole length of the spinal cord and is probably involved in visuomotor coordination. It too is located in the medial part of the ventral funiculus.

Several other small fasciculi run caudally from the brain into the spinal cord, but there is no reason to believe that they are involved in the control of skeletal muscle. The rubrospinal tract provides a pathway of some importance in lower mammals. In humans, however, it is very small, goes no further caudally than the second cervical segment, and is therefore of little significance.

DESCENDING PATHWAYS TO MOTOR NUCLEI OF CRANIAL NERVES

Almost all of the muscles supplied by the cranial nerves participate in voluntarily initiated movements, and some of them are controlled with exquisite precision.

As described in Chapter 8, the oculomotor, trochlear, and abducens nuclei receive afferents through a complicated system of connections involving the cortex of the frontal and occipital lobes, superior colliculus, and various nuclei in the brain stem. It will be recalled that the cerebral cortex controls coordinated movements of the eyes. The frontal eye fields are necessary for changing the direction of gaze voluntarily. The occipital cortex controls involuntary conjugate movements, as when tracking a moving object, and is also necessary for convergence of the eyes to look at a near object.

Knowledge of the afferent connections of the other motor nuclei of cranial nerves is less complete. The nuclei concerned are the trigeminal and facial motor nuclei, nucleus ambiguus, and hypoglossal nucleus. Results of studies in animals indicate that **corticobulbar (corticonuclear) fibers** from the motor areas of the cortex end mainly in the reticular formation near the motor nuclei, with a few contacting the motor neurons directly (see Fig. 23–1). These fibers constitute part of the pyramidal system, and are presumably equivalent to corticospinal fibers. The motor nuclei also receive afferents from the reticular formation that are probably equivalent to the reticulospinal tracts. Therefore, upper motor neuron paralysis or paresis, caused by a lesion in the internal capsule, for example, is due to interruption of both corticobulbar and corticoreticular fibers.

Clinical study of the muscles of the head in patients who have destructive lesions in one cerebral hemisphere has yielded information that is anatomically vague but diagnostically useful. With a unilateral lesion in the motor cortex or in the posterior limb of the internal capsule, the only paralyzed muscles in the head are those of the lower half of the face (moving the lips and cheeks), contralaterally. The contralateral tongue muscles are affected as well, although weak contractions usually persist. The muscles supplied by the trigeminal motor nucleus, rostral portion of the facial motor nucleus, and nucleus ambiguus are not affected on either side by a unilateral lesion in the cerebral hemisphere. It has been deduced that descending pathways are distributed bilaterally to all the motor nuclei of the brain stem except the caudal portion of the facial motor nucleus, which receives only crossed descending afferents. Partial deafferentation of the bilaterally supplied nuclei is evidently compensated for by the intact connections from the ipsilateral hemisphere, with those to the hypoglossal nucleus being least effective.

UPPER MOTOR NEURON LESIONS

The term "upper motor neuron" is unsatisfactory because it refers collectively to descending pathways that make different contributions to the voluntary control of muscle action. The term is still useful in clinical medicine, however, because it is often necessary to determine whether a group of muscles is weakened or paralyzed as a result of denervation or as a consequence of some lesion in the central nervous system. An infarction in the posterior limb of the internal capsule, for example, results in the typical signs of an upper motor neuron lesion. Similar abnormalities occur below the level of a lesion that partly or completely transects the spinal cord. The clinical features of an upper motor neuron lesion are as follows.

1. Voluntary movements of the affected muscles are absent or weak. In the case of the facial muscles only the lower half

of the face is involved; for unknown reasons, muscle action expressing emotional changes is spared.

2. Profound atrophy does not occur in the affected muscles, although there is slow wasting, and contractures may develop over several months if the condition does not improve. The muscles are not denervated, so the myotrophic effect of their motor innervation is preserved. The spasticity (see below) helps to prevent atrophy caused by disuse.

3. The tone of the muscles is increased. This phenomenon, known as **spasticity,** results from the continuous operation of the stretch reflex, which is normally suppressed by the activity of the descending tracts. The tendon jerks are exaggerated. When the examining physician attempts passive extension of a flexed joint, resistance is encountered because of operation of the flexor reflex. When greater force is applied an inhibitory reflex is initiated by the Golgi tendon organs, and the muscles relax suddenly. This phenomenon is known as "clasp knife rigidity."

4. The **plantar reflex** is abnormal. Normally there is plantar flexion of the big toe when the lateral margin of the sole is firmly stroked with a hard object. In the abnormal reflex, known as the Babinski sign or response, the toe is dorsiflexed. Typically this movement is associated with flexion at the knee and hip joints, although similar withdrawal is often seen in normal people with sensitive soles. The descending tracts involved in the normal and abnormal plantar reflexes are unknown. There is no evidence to support the previously held view that a Babinski response is caused by interruption of the pyramidal tract. Indeed, the plantar reflex is normal after transection of corticospinal fibers in the basis pedunculi.

5. The **superficial reflexes** are suppressed or absent. These reflexes are the abdominal reflex (contraction of the anterior abdominal muscles when the overlying skin is firmly stroked) and the cremasteric reflex (withdrawal of the ipsilateral testis when the medial side of the thigh is stroked). The latter reflex is usually sluggish or absent in adult men, but is a useful clinical test in infants. (The plantar reflex is also a superficial one.) These reflexes are presumed to be mediated by long tracts to and from the cerebral cortex, but their anatomical identities are unknown.

SYSTEMS CONTROLLING THE DESCENDING PATHWAYS

Large numbers of pyramidal and corticoreticular fibers originate in the cortex of the frontal and parietal lobes. However, the movements elicited by electrical stimulation of the motor cortical areas (Chap. 15) are much simpler than those that ordinarily occur either in obedience to conscious thoughts or as part of involuntary or habitual patterns of activity. The physiological output of impulses from the motor cortex must therefore be much more complex than its responses to simple, artificial, electrical stimulation. The afferent connections of the motor areas are important with respect to their physiological complexity. The largest of these are the association and commissural fibers from other cortical areas and fibers from the thalamus, especially the ventral lateral nucleus. This thalamic nucleus receives projections from two other systems involved in the control of movement—namely, the cerebellum and basal ganglia.

Cerebellar Circuits

In connection with the motor systems it is appropriate to review the most important of the afferent and efferent connections of the cerebellum (Fig. 23-3). The cortex and central nuclei of the cerebellum receive

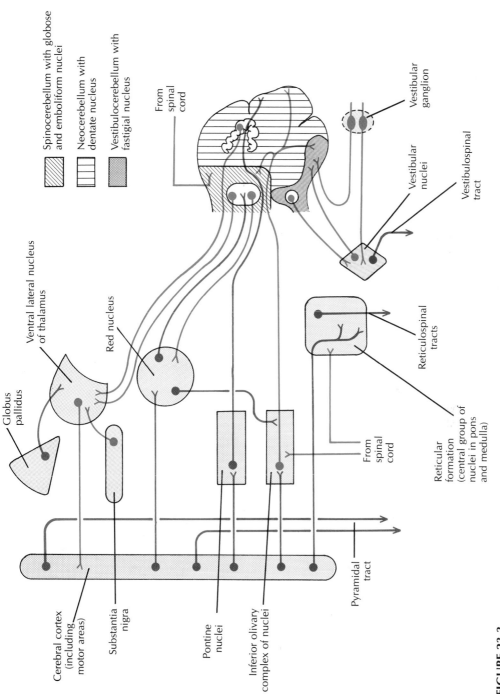

FIGURE 23-3.

Diagram of some neural connections involved in the control of movement, with emphasis on the cerebellum and on the major sources of descending tracts. The figure does not include connections between several reticular nuclei and the spinocerebellum (see Figure 10-15).

input from extensive areas of the contralateral neocortex (by way of corticopontine and pontocerebellar fibers), from ipsilateral proprioceptors in muscles, tendons, and joints (by way of the spinocerebellar tracts), and from the vestibular apparatus. The inferior olivary complex, which receives most of its afferent fibers from the neocortical motor areas, red nucleus, and spinal cord, projects to the entire cerebellar cortex. In addition to these, the precerebellar reticular nuclei relay information from the spinal cord, vestibular nuclei, and cerebral cortex. The cerebellar nuclei send their efferent fibers to the contralateral thalamus (ventral lateral nucleus) and red nucleus, as well as to the reticular formation bilaterally and the ipsilateral vestibular nuclei.

Thus, the cerebellum receives information from the cerebral cortex, including motor areas, and it is also informed of changes in the lengths and tensions of muscles and of the position and angular movements of the head. These large contingents of afferent fibers are supplemented by smaller inputs reporting on cutaneous, visual, and auditory sensations. The output of cerebellar nuclei is brought to bear on the primary motor area through a relay in the posterior division of the ventral lateral thalamic nucleus (VLp). Other cerebellar efferents influence lower motor neurons through connections with reticular and vestibular nuclei.

Electrophysiological investigations indicate that the cerebellum is informed through its olivary afferents of the program of neuronal instructions for any complex movement. The pontocerebellar afferents, which are active earlier than the primary motor area, are involved in the execution of movements. The cerebellar afferents activated by proprioceptive nerve endings enable the program of instructions to be modified in the light of the changes in length and tension of muscles that are occurring.

Basal Ganglia

The basal ganglia, which are not ganglia but nuclei, are the **corpus striatum** of the telencephalon, **subthalamic nucleus** of the diencephalon, and **substantia nigra** of the mesencephalon. The corpus striatum is functionally subdivided into the **neostriatum (striatum)** and **paleostriatum (pallidum)**. The largest of the nuclei that constitute the basal ganglia is the neostriatum. Its afferent fibers come from the whole neocortex, from the intralaminar thalamic nuclei, and from the substantia nigra (Fig. 23-4). The neostriatum projects to the paleostriatum, which influences the premotor and supplementary motor areas through a relay in the anterior division of the ventral nucleus of the thalamus (VLa). The activity of the neostriatum is modulated by a two-way connection with the substantia nigra, and the activity of the paleostriatum is modulated by a two-way connection with the subthalamic nucleus. A small contingent of pallidofugal fibers terminates in the **pedunculopontine nucleus,** one of the lateral group of nuclei of the reticular formation, situated at the junction of the midbrain and pons. The pedunculopontine nucleus sends some fibers to the subthalamic nucleus and some to the pallidum.

The structures mentioned above have other connections, but those noted are the most prominent and therefore are probably the most important. Clearly the basal ganglia comprise a large mass of gray matter influenced directly or indirectly by several parts of the central nervous system. The number and complexity of interconnections within the basal ganglia, which are also reviewed in Chapter 12, indicate that much integrative activity must be occurring. The output of the system is principally to a thalamic nucleus that projects to motor cortical areas, and electrophysiological studies indicate that in the corpus striatum, as in the cerebellar nuclei,

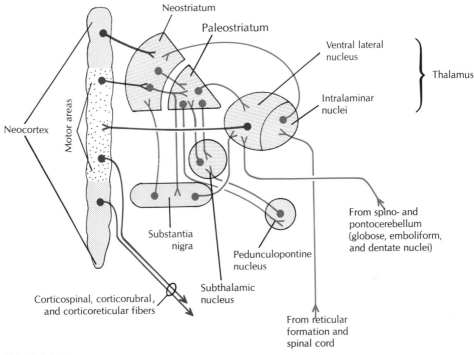

FIGURE 23-4.
Diagram of some neural connections involved in the control of movement, with emphasis on the corpus striatum, thalamus, and motor cortex.

changes in activity precede and accompany movements. It is probable, therefore, that the basal ganglia are involved in the transfer and modification of information from the whole of the neocortex to motor areas, in particular the premotor and supplementary motor areas. The effects of disease indicate a role in remembering encoded instructions for the initiation, control, and cessation of all regularly made movements.

It was once erroneously thought that the pyramidal system controlled all deliberate movements, and that there was a parallel "extrapyramidal" system concerned largely with the habitual or automatic activities of the muscles. Unfortunately, the term *extrapyramidal* has been applied not only to the reticulospinal and vestibular tracts but also to pathways that include the corpus striatum, substantia nigra, and sub-

thalamic nucleus, because some of these structures were once thought to give rise to descending fibers. From anatomical, physiological, and clinical evidence, it is more appropriate to bracket the basal ganglia with the neocerebellum; the activity of both regions is directed through the thalamus to the motor areas of the cerebral cortex. Thus, the term "extrapyramidal system" does not represent any real entity. It is mentioned here because in clinical practice disorders in which there are abnormal spontaneous movements are still often referred to as "extrapyramidal syndromes."

DISORDERS OF MOVEMENT

In cases of disordered movement it is not possible to provide tidy neuroanatomical explanations comparable to those that account for some types of sensory deficit. This is because the normal functions of the parts of the brain involved in the control of movement are imperfectly understood. However, some clinical conditions are caused by circumscribed lesions in certain regions. The best understood condition is the lower motor neuron lesion, described earlier.

Upper Motor Neuron and Cortical Lesions

The clinical signs comprising the upper motor neuron lesion were also identified earlier. The syndrome occurs in its most typical form following infarction of the posterior limb of the internal capsule, resulting in the severance of ascending and descending fibers, including those of the corticospinal, corticopontine, corticoreticular, corticorubral, and thalamocortical pathways. Destruction of both the primary motor and the premotor cortex, such as often follows occlusion of the middle cerebral artery, has similar consequences. Lesions confined to the primary motor area cause a flaccid paralysis affecting that part of the body appropriate to the exact position of the destroyed cortex. As with other lesions in which only small cortical areas are damaged, recovery usually occurs as the functions are taken over by adjacent areas.

Destruction of the premotor area causes contralateral weakness of the muscles that move the shoulder and hip joints. The hand, although its own movements are unimpaired, cannot be brought into a useful position for many ordinary tasks. Locomotion is also impaired. If the supplementary motor area is destroyed, there is a severe contralateral motor disability in which movements cannot be initiated. Bilateral lesions cause permanent akinesia and mutism. These symptoms are consonant with the normal involvement of the supplementary motor area in the initiation of movements (see Chap. 15).

Dyskinesias

Dyskinesias (often referred to as "extrapyramidal syndromes") are diseases in which unwanted superfluous movements occur. **Chorea, athetosis,** and **dystonia musculorum deformans,** which are thought to result from lesions of the corpora striata, were discussed in Chapter 12. **Hemiballismus,** consisting of sudden flailing movements at the proximal joints of limbs, is usually due to a vascular lesion in the contralateral subthalamic nucleus. The most common dyskinesia is **Parkinson's disease,** characterized by muscular rigidity, tremor of distal muscles, and poverty of movement (bradykinesia). The primary lesion is loss of dopaminergic neurons in the pars compacta of the substantiae nigrae. Normally, such neurons are active at all times, irrespective of any movement being made, presumably exerting a continuous modulating influence upon the corpora striata and, indirectly, upon the premotor and supplementary motor areas of the neocortex.

Finally, lesions of the cerebellum lead to a variety of motor disturbances, including a specific type of ataxia, hypotonia, and a characteristic intention tremor (see Chap. 10). Cerebellar lesions may be said in general to lead to errors in the rate, range, force, and direction of willed movements. Unilateral damage to the cerebellum (*e.g.,* vascular occlusion or a tumor) results in symptoms that affect the same side of the body. Bilateral cerebellar dysfunction is a common feature of multiple sclerosis (MS), a disease of unknown etiology in which foci of demyelination develop in white matter throughout the brain and spinal cord. Cerebellothalamic fibers are commonly affected in MS.

SUGGESTED READING

Alexander GE, DeLong MR, Strick PL: Parallel organization of functionally segregated circuits linking basal ganglia and cortex. Annu Rev Neurosci 9:357–381, 1986

Brodal A: Neurological Anatomy in Relation to Clinical Medicine, 3rd ed. New York, Oxford University Press, 1981

Brooks VB (ed): Motor Control. In Handbook of Physiology, 2nd ed. Section I: The Nervous System, Vol 2. Bethesda, American Physiological Society, 1981

Brooks VB: The Neural Basis of Motor Control. New York, Oxford University Press, 1986

Bucy PC, Keplinger JE, Siqueira EB: Destruction of the "pyramidal tract" in man. J Neurosurg 21:385–398, 1964

Davis HL: Trophic effects of neurogenic substances on mature skeletal muscle in vivo. In Fernandez HL, Donoso JA (eds): Nerve–Muscle Cell Trophic Communication. 1987

Dawnay NAH, Glees FP: Mapping the primate corticospinal pathway. J Anat 133:124–126, 1981

FitzGerald MJT: Neuroanatomy Basic and Applied. London, Ballière-Tindall, 1985

Freund H-J, Hummelsheim H: Lesions of premotor cortex in man. Brain 108:697–733, 1985

Gilman S, Marco LA: Effects of medullary pyramidotomy in the monkey. I. Clinical and electromyographic abnormalities. Brain 94:495–514, 1971

Lawrence DG, Kuypers HGJM: The functional organization of the motor system in the monkey, I and II. Brain 91:1–36, 1968

Nathan PH, Smith MC: The rubrospinal and central tegmental tracts in man. Brain 105:223–269, 1982

Penney JB, Young AB: Speculations on the functional anatomy of basal ganglia disorders. Annu Rev Neurosci 6:73–94, 1983

Phillips CG, Porter R: Corticospinal Neurones. Their Role in Movement. Monographs of the Physiological Society, No 34. London, Academic Press, 1977

Schultz W, Ruffieux A, Aebischer P: The activity of pars compacta neurons of the monkey substantia nigra in relation to motor activation. Exp Brain Res 51:377–387, 1983

Sugimoto T, Hattori T: Organization and efferent projections of nucleus tegmenti pedunculopontinus pars compactus with special reference to its cholinergic aspects. Neuroscience 11:931–946, 1984

TWENTY-FOUR

Visceral Innervation

Although viscera are the organs in the thorax and abdomen, the adjective *visceral* is applied in neurobiology to innervated smooth muscle and secretory cells in all parts of the body. The primary role of visceral innervation is to maintain optimal homeostasis in the internal environment (the *"milieu interieur"* of Claude Bernard). This end is attained through regulation of the organs and structures concerned with digestion, circulation, respiration, excretion, and maintenance of normal body temperature. In addition to the regulating role of visceral reflexes, the activity of smooth muscles, glandular elements, and cardiac muscle is altered by influences from the highest levels of the brain, especially in response to emotion and to the external environment.

Afferent impulses of visceral origin reach the central nervous system through primary sensory neurons similar to those for general sensation. Under normal conditions these impulses elicit reflex responses in viscera and a feeling of fullness of hollow organs such as the stomach, large intestine, and urinary bladder. Impulses originating in the viscera also contribute to feelings of well-being or malaise. In the presence of abnormal function and disease, visceral afferents transmit impulses for pain. The painful sensation is often referred to a part of the body wall or a limb supplied by the same segmental nerves as those supplying the affected viscus.

The motor or efferent supply of smooth muscle, cardiac muscle, and gland cells differs from that of voluntary muscles in that the connection between the central nervous system and the viscus consists of a succession of at least two neurons rather than a single motor neuron. The cell body of the first neuron is situated in the brain stem or the spinal cord; its axon terminates on a neuron in an autonomic ganglion, and the axon of the latter neuron ends either on effector cells or on a third neuron. The first and second neurons are called preganglionic and postganglionic neurons, respectively. The third neuron, when present, is part of the plexuses within the wall of the alimentary canal. These plexuses constitute the **enteric nervous system.** Because of its involuntary nature, Langley (1898) assigned the term "autonomic nervous system" to the visceral efferents exclusively. More recently, however, the term has often been used in a wider sense to include also the functionally related afferent neurons.

VISCERAL AFFERENTS

Olfactory neurosensory cells and gustatory neurons transmitting impulses to the brain are classified as **special visceral afferents** because these are special senses eliciting visceral responses. The neurons conveying impulses from the viscera generally constitute the **general visceral afferents,** the main features of which are now discussed.

The cell bodies of general visceral afferent neurons are situated in the inferior ganglia of the glossopharyngeal and vagus nerves, and in the ganglia of spinal nerves. The peripheral processes of visceral afferent neurons traverse autonomic ganglia and plexuses without interruption to reach the viscera. These neurons are functionally of the following types: physiological afferents, and afferents for pain resulting from disturbed function or disease. Physiological afferents accompany both the sympathetic or thoracolumbar division of the autonomic system and the parasympathetic or craniosacral division, although more importantly the latter. The afferents for pain accompany the sympathetic division of the autonomic system exclusively.

Physiological Afferents

The cell bodies of visceral afferent neurons associated with the sympathetic division of the autonomic system are in the dorsal root ganglia of T1 through L2 or L3 spinal nerves. Their peripheral processes reach the sympathetic trunk by way of white communicating rami (Fig. 24-1) and then traverse the cardiac, pulmonary, and splanchnic nerves arising from the sympathetic trunk for distribution to thoracic and abdominal viscera. Except for pacinian corpuscles, most of which are in mesenteries, the sensory endings consist of nonencapsulated terminal branches of the nerve fibers in the viscera. The central branches of these neurons enter the spinal cord through dorsal roots and terminate in the gray matter of segments T1 through L2 or L3. Usually with the intervention of interneurons, impulses reach the intermediolateral cell column in the lateral gray horn, the source of the sympathetic outflow, for visceral reflex action.

Visceral afferents of special physiological importance are associated with the parasympathetic division of the autonomic system. The following examples will serve to illustrate the reflex arcs of which they form the afferent limb.

Cardiovascular System

Terminals of sensory fibers in the aortic arch and carotid sinus at the bifurcation of the common carotid artery serve as **baroreceptors,** signaling changes in arterial blood pressure. The cell bodies of neurons supplying the aortic arch are in the inferior (nodose) ganglion of the vagus nerve, whereas those for the carotid sinus are in the inferior ganglion of the glossopharyngeal nerve. The central processes terminate in the nucleus of the tractus solitarius in the medulla, from which fibers pass to regions of the reticular formation referred to as **cardiovascular "centers."** These in

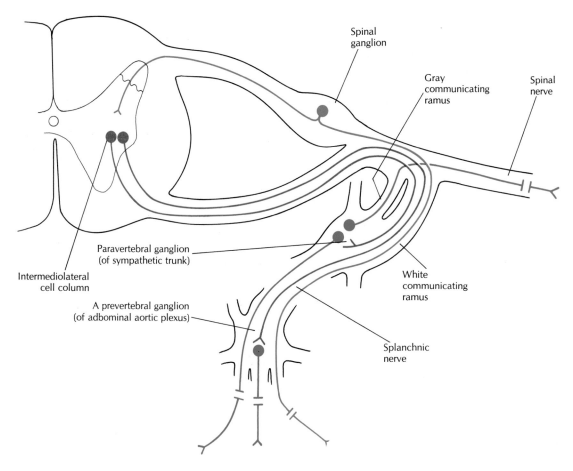

FIGURE 24-1.
Visceral afferent and efferent neurons associated with a thoracic segment of the spinal cord.

turn project to the nucleus ambiguus and intermediolateral cell column of the spinal cord. Through the reflex pathways thereby established, a rapid increase in arterial pressure causes a decrease in heart rate (vagus nerve) and vasodilation through inhibition of the vasoconstrictor action of the sympathetic outflow. A fall in arterial pressure, such as occurs following hemorrhage, initiates reflex responses that are the reverse of those caused by a rise in arterial pressure. Visceral afferents in the glossopharyngeal and vagus nerves therefore participate in the maintenance of normal arterial blood pressure.

The cardiac output is also regulated by the **Bainbridge reflex,** which is triggered by vagally innervated receptors in the right atrium; these monitor the central venous pressure. The central connections involved are unknown, but efferent limbs of the reflex include provisions for stimulation of the sympathetic nervous system and inhibition of the vagal supply to the heart. Thus, the cardiac output is increased as the volume of the venous return rises.

Respiratory System

There are **respiratory "centers"** in the brain stem for automatic control of respiratory movements. Two such regions are situated in the reticular formation of the medulla, an inspiratory center medially and dorsolateral to it an expiratory center. In addition a pneumotaxic center in the pontine reticular formation regulates the rhythmicity of inspiration and expiration. (These "centers," as well as those for the cardiovascular system, are probably fields within the network of long dendrites in the reticular formation, rather than compact collections of cell bodies.) Inspiration is initiated by stimulation of neurons in the inspiratory center by carbon dioxide of the circulating blood, the impulses reaching lower motor neurons supplying the diaphragm and intercostal muscles by means of reticulospinal connections.

Sensory neurons in the vagus nerve constitute the afferent limb of the **Hering–Breuer reflex,** through which expiration is initiated. Nerve terminals in the bronchial tree, especially the smaller branches, discharge at an increasing rate as the lungs are inflated. Impulses reach the expiratory center through a relay in the nucleus of the tractus solitarius. Neurons in the expiratory center then inhibit those of the inspiratory center, and expiration ensues as a passive (elastic) process.

Respiratory movements are also influenced by nerve impulses conducted centrally from the carotid bodies situated near the bifurcation of the common carotid arteries and from small aortic bodies adjacent to the aortic arch. The glomus cells of these bodies function as **chemoreceptors** that are sensitive to a decrease in oxygen tension in the circulating blood. The resulting impulses reach the nucleus of the tractus solitarius through neurons with cell bodies in the inferior ganglia of the glossopharyngeal and vagus nerves. Further connections with respiratory centers in the brain stem bring about an increase in the rate and depth of respiratory movements. This reflex operates in vigorous exercise, when a person is exposed to a lowered oxygen tension such as at high altitudes, or in any circumstances that produce asphyxia.

Other Systems

Sensory fibers in the vagus nerve are distributed to the gastrointestinal tract as far as the splenic flexure at the junction of the transverse colon and descending colon. The nerve terminals are stimulated by distention of the stomach and intestine, contraction of the smooth musculature, and irritation of the mucosa. Although motility and secretion are not dependent on the extrinsic nerves, they are modified by reflex action involving vagal afferent and efferent neurons. The distal colon, rectum, and urinary bladder are supplied by splanchnic branches of the second, third, and fourth sacral nerves. Reflexes involving the corresponding segments of the spinal cord and the sacral portion of the parasympathetic system function in emptying the large bowel and urinary bladder, subject to voluntary control.

Ascending Pathways

There are ascending visceral pathways distinct from the pathway for pain (described in the next section). One such pathway originates in the nucleus of the tractus solitarius in the medulla, which receives general visceral afferents from the vagus nerve predominantly. A second pathway originates in segments T1 through L2 or L3 of the spinal cord, probably in the intermediomedial cell column of lamina VII, and in segments S2 through S4. These ascending fibers are included in the spinoreticular and spinothalamic tracts. Through the pathways from the medulla and spinal cord, impulses of visceral origin reach the reticular formation of the brain stem, hypothalamus, and ventral posterior nucleus of the thalamus. A thalamocortical projection provides for a feeling of fullness when the stomach is distended and a feeling of hunger when the stomach is empty, as well as a feeling of fullness in the distal colon and urinary bladder.

Pain Afferents

The sensory endings for pain arising in internal organs are stimulated in various ways in the presence of abnormal function or disease. Most commonly the pain is caused by distention of a hollow viscus such as the intestine, which may occur proximal to localized and forcible contraction of the smooth muscle of the intestine. Similarly, distention of a bile duct or the ureter occurs when the lumen is obstructed by a calculus. Visceral pain also results from rapid stretching of the capsule of a solid organ, such as the liver or spleen. Peritoneal irritation contributes to the pain of inflammatory disease. In the case of anginal pain and the pain of coronary thrombosis, the effective stimulus is produced by anoxia of the affected cardiac muscle. The stimulus is probably chemical in nature, perhaps a local lowering of the pH because of accumulation of acid metabolites.

The sensory neurons for pain of visceral origin are associated only with the sympathetic division of the autonomic nervous system. The cell bodies of primary sensory neurons are therefore in the dorsal root ganglia of the thoracic and the upper two or three lumbar nerves. The peripheral processes of these neurons reach the sympathetic trunk by way of white communicating rami; they run in the sympathetic trunk for variable distances and then continue to the viscera by way of the cardiac, pulmonary, and splanchnic nerves. The termination of the corresponding dorsal root fibers in the spinal gray matter is not known precisely; however, the majority probably enter the dorsolateral tract of Lissauer along with somatic pain fibers and end similarly in the dorsal horn. The ascending pathway for visceral pain may coincide, in part, with the pathway for somatic pain—that is, through crossed fibers in the spinothalamic tract. There also appears to be crossed and uncrossed conduction by means of spinoreticular fibers. The impulses reach the thalamus through the spinal lemniscus and extralemniscal relays in the reticular formation, along with impulses for pain from somatic structures.

Referred Pain

Visceral pain has characteristics that distinguish it from pain originating in somatic structures, notably diffuse localization and radiation to somatic areas (referred pain). The zone of reference of the pain for a viscus coincides with the part of the body served by somatic sensory neurons associated with the same segments of the spinal cord as the sensory neurons supplying the affected viscus. The principle of referred pain is illustrated by the following examples.

The **heart** is supplied with sensory fibers for pain by the middle and inferior cervical cardiac branches and by the thoracic cardiac branches of the left sympathetic trunk. Central processes of the primary sensory neurons enter segments T1 through T4 or T5 of the spinal cord; pain of cardiac origin is therefore referred to the left side of the chest and to the inner aspect of the left arm. Deviations from this zone of reference are common, however, and are probably caused by anatomical variations in the laterality and segmental levels of the cardiac innervation.

In the case of pain arising from the **gallbladder** or **bile ducts,** the impulses pass centrally in the greater splanchnic nerve on the right side, entering the spinal cord through the seventh and eighth thoracic dorsal roots. The pain is referred to the upper quadrant of the abdomen and the infrascapular region on the right side. Disease of the liver or gallbladder may irritate the peritoneum covering the **diaphragm.** The resulting pain is often referred to the shoulder because the diaphragm is supplied with sensory fibers (as well as motor fibers) by the phrenic nerve, which originates from the third, fourth, and fifth cervical segments of the spinal cord.

Pain of gastric origin is referred to the epigastrium because the **stomach** is supplied with pain afferents that reach the seventh and eighth thoracic segments of the spinal cord by way of the greater splanchnic nerve. Pain from the **duodenum,** as in duodenal ulcer, is referred to the anterior abdominal wall just above the umbilicus, with both this area and the duodenum being supplied by the ninth and tenth thoracic nerves. Afferent fibers from the **appendix** are included in the lesser splanchnic nerve, and impulses enter the tenth thoracic segment of the spinal cord. The pain of appendicitis is referred initially to the region of the umbilicus, which lies in the tenth thoracic dermatome, shifting to the lower right quadrant of the abdomen if the parietal peritoneum becomes involved in the inflammatory process. (The parietal peritoneum and pleura are supplied by segmental somatic nerves.) Pain afferents supplying the **renal pelvis** and **ureter** are included in the least splanchnic nerve; nerve impulses enter the first and second lumbar segments of the spinal cord, and the pain is referred to the loin and the inguinal region.

There is no entirely satisfactory explanation for the referral of pain of visceral origin. An early proposal was that afferent fibers for visceral and somatic pain synapse with the same tract cells in the spinal cord, with these cells being excited by subliminal somatic stimuli when receiving impulses of visceral origin. A more plausible explanation for referred pain is based on a projection of impulses for both visceral and somatic pain from a specific segment of the spinal cord to the same group of cells in the ventral posterior nucleus of the thalamus. The topographic representation of parts of the body in the thalamus and cerebral cortex provides a basis for recognizing the site of origin of impulses

for the general senses. Localization may be in error when the impulses for pain originate in a viscus, perhaps because pain of somatic origin is a common experience compared with pain caused by visceral malfunction or disease. It is of interest that 200 years ago John Hunter called referred pain a "delusion of the mind." Spinal reflexes are responsible for the **muscle spasm** seen in the rigidity of abdominal muscles when there is inflammatory disease of a viscus.

VISCERAL EFFERENT OR AUTONOMIC SYSTEM

The smooth muscle and secretory cells of viscera, as well as cardiac muscle, come under the dual influence of the sympathetic and parasympathetic divisions of the autonomic nervous system. In some organs they are functionally antagonistic to one another, and a delicate balance between them maintains a more or less constant level of visceral activity under conditions that usually prevail. However, autonomic innervation extends beyond the viscera of the major body cavities to include the muscles of the iris and ciliary body in the eye, smooth muscles in the orbit, the lacrimal and salivary glands, sweat glands and arrector pili muscles of the skin, and blood vessels everywhere. In addition, the alimentary canal contains its own intrinsic nerve supply, the enteric nervous system, which is able to control at least the simpler forms of gastrointestinal motility.

Autonomic Ganglia

An autonomic ganglion receives thin, myelinated (group B) afferent fibers from the brain stem or spinal cord. Its efferent fibers, which supply visceral structures, are the axons of the principal cells of the ganglion. They are unmyelinated (group C) and are more numerous than the afferent fibers. Thus, the synapses in the ganglion provide for divergence in the efferent pathway, so that relatively small numbers of neurons in the central nervous system control large numbers of smooth muscle and gland cells in the periphery. The divergence is enhanced by preterminal branching of the postganglionic fibers and, in the alimentary canal, by further synapses with the neurons of the enteric nervous system.

Divergence cannot be the sole reason for the existence of autonomic ganglia; the same effect could be more simply achieved by further branching of axons. There must also be integration and comparison of the various items of information arriving in a ganglion through its preganglionic neurons. Evidence for such activity is seen in the synaptic organization of the ganglion (Fig. 24-2). Each principal cell is inhibited at the dendrodendritic synapses with nearby principal cells and from the small intrinsic neurons of the ganglion. These interneurons, whose only cytoplasmic processes are short dendrites, are excited by branches of the preganglionic axons, and their activity may also be influ-

enced by substances derived from the blood. This latter possibility is indicated by the proximity of the cells to capillary vessels with fenestrated endothelium, although the same structural arrangement could alternatively reflect an endocrine function of the ganglion. In at least some autonomic ganglia, sensory fibers that are passing through give off branches that synapse with the principal cells. This arrangement may provide for reflexes that do not involve the central nervous system.

The preganglionic neurons are invariably cholinergic. The principal cells are all cholinergic in parasympathetic ganglia, but only a small proportion of them are cholinergic in sympathetic ganglia. Most of the principal cells of sympathetic ganglia are noradrenergic at their peripheral synapses. The synapses between adjacent principal cells are either noradrenergic or electrical in sympathetic ganglia, and either cholinergic or electrical in parasympathetic ganglia. The intrinsic neurons of the ganglia contain dopamine, which they are believed to use as a transmitter. All the

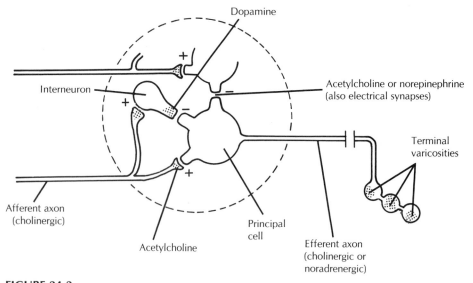

FIGURE 24-2.

Synaptic organization of an autonomic ganglion, showing transmitter substances and their excitatory (+) or inhibitory (−) actions.

neurons in autonomic ganglia also contain two or more peptides, which may serve as additional neurotransmitters or as neuro-modulators. There are several clinically valuable drugs that selectively enhance or inhibit both the synthesis and metabolism of acetylcholine, dopamine, and norepinephrine. Other drugs imitate or block the actions of these transmitters at postsynaptic sites. Information about synaptic connections in autonomic ganglia is therefore valuable in understanding some of the physiological effects, both therapeutic and unwanted, of these drugs.

Parasympathetic Division

The role of the parasympathetic system is to effect changes designed to conserve and restore energy. The responses include a decrease in the rate and force of the heart beat, lowering of the blood pressure, and augmentation of the activity of the digestive system. As previously stated, acetylcholine is the chemical mediator at the synapses between preganglionic and postganglionic neurons and also at the contacts between postganglionic terminals and effector cells, with various peptides also being released. The parasympathetic system is said to be "cholinergic." It acts in localized and discrete regions rather than causing a mass reaction throughout the body. The discrete nature of the response is a result of the fact that there is less divergence between pre- and post-ganglionic neurons and between the latter and effector cells compared with the sympathetic system, and that acetylcholine is rapidly inactivated by cholinesterase—hence, each parasympathetic discharge is of short duration.

Preganglionic parasympathetic neurons, which have long axons, are located in the brain stem and in the sacral portion of the spinal cord (Fig. 24-3). The preganglionic parasympathetic nuclei and the sites of the corresponding postganglionic neurons are as follows: **Edinger–Westphal**

nucleus of the oculomotor complex and ciliary ganglion; **superior salivatory nucleus** of the facial nerve and submandibular ganglion; **lacrimal nucleus** of the facial nerve and pterygopalatine ganglion; **inferior salivatory nucleus** of the glossopharyngeal nerve and otic ganglion; **dorsal nucleus** of the vagus nerve and ganglia in the pulmonary plexus, cells in the myenteric and submucosal plexuses of the gastrointestinal tract (the enteric nervous system), and postganglionic neurons at other sites; **nucleus ambiguus** and cardiac ganglia; and **sacral parasympathetic nucleus** and postganglionic neurons in and near the pelvic viscera.

Sympathetic Division

The sympathetic outflow originates in the **intermediolateral cell column** of all thoracic spinal segments and of the upper two or three lumbar segments (Fig. 24-4). The axons of preganglionic neurons reach the sympathetic trunk by way of the corresponding ventral roots and white communicating rami (see Fig. 24-1). With respect to the sympathetic supply of structures in the head and thorax, the preganglionic fibers terminate in ganglia of the sympathetic trunk. For smooth muscles and glands in the head, the synapses between pre- and post-ganglionic neurons are mainly in the superior cervical ganglion of the sympathetic trunk. In the case of thoracic viscera, the synapses are in the three cervical sympathetic ganglia (superior, middle, and inferior) and in the upper five ganglia of the thoracic portion of the sympathetic trunk.

Preganglionic fibers for abdominal and pelvic viscera proceed without interruption through the sympathetic trunk and its splanchnic branches. The fibers terminate on postganglionic neurons located in plexuses that surround the main branches of the abdominal aorta, notably the celiac plexus and the superior and inferior mesenteric plexuses. The sympathetic supply

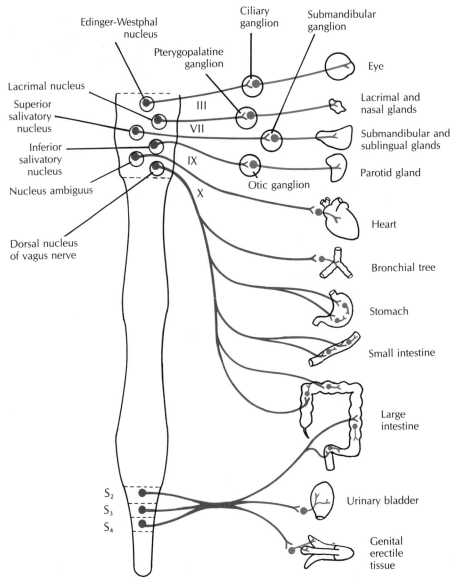

FIGURE 24-3.
The parasympathetic nervous system.

to the adrenal medulla is exceptional. The secretory cells of the medulla, similar to postganglionic sympathetic neurons, are derived from the neural crest of the embryo. The adrenal medulla is consequently supplied directly by preganglionic sympathetic neurons. The glomus cells of the carotid and aortic bodies also receive preganglionic sympathetic innervation, which may control the sensitivity of these chemosensory organs. The alimentary canal is supplied chiefly by the ganglia in the celiac and mesenteric plexuses; the postganglionic fibers do not terminate directly upon smooth muscle and gland cells but within the plexuses constituting the enteric nervous system.

For the body wall and the limbs, pre-

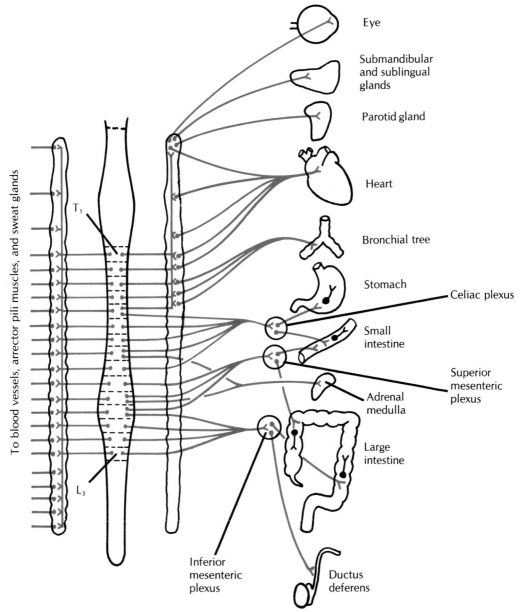

To blood vessels, arrector pili muscles, and sweat glands

T₁

L₃

Eye

Submandibular
and sublingual
glands

Parotid gland

Heart

Bronchial tree

Stomach

Celiac plexus

Small
intestine

Superior
mesenteric
plexus

Adrenal
medulla

Large
intestine

Inferior
mesenteric
plexus

Ductus
deferens

FIGURE 24-4.
The sympathetic nervous system.

ganglionic fibers terminate in all ganglia of the sympathetic trunk, from which postganglionic fibers are distributed by way of gray communicating rami and spinal nerves to blood vessels, arrector pili muscles, and sweat glands.

The sympathetic system stimulates activities that are accompanied by an expenditure of energy. These include acceleration of the heart and increase in force of the heart beat, rise of arterial pressure, elevation of the blood sugar level, and direction of blood flow to skeletal muscles at the expense of visceral and cutaneous circulation. Sympathetic responses are most dramatically expressed during stress and emergency situations (the "flight or fight" response). The neurotransmitter substance between pre- and postganglionic neurons is acetylcholine, as in the parasympathetic system. However, in the case of the sympathetic system, norepinephrine (noradrenaline) is the transmitter substance between postganglionic terminals and effector cells and between postganglionic neurons and neurons of the enteric plexuses. The sympathetic system is said to be "noradrenergic." However, the sympathetic supply to sweat glands is cholinergic, constituting an exception to the general rule. Cutaneous areas lack parasympathetic fibers; this may be related to the fact that sudomotor fibers are anatomically sympathetic but functionally parasympathetic.

Strong sympathetic stimulation produces diffuse effects because of the following factors, which are the converse of those present in the parasympathetic system. Each sympathetic preganglionic neuron synapses with many postganglionic neurons, and each of the latter supplies numerous effector cells or enteric neurons. Hence, there is much divergence of stimuli. Norepinephrine liberated at postganglionic terminals, and epinephrine (adrenaline) and norepinephrine (noradrenaline) secreted by the adrenal medulla on sympathetic stimulation, are deactivated slowly. As expressed by Cannon, "the sympathetics are like the loud and soft pedals, modulating all the tones together, while the parasympathetics are like the separate keys."

Enteric Nervous System

At the beginning of this century Langley recognized the enteric nervous system, consisting of neurons contained within the walls of the alimentary canal, as the third component of the autonomic system, distinct from the sympathetic and parasympathetic divisions. It was realized that well-coordinated peristaltic and related movements could occur in the absence of any extrinsic innervation. The enteric neurons came to be regarded as constituting a very large parasympathetic ganglion, with afferent fibers from the vagus and sacral nerves. Subsequently, however, it was found that the intrinsic neurons of the gut receive input from the sympathetic ganglia as well as from preganglionic parasympathetic neurons. Furthermore, the nervous tissue of the gastrointestinal tract is ultrastructurally and histochemically unlike that of sympathetic or parasympathetic ganglia. Langley's recognition of the enteric nervous system is therefore justified.

From the esophagus to the rectum the walls of the human alimentary canal contain some 10^8 neurons, a population comparable to the number of neurons in the spinal cord. The cell bodies occur in two zones—the **myenteric plexus** (of Auerbach) lies between the longitudinal and circular muscle layers, and the **submucous plexus** (of Meissner) lies in the connective tissue between the circular muscle layer and the muscularis mucosae. Each plexus consists of small groups of neurons, with the groups joined to one another by thin nerves in which most of the axons are unmyelinated. Similar nerves connect the two plexuses across the circular muscle layer and carry branches from the plexuses into the smooth muscle and into the lamina propria of the mucosa. Most of the neurons are multipolar but there are also many bipolar and unipolar ones, especially in the submucous plexus.

In addition to neurons, the enteric nervous system contains neuroglial cells similar to the astrocytes of the central nervous system. The glial cells completely ensheath the neurons and all their processes. The nervous tissue is avascular and receives its nutrients by diffusion from capillary vessels outside the glial sheath. As in the central nervous system and in peripheral nerves, large molecules are

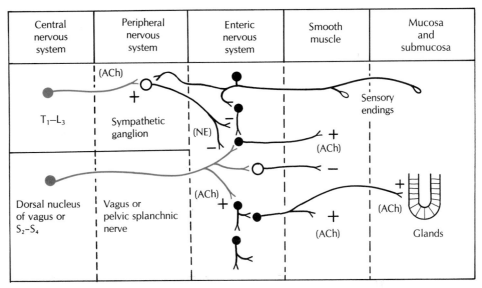

FIGURE 24-5.
Organization of the enteric nervous system. For simplification, the myenteric and submucous plexuses have been combined. The sites of known transmitters are shown, as are sites of synaptic excitation (+) and inhibition (−). **(NE)** Norepinephrine. **(ACh)** acetylcholine.

unable to pass from the blood into the nervous tissue.

The synaptic organization of the enteric nervous system (Fig. 24-5) is still only partly known. Several types of neuron are found in the plexuses. The bipolar and unipolar cells are presumed to have sensory functions, especially in initiating the peristaltic reflex. Neurons of two types have axons that end on smooth muscle and gland cells; the excitatory neurons are cholinergic, whereas the inhibitory neurons probably use either a peptide or nucleotide as their transmitter. Some neurons, whose cytological and chemical characteristics have not been identified, send axons centripetally to the celiac and mesenteric sympathetic ganglia. There are also interneurons within the plexuses. Enteric neurons have been shown to contain many different peptides with pharmacologically demonstrable actions upon the gut, and it is considered probable that at least some of these substances serve as neurotransmitters. The fibers afferent to the enteric nervous system are of two types. Cholinergic axons of preganglionic parasympathetic neurons terminate on the dendrites and cell bodies both of interneurons and of neurons that supply smooth muscle and glands. The noradrenergic axons of sympathetic neurons terminate in axoaxonic synapses upon the boutons of both parasympathetic and intrinsic fibers. They are believed to mediate presynaptic inhibition of the cholinergic neurons that stimulate contraction of the musculature and glandular secretion.

Central Control of the Autonomic Nervous System

The hypothalamus has a diverse afferent input and its efferent connections include projections to neurons that constitute the autonomic outflow. It is therefore an important controlling and integrating center for the autonomic system.

Through afferent connections described in earlier chapters, the hypothalamus is influenced by the neocortex, hippocampal formation, amygdala, septal area, lateral olfactory area, and anterior and mediodorsal thalamic nuclei. The main inputs from these sources are concerned with the emotions (limbic system) and the olfactory sense. Ascending pathways from the spinal cord and brain stem convey information of visceral and gustatory origin. There are also hypothalamic neurons that are sensitive to changes in the temperature, osmolarity, and levels of various substances (including hormones) in the circulating blood. Depending on specific sensitivities, these neurons are related either to the autonomic system or to the pituitary gland.

Impulses originating in the hypothalamus reach autonomic nuclei in the brain stem and spinal cord directly and through relays in the reticular formation. There are also pathways from the limbic and olfactory systems to preganglionic autonomic neurons that do not involve the hypothalamus. The autonomic neurons are influenced as well by visceral "centers" in the medulla and by visceral afferent nuclei, notably the nucleus of the tractus solitarius in the medulla. The autonomic outflow therefore comes under a wide range of influences—visceral (including taste and smell), emotional (both basic drives and moods), and even mental processes at the neocortical level.

SUGGESTED READING

Brooks, CMcC, Koizumi K, Sato AY (eds): Integrative Functions of the Autonomic Nervous System. Amsterdam, Elsevier, 1979

Crosby EC, Humphrey T, Lauer EW: Correlative Anatomy of the Nervous System. New York, Macmillan, 1962

Gershon MD: The enteric nervous system. Annu Rev Neurosci 4:227–272, 1981

Grundy D: Gastrointestinal Motility. Lancaster & Boston, MTP Press, 1985

Karczmar AG, Koketsu K, Nishi S (eds): Autonomic and Enteric Ganglia. New York, Plenum Press, 1986

Nathan PW, Smith MC: The location of descending fibres to sympathetic neurons supplying the eye and sudomotor neurons supplying the head and neck. J Neurol Neurosurg Psychiat 49:187–194, 1986

Shepherd GM: The Synaptic Organization of the Brain, 2nd ed. New York, Oxford University Press, 1979

Smith OA, DeVito JL: Central neural integration for the control of autonomic responses associated with emotion. Annu Rev Neurosci 7:43–65, 1984

Swanson LW, Mogenson GJ: Neural mechanisms for the functional coupling of autonomic, endocrine and somatomotor responses in adaptive behavior. Brain Res Rev 3:1–34, 1981

BLOOD SUPPLY AND THE MENINGES

TWENTY-FIVE

Blood Supply of the Central Nervous System

Lesions of vascular origin are responsible for more neurological disorders than any other category of disease process. Arterial occlusion by a thrombus, which is usually followed by infarction of a portion of the region supplied by the affected artery, is the most common type of cerebral vascular accident. This type of arterial occlusion occurs most frequently in those past middle age because the thrombus usually develops at the site of atheromatous changes in the intima. An embolus originating at some other site in the vascular system is another cause of cerebral arterial occlusion. In addition to intracranial occlusions, impairment of the cerebral circulation is often the result of stenosis of a carotid or vertebral artery extracranially.

The slender, thin-walled arteries that penetrate the ventral surface of the brain to supply the internal capsule and adjacent gray masses are especially prone to rupture. Hypertension and degenerative changes in these arteries are major factors that lead to cerebral hemorrhage. Aneurysms usually occur at the site of branching of one of the larger arteries at the base of the brain. An aneurysm may leak or rupture, in which case the bleeding is typically into the subarachnoid space; however, the hemorrhage may be intracerebral.

There are anastomotic channels between branches of the major arteries on the surface of the brain. There are also communications at the arteriolar level, and the capillary bed is continuous throughout the brain. These anastomoses, however, are usually inadequate to sustain the circulation in the region supplied normally by a major artery. The size of an infarction depends on the caliber of the occluded artery, existing anastomoses, and the time elapsing before complete occlusion.

The calibers of small arteries in the brain are controlled by **autoregulation,** which means that their muscular walls contract if the pressure inside rises, and relax if the pressure falls, so that a constant rate of flow tends to be maintained. The increased blood flow in active areas of gray matter is probably due to vasodilator metabolites, notably carbon dioxide. Noradrenergic axons (from the sympathetic system and from the locus ceruleus) are present in the walls of many cerebral blood vessels, but their functional importance has not yet been ascertained.

The blood supply of the central nervous system is of special interest because of the metabolic demands of nervous tissue. The brain depends on aerobic metabolism of glucose and is one of the most metabolically active organs of the body. Although composing only 2% of the body weight, the brain receives approximately 17% of the cardiac output and consumes about 20% of the oxygen used by the entire body. Unconsciousness follows cessation of cerebral circulation in about 10 sec.

ARTERIAL SUPPLY OF THE BRAIN

Because of the practical importance of cerebral vascular disease, and because the neurological signs depend on the site of the lesion, an understanding of the distribution of the arteries is essential. The brain is supplied by the paired internal carotid and vertebral arteries through an extensive system of branches.

Internal Carotid System

The **internal carotid artery,** a terminal branch of the common carotid artery, traverses the carotid canal in the base of the skull and enters the middle cranial fossa beside the dorsum sellae of the sphenoid bone. Beyond this point the artery undergoes the following sequence of bends that constitute the "carotid siphon" in a cerebral angiogram (see Fig. 25–5). The internal carotid artery first runs forward in the cavernous venous sinus and then turns upward on the medial side of the anterior clinoid process. At this point the artery enters the subarachnoid space by piercing the dura mater and arachnoid, courses backward below the optic nerve, and finally turns upward immediately lateral to the optic chiasma. This brings the artery under the anterior perforated substance, where it divides into the middle and anterior cerebral arteries (Fig. 25-1).

Collateral Branches

The following branches arise from the internal carotid artery before its terminal bifurcation.

Hypophysial Arteries. These arteries originate from the cavernous and postclinoid portions of the internal carotid artery. In addition to supplying the infundibular process of the neurohypophysis, hypophysial arteries enter the median eminence of the hypothalamus. The latter blood vessels break up into capillary loops, into which hypothalamic releasing factors gain access, and the capillary loops drain through small veins into the sinusoids of the adenohypophysis. This constitutes the pituitary portal system through which the hypothalamus influences the output of pituitary hormones.

Ophthalmic Artery. This branch comes off immediately after the internal carotid artery enters the subarachnoid space. The ophthalmic artery passes through the optic foramen into the orbit, supplying the eye and other orbital contents, frontal area of the scalp, frontal and ethmoid paranasal sinuses, and parts of the nose.

Posterior Communicating Artery. This slender artery arises from the internal carotid artery close to its terminal bifurcation. The posterior communicating artery runs backward to join the proximal part of

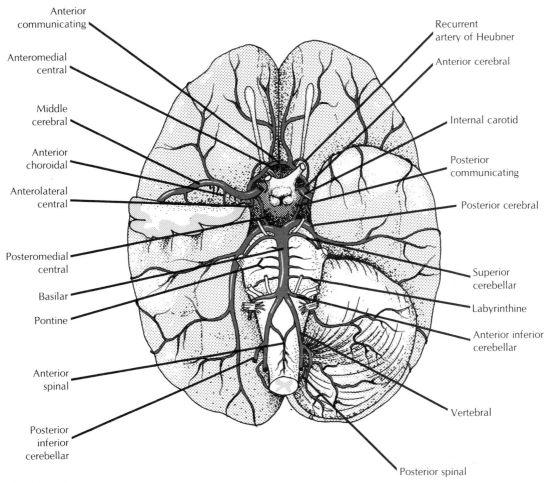

Anterior communicating

Anteromedial central

Middle cerebral

Anterior choroidal

Anterolateral central

Posteromedial central

Basilar

Pontine

Anterior spinal

Posterior inferior cerebellar

Recurrent artery of Heubner

Anterior cerebral

Internal carotid

Posterior communicating

Posterior cerebral

Superior cerebellar

Labyrinthine

Anterior inferior cerebellar

Vertebral

Posterior spinal

FIGURE 25-1.
The blood supply of the brain, as seen on the ventral surface. (The right cerebellar hemisphere and the tip of the right temporal lobe have been removed.)

the posterior cerebral artery, thereby forming part of the arterial circle (circle of Willis).

Anterior Choroidal Artery. This branch comes off the distal part of the internal carotid artery or the beginning of the middle cerebral artery and has a wider distribution than its name suggests. The artery passes back along the optic tract and the choroid fissure at the medial edge of the temporal lobe. In addition to supplying the choroid plexus in the temporal horn of the lateral ventricle, the anterior choroidal artery gives off branches to the optic tract, uncus, amygdala, hippocampus, globus pallidus, lateral geniculate nucleus, and ventral part of the internal capsule. The further distribution of this artery varies considerably, but additional branches have been traced into the subthalamus, ventral portion of the thalamus, and rostral part of the midbrain (including the red nucleus). The anterior choroidal artery is said to be prone to thrombosis because of its small caliber and rather long subarachnoid course. The globus pallidus and the hippocampus, both of which are supplied in part by the anterior choroidal artery, are considered to be favored sites of neuronal degeneration as a result of circulatory deficiency.

Middle Cerebral Artery

Of the terminal branches of the internal carotid artery, the middle cerebral artery is the larger and the more direct continuation of the parent vessel (Fig. 25-1). This artery runs deep in the lateral sulcus between the frontal and temporal lobes. **Frontal, parietal,** and **temporal branches** emerge from the lateral sulcus of the cerebral hemisphere (Fig. 25-2).

The area of distribution of the middle cerebral artery includes motor and general sensory areas, except those for the lower limb and the perineum. Occlusion of the artery therefore results in contralateral paralysis most noticeable in the lower part of the face and in the arm, together with general sensory deficits of the cortical type. The auditory cortex is included in the area of distribution; however, a unilateral lesion causes no demonstrable impairment of hearing because of the bilateral cortical projection from the organ of Corti. Occlusion of a branch of the middle cerebral artery in the left hemisphere is the principal cause of aphasia (Chap. 15). The cortical areas concerned are the sensory language area in the temporal and parietal lobes, especially Wernicke's area in the temporal lobe, and Broca's motor speech area in the inferior frontal gyrus (see Fig. 25-2).

Anterior Cerebral Artery

The smaller terminal branch of the internal carotid artery is the anterior cerebral artery, which is first directed medially above the optic nerve (see Fig. 25-1). The two anterior cerebral arteries almost meet at the midline where they are joined together by the **anterior communicating artery.** The anterior cerebral artery then as-

cends in the longitudinal fissure and bends backward around the genu of the corpus callosum (Fig. 25-3). Branches given off just distal to the anterior communicating artery supply the medial portion of the orbital surface of the frontal lobe, including the olfactory bulb and olfactory tract.

The artery continues along the upper surface of the corpus callosum as the **pericallosal artery,** and a large branch, the **callosomarginal artery,** follows the cingulate sulcus. The anterior cerebral artery supplies the medial portions of the frontal and parietal lobes and the corpus callosum. In addition, branches extend over the dorsomedial border of the hemisphere and supply a strip on the lateral surface (see Fig. 25-2). The dorsal portions of the motor and general sensory areas are included in its territory; occlusion of the anterior cerebral artery therefore causes paralysis and sensory deficits in the contralateral leg and perineum.

A special branch of the anterior cerebral artery is given off just proximal to the anterior communicating artery. This is the **recurrent artery of Heubner,** which penetrates the anterior perforated substance to supply the ventral part of the head of the caudate nucleus, adjacent portion of the putamen, and anterior limb and genu of the internal capsule. The recurrent artery of Heubner is sometimes called the **medial striate artery** because of its contribution to the blood supply of the corpus striatum.

Vertebral System

The **vertebral artery,** a branch of the subclavian artery, ascends in the foramina of the transverse processes of the upper six cervical vertebrae. On reaching the base of the skull, the artery winds around the lateral mass of the atlas, pierces the posterior atlanto-occipital membrane, and enters the subarachnoid space at the level of the foramen magnum by piercing the dura mater and arachnoid. The vertebral artery

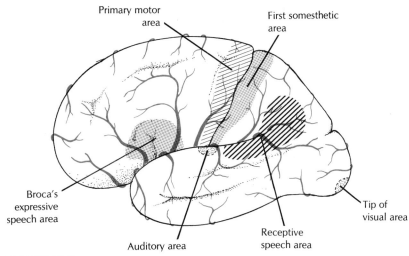

FIGURE 25-2.
Distribution of the middle cerebral artery on the lateral surface of the cerebral hemisphere.

runs forward with a medial inclination beneath the medulla, joining its fellow of the opposite side at the caudal border of the pons to form the **basilar artery.** The latter artery runs forward in the midline of the pons and divides into the **posterior cerebral arteries** (see Fig. 25-1).

Branches of the Vertebral Artery

Spinal Arteries. The upper portion of the cervical cord receives blood through spinal branches of the vertebral arteries. A single **anterior spinal artery** is formed by a contribution from each vertebral artery. A **posterior spinal artery** arises on each side as a branch of either the vertebral or the posterior inferior cerebellar artery (see Fig. 25-1). The anterior and posterior spinal arteries continue throughout the length of the spinal cord. However, except for their proximal portions, the blood comes from reinforcements by the anterior and posterior radicular arteries (described below).

Posterior Inferior Cerebellar Artery. This artery, the largest branch of the vertebral artery, pursues an irregular course between the medulla and cerebellum. Branches are distributed to the posterior part of the cerebellar hemisphere, inferior vermis, central nuclei of the cerebellum, and choroid plexus of the fourth ventricle. There are also medullary branches to the dorsolateral region of the medulla. Occlusion of the posterior inferior cerebellar artery therefore results in the lateral medullary or Wallenberg's syndrome (Chap. 7). In addition to branches from the posterior inferior cerebellar artery, fine branches arising directly from the vertebral artery supply the medulla.

Branches of the Basilar Artery

The basilar artery gives off the following branches before dividing into the posterior cerebral arteries at the rostral border of the pons.

Anterior Inferior Cerebellar Artery. Arising from the caudal end of the basilar artery, the anterior inferior cerebellar artery supplies the cortex of the inferior surface of the cerebellum anteriorly and the underlying white matter; it assists in the supply

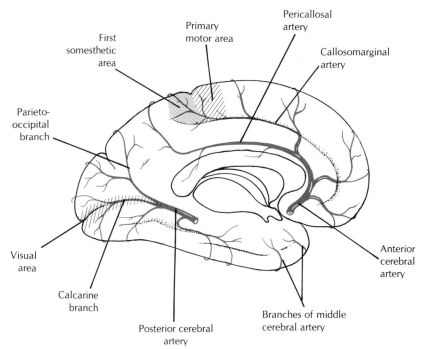

FIGURE 25-3.
Distribution of the anterior and posterior cerebral arteries on the medial surface of the cerebral hemisphere.

of the central cerebellar nuclei. In addition slender twigs from the artery penetrate the upper medulla and lower pons.

Labyrinthine Artery. This artery, a branch of either the basilar artery or the anterior inferior cerebellar artery, traverses the internal acoustic meatus and ramifies throughout the membranous labyrinth of the internal ear. Although of rare occurrence, occlusion of the labyrinthine artery results in the expected deafness in the corresponding ear and vestibular dysfunction (vertigo, with a tendency to fall toward the side of the lesion).

Pontine Arteries. These are slender branches arising from the basilar artery along its length. They penetrate the pons and ramify in both the ventral portion of the pons and pontine tegmentum. Infarction of the ventral part of the pons causes paralysis of all voluntary movement, ex-

cept of the eyes. The general and special sensory pathways are spared. This condition is called the "locked-in" syndrome.

Superior Cerebellar Artery. This branch arises close to the terminal bifurcation of the basilar artery, ramifies over the dorsal surface of the cerebellum, and supplies the cortex, medullary center, and central nuclei. Branches from the proximal part of the superior cerebellar artery are distributed to the pons, superior cerebellar peduncle, and inferior colliculus of the midbrain.

Posterior Cerebral Artery

Each posterior cerebral artery curves around the midbrain and reaches the medial surface of the cerebral hemisphere beneath the splenium of the corpus callosum (see Fig. 25-3). The artery gives off **temporal branches,** which ramify over the inferior surface of the temporal lobe, and **calcarine** and **parieto-occipital branches,** which run along the corresponding sulci. All these arteries send branches around the border of the cerebral hemisphere to supply a peripheral strip on the lateral surface (see Fig. 25-2). The calcarine branch is of special significance because it supplies the visual area of cortex, and occlusion causes blindness in the contralateral field of vision. Central or macular vision is usually spared, although this may be an artifact caused by the subject being tested shifting his fixation point slightly during examination of the visual field.

The **posterior choroidal artery** comes off the posterior cerebral artery in the region of the splenium and runs forward in the transverse fissure beneath the corpus callosum. The posterior choroidal artery supplies the choroid plexus of the central part of the lateral ventricle, choroid plexus of the third ventricle, posterior part of the thalamus, fornix, and tectum of the midbrain.

Cortical Branches of the Cerebral Arteries

Anastomoses between branches of the anterior, middle, and posterior cerebral arteries are concealed in the sulci. The caliber of an anastomotic vessel may be sufficient to sustain a portion of the territory of another artery if the latter is occluded. The cerebral arteries are also interconnected through an arteriolar network in the pia mater. Short cortical branches from the pial plexus supply the rich capillary network of the cortex, whereas longer branches of arteries in the subarachnoid space penetrate into the white matter and form a less profuse capillary network.

Arterial Circle (Circle of Willis)

The major arteries supplying the cerebrum are joined to one another at the base of the brain in the form of an arterial circle or the circle of Willis (see Fig. 25-1). Starting from the midline in front, the circle consists of the anterior communicating, anterior cerebral, internal carotid (a short segment), posterior communicating, and posterior cerebral arteries; then it continues to the starting point in reverse order. There is normally little exchange of blood between the main arteries through the slender anterior and posterior communicating arteries. However, the arterial circle provides alternative routes when one of the major arteries leading into it is occluded. These anastomoses are frequently inadequate, especially in the elderly, in whom the communicating arteries may be narrowed because of vascular disease.

There are frequent variants of the conventional configuration of the arterial circle. The posterior cerebral artery is a branch of the internal carotid artery in the embryo. In the course of development the posterior cerebral artery becomes a terminal branch of the basilar artery, the vestige of the embryonic condition being seen in the posterior communicating artery. The embryonic condition persists in about a third of all individuals, in whom one of the posterior cerebral arteries is a major branch of the internal carotid artery. This type of connection of the posterior cerebral artery occurs bilaterally very rarely. One of the anterior cerebral arteries may be unusually small in the first part of its course, in which case the anterior communicating artery has a larger than usual caliber.

Central Arteries

Numerous central arteries arise from the region of the arterial circle as four groups (see Fig. 25-1). These slender, thin-walled blood vessels, also known as ganglionic or nuclear arteries, supply portions of the corpus striatum, internal capsule, diencephalon, and midbrain. The recurrent artery of Heubner is similar to the central arteries with respect to its distribution, as are the anterior and posterior choroidal arteries with respect to portions of their distribution.

Anteromedial Group

These central arteries arise from the anterior cerebral arteries and from the anterior communicating artery. They penetrate the medial part of the anterior perforated substance and are distributed mainly to the preoptic and suprachiasmatic regions of the hypothalamus.

Anterolateral Group

This group of central arteries consists mainly of branches of the middle cerebral artery. They enter the anterior perforated substance and are also called **striate arteries** (or lateral striate arteries) because they supply a major portion of the corpus striatum. The region of distribution of the anterolateral central arteries includes the head of the caudate nucleus, putamen, lateral part of the globus pallidus, much of the internal capsule (anterior limb, genu, and dorsal portion of the posterior limb), external capsule, and claustrum. Several of these arteries also send twigs into the lateral area of the hypothalamus.

Posteromedial Group

The posteromedial central arteries are branches of the posterior cerebral and posterior communicating arteries. After penetrating the posterior perforated substance between the cerebral peduncles, they are distributed to the anterior and medial portions of the thalamus, subthalamus, middle and posterior regions of the hypothalamus, and medial parts of the cerebral peduncles of the midbrain.

Posterolateral Group

These central arteries come off the posterior cerebral artery as it curves around the midbrain. They are distributed to the posterior portion of the thalamus (including the medial and lateral geniculate bodies), tectum of the midbrain, and lateral part of the cerebral peduncle.

Distribution of Central Arteries

The following summary identifies the blood supply of structures situated within the region of the brain that is nourished by the central arteries.

Head of caudate nucleus and putamen (striatum): anterolateral central arteries; recurrent artery of Heubner

Globus pallidus (pallidum): anterolateral central arteries; anterior choroidal artery

Thalamus: posteromedial and posterolateral central arteries; anterior and posterior choroidal arteries

Subthalamus: posteromedial central arteries; anterior choroidal artery

Hypothalamus: anteromedial, posteromedial, and anterolateral central arteries

Pineal gland: posterolateral central arteries

Internal capsule: anterolateral and posterolateral central arteries; anterior choroidal artery; recurrent artery of Heubner

Amygdala, uncus, and hippocampal formation: anterior choroidal artery; temporal branches of posterior cerebral artery

External capsule and claustrum: anterolateral central arteries

Tectum of midbrain: posterolateral central arteries; posterior choroidal artery; superior cerebellar artery

Cerebral peduncle: posteromedial and posterolateral central arteries; anterior choroidal artery

VENOUS DRAINAGE OF THE BRAIN

The capillary bed of the brain stem and the cerebellum is drained by unnamed veins that empty into dural venous sinuses situated adjacent to the posterior cranial fossa. The cerebrum has an external and an internal venous system. The external cerebral veins lie in the subarachnoid space on all surfaces of the hemispheres, whereas the central core of the cerebrum is drained by internal cerebral veins situated beneath the corpus callosum in the transverse fissure. Both sets of cerebral veins empty into dural venous sinuses, which are identified in the following chapter.

External Cerebral Veins

The **superior cerebral veins**, eight to twelve in number, course upward over the lateral surface of the hemisphere. On nearing the midline they pierce the arachnoid, run between the arachnoid and the dura mater for 1 cm to 2 cm, and empty into the superior sagittal sinus or into venous lacunae adjacent to the sinus. Trauma to the head may tear a superior cerebral vein as it lies between the arachnoid and dura mater, resulting in a subdural hemorrhage.

The **superficial middle cerebral vein** runs downward and forward along the lateral sulcus and empties into the cavernous sinus. However, anastomotic channels allow for drainage in other directions. These are the superior anastomotic vein (of Trolard), which opens into the superior sagittal sinus, and the inferior anastomotic vein (of Labbé), which opens into the transverse sinus.

The **deep middle cerebral vein** runs downward and forward in the depths of the lateral sulcus to the ventral surface of the brain; the **anterior cerebral vein** accompanies the anterior cerebral artery. These veins unite in the region of the anterior perforated substance to form the **basal vein** (of Rosenthal), which runs backward at the base of the brain, curves around the midbrain, and empties into the great cerebral vein (see Internal Cerebral Veins). The basal vein receives tributaries from the optic tract, hypothalamus, temporal lobe, and midbrain.

In addition to the named veins just noted, there are numerous small veins that drain limited areas. These have no consistent pattern and empty into adjacent dural sinuses.

Internal Cerebral Veins

The internal venous system forms adjacent to each lateral ventricle and continues through the transverse cerebral fissure beneath the corpus callosum (Fig. 25-4). The **thalamostriate vein (vena terminalis)** begins in the region of the amygdaloid body in the temporal lobe and follows the curve of the tail of the caudate nucleus on its medial side. The thalamostriate vein receives tributaries from the corpus striatum, internal capsule, thalamus, fornix, and septum pellucidum. The **choroidal vein,** which is rather tortuous, runs along the choroid plexus of the lateral ventricle. In addition to draining the plexus, the choroidal vein receives tributaries from the hippocampus, fornix, and corpus callosum. The thalamostriate vein and choroidal vein unite immediately behind the interventricular foramen to form the **internal cerebral vein.** The paired internal cerebral veins run posteriorly in the transverse fissure, uniting beneath the splenium of the corpus callosum to form the **great cerebral vein** (of Galen). The latter vein, which is no more than 2 cm in length, receives the basal veins and tributaries from the cerebellum. The great cerebral vein empties into the straight sinus, situated in the midline of the tentorium cerebelli.

BLOOD SUPPLY OF THE SPINAL CORD

Spinal Arteries

Three arterial channels, the **anterior spinal artery** and paired **posterior spinal arteries**,

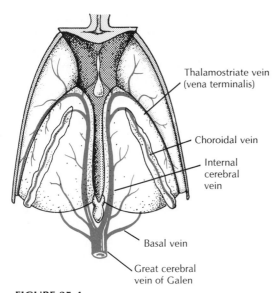

FIGURE 25-4.
The internal cerebral system of veins, as seen from above after removal of the corpus callosum and fornix.

run longitudinally throughout the length of the spinal cord. The anterior spinal artery originates in a Y-shaped configuration from the vertebral arteries, as already described, and runs caudally along the ventral median fissure. Each posterior spinal artery is a branch of either the vertebral artery or the posterior inferior cerebellar artery and consists of multiple anastomosing channels along the line of attachment of the dorsal roots of the spinal nerves.

The blood received by the spinal arteries from the vertebral arteries is sufficient for only the upper cervical segments of the spinal cord. The arteries are therefore reinforced at intervals in the following manner. The vertebral artery in the cervical region, the posterior intercostal branches of the thoracic aorta, and the lumbar branches of the abdominal aorta give off segmental **spinal arteries**, which enter the vertebral canal through the intervertebral foramina. In addition to supplying the vertebrae, these segmental spinal arteries give rise to **anterior** and **posterior radicular arteries**, which run along the ventral and dorsal roots of the spinal nerves. Most of

the radicular arteries are of small caliber, sufficient only to supply the nerve roots and contribute to a vascular plexus in the pia mater covering the spinal cord. A variable number of anterior radicular arteries of substantial size, approximately 12 including both sides, join the anterior spinal artery. Similarly, a variable number of posterior radicular arteries, approximately 14 including both sides, join the anastomosing channels composing the posterior spinal arteries. These radicular arteries are situated mainly in the lower cervical, lower thoracic, and upper lumbar regions; the largest, an anterior radicular artery known as the spinal artery of Adamkiewicz, is usually in the upper lumbar region. The spinal cord is vulnerable to circulatory impairment if the important contribution by a major radicular artery is compromised by injury or by the placing of a ligature.

Sulcal branches arise in succession from the anterior spinal artery and enter the right and left sides of the spinal cord alternately from the ventral median fissure. The sulcal arteries are least frequent in the thoracic part of the spinal cord. The anterior spinal artery supplies the ventral gray horns, part of the dorsal gray horns, and the ventral and lateral white funiculi. Penetrating branches from the posterior spinal arteries supply the remainder of the dorsal gray horns and the dorsal funiculi of white matter. A fine plexus (the vasocorona) derived from the spinal arteries is present in the pia mater on the lateral and ventral surfaces of the cord. Penetrating branches from the vasocorona supply a narrow zone of white matter beneath the pia mater.

Spinal Veins

Although the pattern of spinal veins is irregular, there are essentially six of them. **Anterior spinal veins** run along the midline and each ventrolateral sulcus; **posterior spinal veins** are situated in the midline and along the dorsolateral sulci. The spinal veins are drained at intervals by up to 12 **anterior radicular veins** and by a similar number of **posterior radicular veins.** The radicular veins empty into an epidural venous plexus, which in turn drains into an external vertebral plexus through channels in the intervertebral foramina. Blood from the external vertebral plexus empties into the vertebral, intercostal, and lumbar veins.

BLOOD–BRAIN BARRIER

Certain substances fail to pass from capillary blood into the central nervous system, although the same substances gain access to nonnervous tissues. They include dyes used in animal experimentation and, more importantly, some agents that would otherwise be of therapeutic value. In the blood, these substances are bound to plasma protein molecules, which are unable to leave normal cerebral blood vessels. The lumen of a capillary and the parenchyma of the brain and spinal cord are separated by endothelium, a basal lamina, and perivascular end feet of astrocytic processes. Much

research has been directed toward the identification of the blood–brain barrier in an anatomical or physical sense. The best evidence points to the tight junctions between endothelial cells and special properties of the internal plasma membrane of these cells. In a few small regions—for example, the area postrema in the medulla, the subfornical organ, and the neurohypophysis—the classical blood–brain barrier is lacking.

There is a similar blood–tissue barrier to large molecules in the myenteric and submucous plexuses of the digestive tract and within the endoneurium in peripheral nerves, but not in sensory and autonomic ganglia. The blood–brain and other barriers are defective after injury and in various pathological states.

CEREBRAL ANGIOGRAPHY

In 1927 de Egas Moniz introduced the technique of cerebral angiography, which developed into a valuable diagnostic aid in the hands of neuroradiologists. Briefly stated, the method consists of injecting a

FIGURE 25-5.
Carotid angiogram (lateral view).   **(A)** Carotid siphon. **(B)** Branches of the middle cerebral artery.   **(C)** Anterior cerebral artery. (Courtesy of Dr. J. M. Allcock)

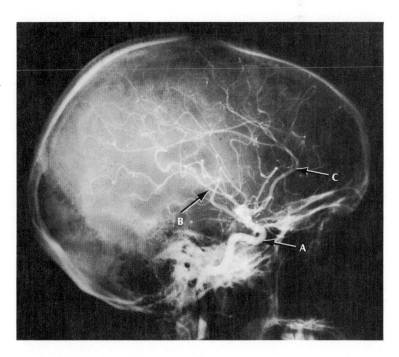

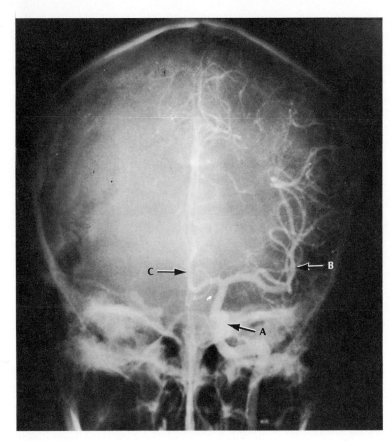

FIGURE 25-6.
Carotid angiogram
(anteroposterior view).
(A) Carotid siphon.
(B) Branches of the middle
cerebral artery.   **(C)**
Anterior cerebral artery.
(Courtesy of Dr. J. M. Allcock)

radiopaque solution into the artery, followed by serial x-ray photography at approximately 1-sec intervals. The roentgenograms show the contrast medium in progressive stages of its passage through the arterial tree and the venous return. Injection into the common carotid artery or the internal carotid artery shows the distribution of the middle and anterior cerebral arteries (Figs. 25-5 and 25-6). Similarly, injection of the vertebral artery, which is approached with a long catheter passed through the femoral artery and aorta, permits visualization of the vertebral, basilar, and posterior cerebral arteries, together with their larger branches. The cerebral veins are seen in later roentgenograms of a series.

The technique of cerebral angiography is especially useful in identifying vascu-

lar malformations and aneurysms. The method often provides valuable information concerning occlusive vascular disease and space-occupying lesions. The cerebral vessels can also be demonstrated by computed tomography after intravenous injection of a contrast medium, and by nuclear magnetic resonance imaging.

SUGGESTED READING

FitzGerald MJT: Neuroanatomy Basic and Applied. London, Ballière-Tindall, 1985

Gillilan LA: The blood supply of the human spinal cord. J Comp Neurol 110:75–103, 1958

Montemurro DG, Bruni JE: The Human Brain in Dissection. Philadelphia, WB Saunders, 1981

Netter FH: The Ciba Collection of Medical Illustrations. Vol I: The Nervous System,

Part I: Anatomy and Physiology. West Caldwell, NJ, CIBA-GEIGY Corporation, 1983

Raichle ME, Eichling GO, Grubb RL, Hartman BK: Central noradrenergic regulation of the brain microcirculation. In Pappius HM, Feindel W (eds): Dynamics of Brain Edema, pp 11–17. Berlin, Springer-Verlag, 1976

Rapoport SI: Blood–Brain Barrier in Physiology and Medicine. New York, Raven Press, 1976

Thomas DJ, Bannister R: Preservation of autoregulation of cerebral blood flow in autonomic failure. J Neurol Sci 44:205–212, 1980

TWENTY-SIX

Meninges and Cerebrospinal Fluid

The consistency of the brain is soft and gelatinous, although the spinal cord is slightly firmer. The meninges provide protection for the central nervous system in addition to the protection provided by the skull and the vertebral column and its ligaments. They consist of the thick dura mater externally, the delicate arachnoid lining the dura, and the thin pia mater adhering to the brain and spinal cord. The latter two layers, constituting the pia-arachnoid, bound the subarachnoid space filled with cerebrospinal fluid. The main support and protection provided by the meninges come from the dura mater and the cushion of cerebrospinal fluid in the subarachnoid space.

DURA MATER AND ASSOCIATED STRUCTURES

The internal surfaces of the bones enclosing the cranial cavity are clothed by peri-osteum, such as covers bones elsewhere. This periosteum is continuous with the periosteum on the external surface of the cranium at the margins of the foramen magnum and smaller foramina for nerves and blood vessels. The cranial dura mater is attached intimately to the periosteum, which is sometimes referred to incorrectly as the external layer of the dura mater.

Periosteum and Meningeal Blood Vessels

The periosteum consists of collagenous connective tissue and contains arteries, somewhat inappropriately called meningeal arteries, which mainly supply the adjoining bone. Of these the largest is the **middle meningeal artery,** a branch of the maxillary artery that enters the cranial cavity through the foramen spinosum in the floor of the middle cranial fossa. The artery divides into anterior and posterior branches soon after entering the middle cranial fossa; these branches ramify over the lateral surface of the cranium, producing grooves on the bones. A fracture in the temporal region of the skull may tear a branch of the middle meningeal artery. The extravasated blood accumulates between the bone and the periosteum, forming an extradural hematoma. As in the case of any space-occupying lesion in the nonexpansile cranial cavity, intracranial pressure rises and prompt surgical intervention is usually necessary. Less extensive areas of the cranium and dura are supplied by several small arteries. These include meningeal branches of the ophthalmic artery, branches of the occipital artery traversing the jugular foramen and hypoglossal canal, and small twigs arising from the vertebral artery at the foramen magnum.

The meningeal arteries are accompanied by **meningeal veins,** which are also subject to tearing in fractures of the skull. The largest meningeal veins accompany the middle meningeal artery, leave the cranial cavity through the foramen spinosum or the foramen ovale, and drain into the pterygoid venous plexus. **Diploic veins,** within the cancellous bone of the vault of the skull, drain into the veins of the scalp and into the dural venous sinuses described below.

Dura Mater

The dura mater or pachymeninx (thick membrane) is a dense, firm layer consisting of collagenous connective tissue. The **spinal dura mater** takes the form of a tube, pierced by the roots of spinal nerves, that extends from the foramen magnum to the second segment of the sacrum. The spinal dura mater is separated from the wall of the spinal canal by an epidural space containing adipose tissue and a venous plexus. The **cranial dura mater** is firmly attached to the periosteum, as previously described, from which it receives small blood vessels. The smooth inner surface of the dura mater consists of simple squamous epithelium, and a film of fluid oc-

cupies the subdural space between the dura and arachnoid. The cranial dura mater has several features of importance, notably the dural reflections and dural venous sinuses.

Dural Reflections

The dura mater is reflected along certain lines to form the dural reflections or dural septa. The intervals between the periosteum and dura along the lines of attachment of the septa accommodate dural venous sinuses (Fig. 26-1). The largest septa, the falx cerebri and the tentorium cerebelli, form incomplete partitions dividing the cranial cavity into three compartments (Fig. 26-2).

The **falx cerebri,** so-named because of its sickle shape, is a vertical partition in the longitudinal fissure between the cerebral hemispheres. This dural reflection is attached to the crista galli of the ethmoid bone in front, to the midline of the vault as far back as the internal occipital protuberance, and to the tentorium cerebelli. The free edge is close to the splenium of the corpus callosum, but some distance from the corpus callosum further forward. The anterior portion of the falx cerebri is often fenestrated.

The **tentorium cerebelli** intervenes between the occipital lobes of the cerebral hemispheres and the cerebellum. The attachment of the falx cerebri along the midline draws the tentorium upward, giving it a shallow tentlike configuration. The peripheral border of the tentorium is attached to the upper edges of the petrous portion of the temporal bones and to the margins of the sulci on the occipital bone for the transverse sinuses. The free border bounds the **incisura of the tentorium** (tentorial notch); the incisura is completed by the sphenoid bone and accommodates the midbrain.

The narrow interval between the midbrain and the boundary of the tentorial incisura is the only communication between the subtentorial and supratentorial regions

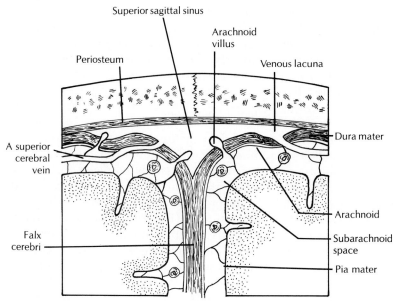

Superior sagittal sinus

Arachnoid villus

Periosteum

Venous lacuna

Dura mater

A superior cerebral vein

Arachnoid

Subarachnoid space

Falx cerebri

Pia mater

FIGURE 26-1.
Coronal section at the vertex of the skull, including the superior sagittal sinus and the attachment of the falx cerebri.

of the subarachnoid space. The cerebrospinal fluid produced in the ventricles enters the subarachnoid space of the posterior cranial fossa and then moves slowly upward around the midbrain to be absorbed into venous blood along the attached border of the falx cerebri. Obstruction of the subarachnoid space around the midbrain results in dilation of the ventricles and of the subarachnoid space in the posterior cranial fossa. An expanding lesion in a cerebral hemisphere may cause the medial part of the temporal lobe to herniate into the incisura of the tentorium. The midbrain is displaced toward the opposite side, and the pressure of the firm edge of the tentorium on the basis pedunculi may result in the unusual finding of voluntary motor paresis on the same side of the body as the cerebral lesion.

The **falx cerebelli** is a small dural fold in the posterior cranial fossa, extending vertically for a short distance between the cerebellar hemispheres. The **diaphragma sellae** roofs over the pituitary fossa or sella turcica of the sphenoid bone and has an opening for passage of the infundibular stem of the neurohypophysis.

Nerve Supply of the Dura Mater

The cranial dura mater has a plentiful supply of sensory nerve fibers, mainly from the trigeminal nerve. The fibers terminate as nonencapsulated endings, for the most part, and are of significance in certain types of headache.

The dura lining the anterior cranial fossa is supplied by ethmoid branches of the ophthalmic nerve. The mandibular nerve supplies a large area through the nervus spinosum, which enters the middle cranial fossa with the middle meningeal artery and ramifies with the arterial branches. A meningeal branch comes off the maxillary nerve while it is still in the cranial cavity and joins the fibers of the nervus spinosum that accompany the anterior branch of the middle meningeal artery. The tentorium cerebelli and the dura mater lining the vault above it are supplied by several large branches coming off the first part of the ophthalmic nerve. These nerves run backward in the tentorium, spreading out over the vault and in the falx cerebri. The dura lining the floor of the posterior cranial fossa is supplied by the vagus nerve and upper cervical nerves. The meningeal branch of the vagus nerve arises from the superior ganglion at the level of the jugular foramen, through which it enters the posterior fossa. Sensory twigs from the first three cervical spinal nerves enter the posterior fossa through the hypoglossal canal. (The first cervical nerve lacks a sensory component in about half of individuals.) Recurrent branches of all spinal nerves enter the vertebral canal through the intervertebral foramina and give off meningeal branches to the spinal dura mater.

Dural Venous Sinuses

The veins draining the brain empty into the venous sinuses of the dura mater, from which blood flows into the internal jugular veins. The walls of the sinuses consist of dura mater and periosteum, lined by endothelium. The location of most of the dural venous sinuses is shown in Figure 26-2.

The **superior sagittal sinus** lies along the attached border of the falx cerebri. It begins in front of the crista galli of the ethmoid bone, where there may be a narrow communication with nasal veins. Venous lacunae lie alongside the superior sagittal sinus and open into it. The superior cerebral veins drain into the sinus or into the lacunae. The superior sagittal si-

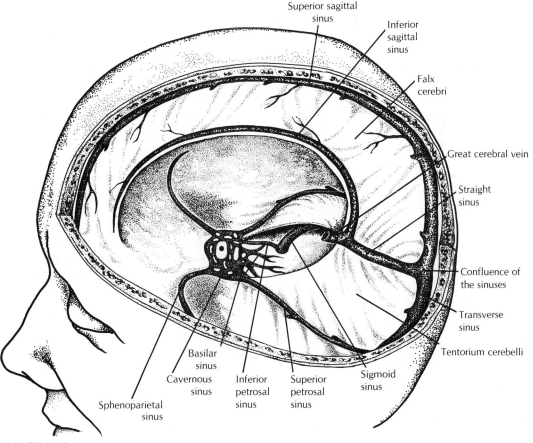

FIGURE 26-2.
Dural reflections and dural venous sinuses.

nus is usually continuous with the right transverse sinus.

The **inferior sagittal sinus** is smaller than the one just described; it runs along the free border of the falx cerebri and receives veins from the medial aspects of the cerebral hemispheres. The inferior sagittal sinus opens into the **straight sinus,** which lies in the attachment of the falx cerebri to the tentorium cerebelli. The straight sinus receives the great cerebral vein; it therefore drains the system of internal cerebral veins and the territories of the cerebral hemispheres drained by the basal vein, formed by the union of the deep middle cerebral and anterior cerebral veins. The straight sinus is usually continuous with the left transverse sinus. Venous channels connect the transverse sinuses at the internal occipital protuberance; the configuration of sinuses in this location is called the **confluence of the sinuses** (torcular Herophili).

Each **transverse sinus** lies in a groove on the occipital bone along the attached margin of the tentorium cerebelli. On reaching the petrous portion of the temporal bone, the transverse sinus continues as the **sigmoid sinus;** the latter follows a curved course in the posterior fossa on the mastoid portion of the petrous bone and becomes continuous with the internal jugular vein at the jugular foramen.

The **cavernous sinuses** are situated one on each side of the body of the sphenoid bone; each sinus receives the ophthalmic vein and the superficial middle cerebral vein. Venous channels in the anterior and posterior margins of the diaphragma sellae connect the cavernous sinuses; these channels and the cavernous sinuses constitute the **circular sinus.** The cavernous sinus drains into the transverse sinus through the **superior petrosal sinus,** running along the attachment of the tentorium cerebelli to the petrous portion of the temporal bone. The **inferior petrosal sinus** lies in the groove between the petrous portion of the temporal bone and the basilar portion of the occipital bone, providing a communication between the cavernous sinus and the internal jugular vein. Small venous channels posterior to the circular sinus constitute the **basilar sinus,** which is connected with the cavernous and inferior petrosal sinuses. Finally the **sphenoparietal sinus** is a small venous channel under the lesser wing of the sphenoid bone draining into the cavernous sinus, and the small **occipital sinus** in the falx cerebelli drains into the confluence of the sinuses. The sinuses at the base of the cranium receive veins from adjacent parts of the brain.

Emissary veins connect dural venous sinuses with veins outside the cranial cavity. Blood may flow in either direction, depending on venous pressure relationships. The parietal and mastoid emissary veins are the largest of these connecting channels. The parietal emissary vein traverses the parietal foramen, joining the superior sagittal sinus with tributaries of the occipital veins. The mastoid emissary vein traverses the mastoid foramen and joins the sigmoid sinus with the occipital and posterior auricular veins.

PIA–ARACHNOID

The **pia mater** and the **arachnoid** develop initially as a single layer from the mesodermal tissue surrounding the embryonic brain and spinal cord. Fluid-filled spaces appear within the layer; these become the subarachnoid space, and the origin of the membranes from a single layer is reflected in the numerous trabeculae passing between them. Histologically the pia and arachnoid consist of collagenous fibers and some elastic fibers. Both surfaces of the arachnoid and the external surface of the pia mater are covered by simple squamous epithelium. The trabeculae crossing the subarachnoid space consist of delicate strands of connective tissue with squamous epithelial cells on their surfaces. Tight junctions connect adjacent arachnoid epithelial cells, preventing exchange

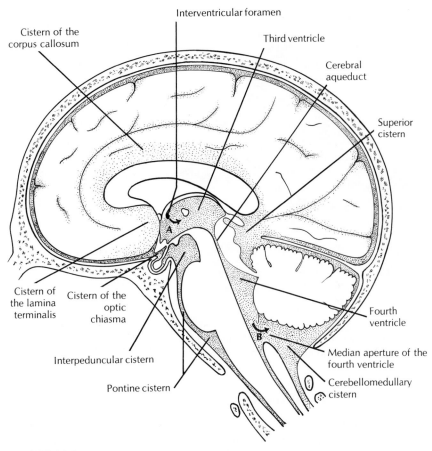

FIGURE 26-3.
Subarachnoid cisterns. **(A)** Cerebrospinal fluid entering the third ventricle from the right lateral ventricle through an interventricular foramen. **(B)** Cerebrospinal fluid entering the cerebellomedullary cistern from the fourth ventricle through the median aperture.

of large molecules between the cerebrospinal fluid and the blood in the dural vasculature. There are no tight junctions between the pial cells, so there is free exchange of macromolecules between the cerebrospinal fluid and the central nervous tissue. The pia mater and arachnoid together constitute the leptomeninges (slender membranes).

The avascular arachnoid is separated from the dura mater by a film of fluid in the subdural space. The pia mater, which contains a network of fine blood vessels, adheres to the surface of the brain and spinal cord, following all their contours. The connective tissue fibers in the spinal pia mater tend to run in a longitudinal direction. This is accentuated along the ventromedian line of the spinal cord, where a thickened strand of fibers superficial to the anterior spinal artery is known as the **linea splendens.** The **denticulate ligament,** described in Chapter 5, is derived from the pia mater.

The larger arteries and veins entering and leaving the substance of the brain are surrounded by a sleeve of pia mater. There are thus formed **perivascular spaces** (Virchow–Robin spaces), continuous with the subarachnoid space and extending in increasingly attentuated form as far as arterioles and venules in the brain.

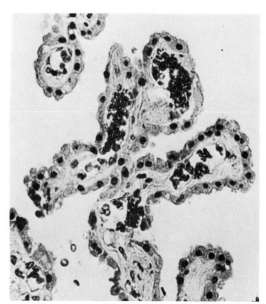

FIGURE 26-4.
A fragment of choroid plexus showing the large capillaries and choroid epithelium. (Stained with alum-hematoxylin and eosin, × 400)

SUBARACHNOID CISTERNS

The width of the subarachnoid space varies because the arachnoid rests on the dura mater, whereas the pia mater adheres to the irregular contours of the brain. The space is narrow over the summits of gyri, wider in the regions of major sulci, and wider yet at the base of the brain and in the lumbosacral region of the spinal canal. Regions of the subarachnoid space containing more substantial amounts of cerebrospinal fluid are called **subarachnoid cisterns** (Fig. 26-3).

The **cerebellomedullary cistern (cisterna magna)** occupies the interval between the cerebellum and medulla and receives cerebrospinal fluid through the median aperture of the fourth ventricle. The basal cisterns beneath the brain stem and diencephalon include the **pontine** and **interpeduncular cisterns** and the **cistern of the optic chiasma.** The last-named cistern is continuous with the **cistern of the lamina terminalis**, which in turn continues into the **cistern of the corpus callosum**

above this commissure. The subarachnoid space dorsal to the midbrain is called the **superior cistern** or, alternatively, the **cistern of the great cerebral vein.** This cistern and subarachnoid space on the sides of the midbrain constitute the **cisterna ambiens.** The **cistern of the lateral sulcus** corresponds with that sulcus. The **lumbar cistern** of the spinal subarachnoid space is especially large, extending from the second lumbar vertebra to the second segment of the sacrum. It contains the cauda equina, formed by lumbosacral spinal nerve roots.

The meningeal layers and subarachnoid space extend around cranial nerves and spinal nerve roots for a distance, approximately to the level of sensory ganglia when these are present. For example, an extension of the subarachnoid space, enclosed by dura mater, around the proximal part of the trigeminal ganglion in the middle cranial fossa at the tip of the petrous portion of the temporal bone constitutes the trigeminal cave (Meckel's cave). The most important meningeal extension clinically surrounds the optic nerve to its attachment to the eyeball. The central artery and central vein of the retina run within the anterior part of the optic nerve and cross the extension of the subarachnoid space to join the ophthalmic artery and ophthalmic vein. An increase of cerebrospinal fluid pressure slows the return of venous blood, causing edema of the retina. This is most apparent on ophthalmoscopic examination as swelling of the optic papilla or disk (papilledema). Dilation of the axons of the optic nerve, caused by impairment of the slow component of anterograde axoplasmic transport, also contributes to the swelling. Inspection of the ocular fundi is an important part of the neurological examination.

CEREBROSPINAL FLUID

The cerebrospinal fluid is produced mainly by the choroid plexuses of the lat-

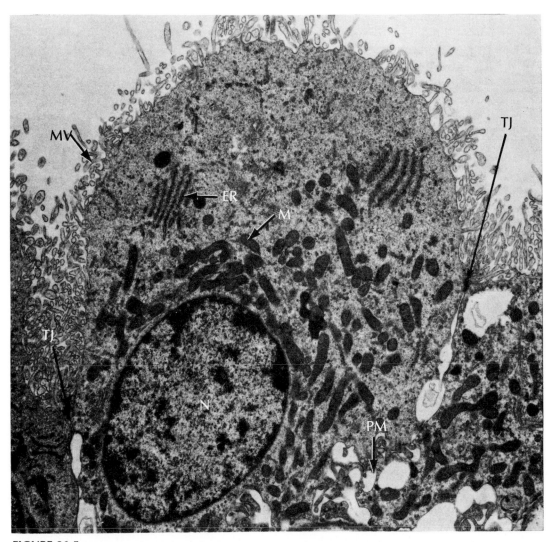

FIGURE 26-5.
Electron micrograph of a choroid epithelial cell.   **(ER)** Endoplasmic reticulum.   **(M)** Mitochondria.
(MV) Microvilli.   **(N)** Nucleus.   **(PM)** Folds of plasma membrane;   **(TJ)** Tight junctions (zonulae
occludentes). (× 8800; courtesy of Dr. D. H. Dickson)

eral, third, and fourth ventricles, with
those in the lateral ventricles being the
largest and most important.

The **choroid plexus** of each lateral ventricle is formed by an invagination of vascular pia mater (the tela choroidea) on the
medial surface of the cerebral hemisphere.
The vascular connective tissue picks up a
covering layer of epithelium from the

ependymal lining of the ventricle. The
choroid plexuses of the third and fourth
ventricles are similarly formed by invaginations of the tela choroidea attached to
the roofs of these ventricles. The choroid
plexuses, which have a minutely folded
surface, therefore consist of a core of connective tissue containing many wide capillaries and a surface layer of simple cu-

boidal or low columnar epithelium (the choroid epithelium; Fig. 26-4). The surface area of the choroid plexuses of the two lateral ventricles combined is about 40 cm^2.

Several features of the choroid epithelium as seen in electron micrographs are of functional interest (Fig. 26-5). The large spherical nucleus, abundant cytoplasm, and numerous mitochondria indicate that the production of cerebrospinal fluid is at least partly an active process requiring expenditure of energy on the part of these cells. The plasma membrane at the free surface is greatly increased in area by irregular microvilli. The membranes of adjoining cells are thrown into complicated folds at the base of the cells. The choroid epithelial cells bear motile cilia in the embryo, and patches of ciliated epithelium persist for varying periods postnatally. A basement membrane separates the epithelium from the subjacent stroma with its rich vascular network. The capillaries are unlike those supplying nervous tissue generally in that the endothelial cells have fenestrations or pores closed by thin diaphragms and are permeable to large molecules. The blood–cerebrospinal fluid barrier to macromolecules is formed by the cells of the choroid epithelium and the tight junctions (zonulae occludentes) between adjacent cells.

Production of cerebrospinal fluid is a complex process, the details of which are still being studied. Some components of the blood plasma enter the cerebrospinal fluid readily by diffusion. Others negotiate the capillary wall and the choroid epithelium with difficulty, and still others reach the fluid with the assistance of metabolic activity on the part of the choroid epithelial cells. An important factor appears to be active transport of certain ions (notably sodium ions) through the epithelial cells, followed by passive movement of water to maintain the osmotic equilibrium between cerebrospinal fluid and blood plasma.

The flow of cerebrospinal fluid is from the lateral ventricles into the third ventricle through the interventricular foramina, and then into the fourth ventricle by way of the cerebral aqueduct. Cerebrospinal fluid leaves the ventricular system through the median and lateral apertures of the fourth ventricle, with the former opening into the cerebellomedullary cistern and the latter into the pontine cistern. From these sites there is a sluggish movement of fluid through the spinal subarachnoid space, determined in part by movements of the vertebral column. More importantly, the cerebrospinal fluid flows slowly forward through the basal cisterns and then upward over the medial and lateral surfaces of the cerebral hemispheres. Movement of cerebrospinal fluid is assisted by the pulsation of arteries in the subarachnoid space, especially in the subarachnoid space around the spinal cord.

The main site of absorption of the cerebrospinal fluid into venous blood is through the **arachnoid villi** projecting into dural venous sinuses, especially the superior sagittal sinus and adjacent venous lacunae (see Fig. 26-1). Each arachnoid villus consists of a thin cellular layer, derived from the epithelium of the arachnoid and the endothelium of the sinus, which encloses an extension of the subarachnoid space containing trabeculae. The absorptive mechanism depends on the higher hydrostatic pressure of the cerebrospinal fluid compared with venous blood in the dural sinuses, the difference of colloidal osmotic pressure between the virtually protein-free cerebrospinal fluid and the blood, and active transport by cells forming the walls of the arachnoid villi. The arachnoid cells of the villus are joined by tight junctions, and the movement of fluid occurs in large vesicles that are transported through the cytoplasm. The arachnoid villi become hypertrophied with age, when they are called **arachnoid granulations** or **pacchionian bodies;** these may be sufficiently large to produce erosion or pitting of the cranial bones.

Although the choroid plexuses are the main source of cerebrospinal fluid and the arachnoid villi of its absorption, there are exchanges between blood plasma and cerebrospinal fluid elsewhere. Results of studies using radioactive isotopes in experimental animals show that the chemical composition of cerebrospinal fluid is determined in part by passive two-way transfer of water and solutes across the ependymal lining of the ventricles and walls of small blood vessels in the pia mater. Some cerebrospinal fluid is absorbed into arachnoid villi that protrude into veins that pass alongside the spinal nerve roots before emptying into the epidural venous plexus, and a small proportion of the fluid enters lymphatic vessels adjacent to the extensions of the subarachnoid space around cerebrospinal nerves.

The volume of the cerebrospinal fluid varies from 80 to 150 ml; these figures include the fluid in both the ventricles and subarachnoid space. The ventricular system alone contains from 15 to 40 ml fluid. The rate of production of fluid is thought to be sufficient to effect a total replacement several times daily. The pressure of cerebrospinal fluid is from 80 to 180 mm water when a subject is recumbent; the pressure in the lumbar cistern is approximately twice these values when measured in a sitting position. Venous congestion in the closed space of the cranial cavity and the spinal canal, as produced by straining or coughing, is reflected in a prompt rise of cerebrospinal fluid pressure.

Cerebrospinal fluid is clear and colorless, with a specific gravity of 1.003 to 1.008. The few cells present are mainly lymphocytes. These vary in number from one to eight in each cubic millimeter; a count of over ten cells is indicative of disease. The glucose level is about half that of blood, and the protein content is very low (15 to 45 mg/dl).

When there is an excess of cerebrospinal fluid the condition is known as **hydrocephalus,** of which there are several types.

External hydrocephalus, in which the excess fluid is mainly in the subarachnoid space, is found in senile atrophy of the brain. **Internal hydrocephalus** refers to dilation of the ventricles. All the ventricles are enlarged if the apertures of the fourth ventricle are occluded, the third and lateral ventricles if the obstruction is in the cerebral aqueduct, and one lateral ventricle only in the rare occurrence of occlusion of an interventricular foramen. The term **communicating hydrocephalus** refers to a combination of internal and external hydrocephalus. The commonest cause is obstruction of the arachnoid villi by blood, following a subarachnoid hemorrhage. If the flow of cerebrospinal fluid through the incisura of the tentorium around the midbrain is obstructed, the excess fluid accumulates in the ventricles and in the part of the subarachnoid space below the tentorium.

SUGGESTED READING

Agnew WF, Yuen TGH, Achtyl TR: Ultrastructural observations suggesting apocrine secretion in the choroid plexus. A comparative study. Neurol Res 1:313–332, 1980

Alksne JF, Lovings ET: Functional ultrastructure of the arachnoid villus. Arch Neurol 27:371–377, 1972

Baumbach GL, Cancilla PA, Hayreh MS, Hayreh SS: Experimental injury of the optic nerve with optic disc swelling. Lab Invest 39:50–60, 1978

Bradbury MWB: The structure and function of the blood–brain barrier. Fed Proc 43:186–190, 1984

Crosby EC, Humphrey T, Lauer EN: Correlative Anatomy of the Nervous System. New York, Macmillan, 1962

Cserr HF: Physiology of the choroid plexus. Physiol Rev 51:273–311, 1971

Dandy WE: Experimental hydrocephalus. Trans Am Surg Assoc 37:397–428, 1919

Davson H: Formation and drainage of the cerebrospinal fluid. In Shapiro K, Marmarou A, Portnoy H (eds): Hydrocephalus, pp 3–40. New York, Raven Press, 1984

Somjen GG: Neurophysiology—the Essentials. Baltimore, Williams & Wilkins, 1983

APPENDICES

Investigators Mentioned in the Text

Adamkiewicz, Albert (1850–1921) Polish pathologist. Described the blood supply of the human spinal cord (an anterior radicular artery supplying the lumbar region of the spinal cord is known as the artery of Adamkiewicz).

Alzheimer, Alois (1864–1915) German neuropsychiatrist; also made important contributions to neuropathology. Studied presenile and senile dementia, describing in 1907 the condition now known as Alzheimer's disease.

Argyll Robertson, Douglas Moray Cooper Lamb (1837–1909) Scottish ophthalmologist. The Argyll Robertson pupil includes, among other signs, pupillary constriction in accommodation, but not in response to light.

Auerbach, Leopold (1828–1897) German anatomist. Auerbach's plexus (myenteric plexus) in the gastrointestinal tract; end bulbs of Held–Auerbach (synaptic end bulbs or boutons terminaux).

Babinski, Joseph François Félix (1857–1932) French neurologist of Polish origin. The Babinski sign, which consists of up-turning of the great toe and spreading of the toes on stroking the sole, is characteristic of an upper motor neuron lesion.

Baillarger, Jules Gabriel François (1806–1891) French psychiatrist. The lines of Baillarger consist of two transverse strata of nerve fibers in the cerebral cortex.

Bainbridge, Francis Arthur (1874–1921) British physiologist. Found that an increase of pressure on the venous side of the heart accelerates the heart rate.

Beevor, Charles Edward (1854–1908) English neurologist. Contributed to our knowledge of neurology, especially with respect to localization of function in the cerebral cortex.

Bell, Sir Charles (1774–1842) Scottish anatomist, neurologist, and surgeon. Bell's palsy is a form of facial paralysis caused by interruption of conduction by the facial nerve. The Bell–Magendie law states that dorsal spinal roots are sensory, whereas ventral roots are motor.

Bernard, Claude (1813–1878) French physiologist and one of the great investigators of the 19th century. Established experimental physiology as an exact science. One of his contributions was the demonstration of vasomotor mechanisms.

Betz, Vladimir A. (1834–1894) Russian anatomist. Discovered and described the giant pyramidal cells (Betz cells) in the motor area of the cerebral cortex.

Bielschowsky, Max (1869–1940) German neuropathologist and neurologist. Developed Bielschowsky's silver staining method for nerve cells and fibers.

Bodian, David (b. 1910) Contemporary American anatomist who has made important contributions to neurology. Developed Bodian's stain for nerve cells and fibers, using the organic silver compound protargol.

Bowman, Sir William (1816–1892) English anatomist and ophthalmologist. His name is associated with glands in the olfactory mucosa, the capsule of the renal glomerulus, and a layer in the cornea.

Breuer, Josef (1842–1925) Austrian physician and psychologist. Contributed to our knowledge of reflexes controlling respiratory movements.

Broca, Pierre Paul (1824–1880) French pathologist and anthropologist. Localized the cortical motor speech area in the inferior frontal gyrus; also described a band of nerve fibers (the diagonal band of Broca) in the anterior perforated substance on the ventral surface of the cerebral hemisphere.

Brodal, Alf (b. 1910) Contemporary Norwegian neuroanatomist. Has made numerous contributions to our knowledge of the reticular formation, cranial nerves, cerebellum, and other aspects of neuroanatomy, including the nucleus Z of Brodal and Pompeiano (in the medulla).

Brodmann, Korbinian (1868–1918) German neuropsychiatrist. Brodmann's cytoarchitectural map of the cerebral cortex is used frequently when referring to specific regions of the cortex.

Brown–Séquard, Charles Edouard (1817–1894) Physiologist and neurologist. Born in the Crown Colony of Mauritius of American and French parents; he retained British citizenship even though his professional life was spent in several countries. The Brown–Séquard syndrome consists of the sensory and motor abnormalities that follow hemisection of the spinal cord.

Bruch, Karl Wilhelm Ludwig (1819–1884) German anatomist. Bruch's membrane is the innermost layer of the choroid of the eye, separating the capillary layer of the choroid from the retina.

Bucy, Paul C. (b. 1904) Contemporary American neurosurgeon. The Klüver–Bucy syndrome is caused by extensive bilateral lesions of the temporal lobes.

Büngner, Otto von (1858–1905) German neurologist. Described the endoneurial tubes containing modified Schwann cells in the distal portion of a sectioned peripheral nerve (bands of von Büngner).

Cajal See Ramón y Cajal.

Cannon, Walter Bradford (1871–1945) American physiologist who contributed much to our understanding of autonomic regulation of visceral functions. Among other contributions he developed the concept of homeostasis of the internal environment and demonstrated the "fight or flight" reactions of the body to stress.

Clark, Sir Wilfrid Edward Le Gros (1895–1971) English anatomist. Made important contributions to comparative anatomy and neuroanatomy, especially of sensory systems, and to primate paleontology.

Clarke, Jacob Augustus Lockhard (1817–1880) English anatomist and neurologist. Among numerous contributions, described the nucleus dorsalis (thoracicus) of the spinal cord, which is also known as Clarke's column.

Corti, Marchese Alfonso (1822–1888) Italian histologist. Described the sensory epithelium of the cochlea (organ of Corti).

Cushing, Harvey (1869–1939) Pioneer American neurosurgeon. Contributed to many basic aspects of neurology, including the function of the pituitary gland, pituitary tumors, tumors of the eighth cranial nerve, and classification of brain tumors.

Darkschewitsch, Liverij Osipovich (1858–1925) Russian neurologist. Discovered nucleus of Darkschewitsch, one of the accessory oculomotor nuclei in the midbrain.

de Egas Moniz, Antônio Caetano de Abreau Friere (1874–1955) Portuguese physician. Awarded the Nobel Prize for Medicine and Physiology in 1949 for demonstration of the therapeutic value of prefrontal leukotomy; introduced the technique of cerebral angiography in 1927.

Deiters, Otto Friedrich Karl (1834–1863) German anatomist. The lateral vestibular nucleus, the origin of the vestibulospinal tract, is known as Deiters' nucleus.

Dusser de Barenne, Johannes Gregorius (1885–1940) Dutch neurophysiologist. Studied cortical function and introduced the technique of physiological neuronography.

Edinger, Ludwig (1855–1918) German neuroanatomist and neurologist. An outstanding teacher of functional neuroanatomy and a pioneer in comparative neuroanatomy. The Edinger–Westphal nucleus is the parasympathetic component of the oculomotor nucleus.

Eustachio, Bartolemeo (1524–1574) Italian physician, surgeon, and anatomist. The auditory tube bears his name.

Ferrier, Sir David (1843–1928) Scottish neuropathologist, neurophysiologist, and neurologist. Best known for his studies of the motor and sensory areas of the cerebral cortex.

Foerster, Otfrid (1873–1941) German neurologist and neurosurgeon. Made important contributions to the study of epilepsy, pain, the dermatomes, brain tumors, and the cytoarchitecture and functional localization of the cerebral cortex; introduced the chordotomy (tractotomy) operation for intractable pain.

Forel, Auguste Henri (1848–1931) Swiss neuropsychiatrist. Described certain fiber bundles in the subthalamus, which are known as the fields of Forel. The ventral tegmental decussation of Forel in the midbrain consists of crossing rubrospinal fibers. Forel proposed the Neuron Theory on the basis of the response of nerve cells to injury.

Fritsch, Gustav Theodor (1838–1927) German anthropologist and anatomist. With Hitzig, he studied localization of motor function in the dog's cerebral cortex by electrical stimulation.

Frölich, Alfred (1871–1953) Austrian pharmacologist and neurologist. Described the adiposogenital syndrome, which is caused by a lesion involving the hypothalamus.

Galen, Claudius (129-200) Hellenistic physician, who practiced mainly in Rome and Pergamon. Galen was the leading medical authority of the Christian world for 1400 years. His name is attached to the great cerebral vein.

Gasser, Johann Laurentius Austrian anatomist of the 18th century. The sensory ganglion of the trigeminal nerve was named for him by one of his students, A.B.R. Hirsch, in 1765.

Gennari, Francesco (1750–1796?) Italian physician. Described the white line in the visual cortex, now known as the line of Gennari, while still a medical student in Parma, Italy.

Golgi, Camillo (1843–1926) Italian histologist. Introduced a silver staining method that provided the basis of numerous advances in neurohistology. Described type I and type II neurons and the tendon spindles. Awarded the Nobel Prize for Medicine and Physiology in 1906 (with Santiago Ramón y Cajal).

Gray, Edward George (b. 1924) Contemporary English biologist. Has made numerous contributions to an appreciation of the ultrastructure of the nervous system. Gray's type I and type II synapses are named for him.

Grünbaum, Albert S.F. (later Leyton, A.S.F.) (1869–1921) British bacteriologist and physiologist. Worked with Sir Charles Sherrington on functional localization of the cerebral cortex.

Gudden, Bernhard Aloys von (1824–1886) German neuropsychiatrist. Described the partial crossing of optic nerve fibers in the optic chiasma together with certain small commissural bundles adjacent to the chiasma. Gudden also studied connections in the brain by observing changes subsequent to lesions made in the brains of young animals.

Head, Sir Henry (1861–1940) English neurologist. Studied the dermatomes (Head's areas), cutaneous sensory physiology, and especially sensory disturbances and aphasia following cerebral lesions.

Held, Hans (1866–1942) German anatomist. Made extensive studies of interneuronal relationships (axonal synaptic terminals or end bulbs of Held–Auerbach).

Henle, Friedrich Gustav Jacob (1809–1885) German anatomist and a pioneer in histology. The endoneurial sheath surrounding individual fibers of a peripheral nerve is known as the sheath of Henle.

Hensen, Victor (1835–1924) German embryologist and physiologist. Studied the anatomy and physiology of the sense organs (cells of Hensen in the organ of Corti).

Hering, Heinrich Ewald (1866–1948) German physiologist. Best known for his study of the reflex that initiates expiration.

Herophilus (*ca.* 300–250 BC) Greek physician in Alexandria. Made early observations on the anatomy of the brain and other organs. The confluence of the dural venous sinuses at the internal occipital protuberance is known as the torcular Herophili.

Herrick, Charles Judson (1868–1960) American neuroanatomist. Made many contributions to the embryology and comparative anatomy of the nervous system. Founder of the Journal of Comparative Neurology.

Heschl, Richard (1824–1881) Austrian anatomist and pathologist. Described the anterior transverse temporal gyri (Heschl's convolutions), which serve as a landmark for the auditory area of the cerebral cortex.

Heubner, Johann Otto Leonhard (1843–1926) German pediatrician. Described the recurrent branch of the anterior cerebral artery.

Hilton, John (1804–1878) English surgeon. Hilton's law states that the nerve supplying a joint also supplies the muscles that move the joint and the skin covering the articular insertion of those muscles.

His, Wilhelm (1831–1904) Swiss anatomist and a founder of human embryology. Proposed the Neuron Theory on the basis of his embryological studies of the development of nerve cells.

Hitzig, Eduard (1838–1907) German physiologist and neurologist. Studied localization of motor function in the cerebral cortex of dogs and monkeys by electrical stimulation.

Holmes, William Contemporary British zoologist. Developed the Holmes silver staining method for axons. Has also contributed to knowledge of axonal regeneration and comparative histology of the peripheral nervous system.

Horner, Johann Friedrich (1831–1886) Swiss ophthalmologist. Described Horner's syndrome, caused by interruption of the sympathetic innervation of the eye; includes pupillary constriction and ptosis of the upper eyelid.

Horsley, Sir Victor Alexander Haden (1857–1916) A founder of neurosurgery in England. Studied the motor cortex and other parts of the brain by electrical stimulation; introduced the Horsley–Clarke stereotaxic apparatus.

Hubel, David Hunter (b. 1926) Contemporary American neurophysiologist (born and educated in Canada). With T.N. Wiesel, mapped the columnar organization of the monkey's visual cortex.

Hunter, John (1728–1793) British anatomist and pioneer surgeon of the 18th century. His collection of anatomical and pathological specimens formed the basis of the Hunterian Museum of the Royal College of Surgeons.

Huntington, George Sumner (1850–1916) American general medical practitioner. Described a hereditary form of chorea resulting from neuronal degeneration in the corpus striatum and the cerebral cortex.

Jackson, John Hughlings (1835–1911) English neurologist and pioneer of modern neurology. Gave a thorough description of focal epilepsy (jacksonian seizures) resulting from local irritation of the motor cortex.

Kappers, C.U. Ariëns (1878–1946)   Dutch neuroanatomist and Director of the Central Brain Institute in Amsterdam. His many contributions include the theory of neurobiotaxis, anthropological studies of the brain, and cytoarchitectonics of the cerebral cortex in relation to cortical function.

Klüver, Heinrich (1897–1979)   American psychologist. The Klüver–Bucy syndrome is caused by bilateral lesions of the temporal lobes.

Korsakoff, Sergei Sergeievich (1854–1900)   Russian psychiatrist. Korsakoff's psychosis or syndrome, which is usually a sequel of chronic alcoholism, includes a memory defect, fabrication of ideas, and polyneuritis.

Krause, Wilhelm Johann Friedrich (1833–1910)   German anatomist. Described sensory endings in the skin, including the end bulbs of Krause.

Labbé, Léon (1832–1916)   French surgeon. Studied the veins of the brain (lesser anastomotic veins of Labbé).

Lancisi, Giovanni Maria (1654–1720)   Italian physician, who was physician to three successive popes. The longitudinal striae in the indusium griseum are known as the striae of Lancisi.

Langley, John Newport (1852–1925)   English physiologist. Best known for his studies of the autonomic nervous system, a term that he introduced in 1898.

Lanterman, A. J.   American anatomist of the 19th century. Described the incisures of Schmidt–Lanterman in myelin sheaths of peripheral nerve fibers.

Lewis, Sir Thomas (1881–1945)   British physician. Noted for studies of human physiology, especially as related to the heart and blood vessels, and of referred pain.

Lissauer, Heinrich (1861–1891)   German neurologist. Described the dorsolateral fasciculus of the spinal cord (Lissauer's tract or zone).

Luschka, Hubert von (1820–1875)   German anatomist. Among other contributions to anatomy, described the lateral apertures of the fourth ventricle (foramina of Luschka).

Luys, Jules Bernard (1828–1895)   French neurologist. Described the subthalamic nucleus (nucleus of Luys), whose degeneration causes hemiballismus.

Magendie, François (1783–1855)   French physiologist and pioneer of experimental physiology. The sensory function of dorsal spinal nerve roots and motor function of ventral roots constitute the Bell–Magendie law. Also described the median aperture of the fourth ventricle (foramen of Magendie).

Marchi, Vittorio (1851–1908)   Italian physician and histologist. Developed the Marchi staining method for tracing the course of degenerating myelinated fibers.

Martinotti, Giovanni (1857–1928)   Italian physician and student of Golgi. Described a type of neuron known as the cell of Martinotti in the cerebral cortex.

Mazzoni, Vittorio   Italian physician of the 19th century. The Golgi–Mazzoni ending is a type of sensory receptor.

Meckel, Johann Friedrich (1714–1774)   German anatomist. Especially known for his careful description of the trigeminal nerve. The trigeminal ganglion is situated in an extension of the meninges called Meckel's cave.

Meissner, Georg (1829–1905)   German anatomist and physiologist. His name is associated with touch corpuscles in the dermis and the submucous nerve plexus of the gastrointestinal tract.

Ménière, Prosper (1801–1862)   French otologist. Described the syndrome characterized by episodes of vertigo, nausea, and vomiting, occurring in some diseases of the internal ear.

Merkel, Friedrich Siegmund (1845–1919)   German anatomist. Described tactile endings in the epidermis, known as Merkel's disks.

Meyer, Adolph (1866–1950)   American psychiatrist. The fibers of the geniculocalcarine tract that loop forward in the temporal lobe constitute Meyer's loop.

Meynert, Theodor Hermann (1833–1892) Austrian neuropsychiatrist. The habenulointerpeduncular fasciculus is also called the fasciculus retroflexus of Meynert. The dorsal tegmental decussation of Meynert in the midbrain consists of crossing tectospinal fibers. The nucleus basalis of Meynert is in the substantia innominata of the forebrain.

Monakow, Constatin von (1853–1930) Neurologist of Russian birth who lived in Switzerland. Made fundamental contributions to knowledge of the thalamus, red nucleus, and rubrospinal tract. The dorsolateral region of the medulla is known as Monakow's area.

Moniz See de Egas Moniz.

Monro, Alexander (1733–1817) Scottish anatomist, also known as Alexander Monro (Secundus). Including tenure by his father (Primus) and son (Tertius), the Chair of Anatomy in the University of Edinburgh was occupied by Alexander Monros for over a century. The interventricular foramen between the lateral and third ventricles is known as the foramen of Monro.

Müller, Heinrich (1820–1864) German anatomist. Müller's orbital muscle and cells of Müller in the retina.

Nissl, Franz (1860–1919) German neuropsychiatrist. Made important contributions to neurohistology and neuropathology. Introduced a method of staining gray matter with cationic dyes to show the basophil material (Nissl bodies) of nerve cells.

Pacchioni, Antonio (1665–1726) Italian anatomist. The arachnoid villi become hypertrophied with age and are then known as arachnoid granulations or pacchionian bodies.

Pacini, Filippo (1812–1883) Italian anatomist and histologist. Described the sensory endings known as the corpuscles of Vater–Pacini.

Papez, John Wenceslas (1883–1958) American anatomist. Made important contributions to comparative neuroanatomy, and in 1937 postulated the involvement of the circuitry of the limbic system in emotional feeling and expression.

Parkinson, James (1775–1824) English physician, surgeon, and paleontologist. Described "shaking palsy" or paralysis agitans, which is frequently referred to as Parkinson's disease.

Penfield, Wilder Graves (1891–1976) Canadian neurosurgeon. Made fundamental contributions to neurocytology and neurophysiology, including functions of the cerebral cortex, speech mechanisms, and factors underlying epilepsy.

Perroncito, Aldo (1882–1929) Italian histologist. Described the whorls of regenerating fibers (spirals of Perroncito) in the central stump of a sectioned peripheral nerve.

Pompeiano, Ottavio (b. 1927) Contemporary Italian physiologist. Has contributed to knowledge of the physiology of the cerebellum, vestibular nuclei, and nucleus Z of Brodal and Pompeiano (in the medulla).

Purkinje, Johannes (Jan) Evangelista (1787–1869) Bohemian physiologist, pioneer in histological techniques, and accomplished histologist. Described the Purkinje cells of the cerebellar cortex and Purkinje fibers in the heart, among others.

Ramón y Cajal, Santiago (1852–1934) Spanish histologist who is acknowledged as the foremost among neurohistologists. Awarded the Nobel Prize for Medicine and Physiology (with Camillo Golgi) in 1906. Among innumerable contributions Cajal vigorously championed the Neuron Theory on the basis of his observations with silver staining methods.

Ranvier, Louis–Antoine (1835–1922) French histologist and a founder of experimental histology. Described the nodes of Ranvier in the myelin sheaths of nerve fibers.

Rasmussen, Grant Litster (b. 1904) Contemporary American neuroanatomist. Has made numerous contributions to neuroanatomy, including a description of the olivocochlear bundle (of Rasmussen).

Reil, Johann Christian (1759–1813) German physician. The insula, lying in the depths of the lateral sulcus of the cerebral hemisphere, is known as the island of Reil.

Reissner, Ernst (1824–1878)   German anatomist. The vestibular membrane of the cochlea is known as Reissner's membrane.

Renshaw, Birdsey (1911–1948)   American neurophysiologist. Certain interneurons in the ventral gray horn of the spinal cord are called Renshaw cells.

Rexed, Bror (b. 1914)   Contemporary Swedish neuroanatomist. Divided the gray matter of the spinal cord into regions (laminae of Rexed) on the basis of differences in cytoarchitecture.

Rio Hortega, Pio Del (1882–1945)   Spanish histologist who worked in his later years in England and Argentina. Best known for his studies of neuroglial cells, especially the microglia.

Robin, Charles Philippe (1821–1885)   French anatomist. The perivascular spaces of the brain are known as Virchow–Robin spaces.

Rolando, Luigi (1773–1831)   Italian anatomist. Among various contributions to neurology, described the central sulcus of the cerebral hemisphere and the substantia gelatinosa of the spinal cord.

Roller, Christian Friedrich Wilhelm (1802–1878)   German psychiatrist. One of the perihypoglossal nuclei is known as the nucleus of Roller.

Romberg, Moritz Heinrich (1795–1873)   German neurologist. Romberg's sign of impaired proprioceptive conduction in the spinal cord consists of abnormal unsteadiness when standing with the feet together and the eyes closed.

Rosenthal, Friedrich Christian (1779–1829)   German anatomist. Studied the veins of the brain (basal vein of Rosenthal).

Ruffini, Angelo (1864–1929)   Italian anatomist. Described sensory endings, especially those known as the end bulbs of Ruffini.

Russell, James Samuel Risien (1863–1939)   British physician and neurologist. Published on diseases of the nervous system and described the uncinate fasciculus of efferent cerebellar fibers.

Scarpa, Antonio (1747–1832)   Italian anatomist and surgeon. Made numerous contributions to anatomy, including a description of the vestibular ganglion.

Schmidt, Henry D. (1823–1888)   American anatomist and pathologist. Described the incisures of Schmidt–Lanterman in myelin sheaths of peripheral nerve fibers.

Schütz, H.   German anatomist. Described the dorsal longitudinal fasciculus of the brain stem in 1891.

Schwann, Theodor (1810–1882)   German anatomist. Formulated the Cell Theory (with M. J. Schleiden) and described the neurolemmal cells (Schwann cells) of peripheral nerve fibers.

Sherrington, Sir Charles Scott (1856–1952)   English neurophysiologist. A foremost contributor to basic knowledge of the function of the nervous system. His researches included studies of reflexes, decerebrate rigidity, reciprocal innervation, the synapse, and the concept of the integrative action of the nervous system.

Sperry, Roger Wolcott (b. 1913)   Contemporary American neurobiologist. Made major contributions to knowledge of development of specific connections in the brains of fishes and amphibians, and of the functions of the human corpus callosum.

Sydenham, Thomas (1624–1689)   English physician, known as the English Hippocrates. Described the form of chorea to which his name is attached.

Sylvius, Francis De La Boe (1614–1672)   French anatomist. Gave the first description of the lateral sulcus of the cerebral hemisphere.

Sylvius, Jacobus (also known as Jacques Dubois) (1478–1555)   French anatomist. Described the cerebral aqueduct of the midbrain (aqueduct of Sylvius).

Trolard, Paulin (1842–1910)   French anatomist. Described the venous drainage of the brain (greater anastomotic vein of Trolard).

Vater, Abraham (1684–1751)   German anatomist. Among other contributions to anatomy, described the sensory endings known as the corpuscles of Vater–Pacini.

Vicq D'Azyr, Felix (1748–1794)   French anatomist and a leading comparative anatomist. The mamillothalamic fasciculus bears his name.

Virchow, Rudolph Ludwig Karl (1821–1902) German pathologist. Founder of cellular pathology, or modern pathology. The perivascular spaces of the brain are known as Virchow–Robin spaces.

Waldeyer, Heinrich Wilhelm Gottfried (1836–1921) German anatomist. Popularized the Neuron Theory on the basis of studies by Cajal, Forel, His, and others. Waldeyer cells in the dorsal horn of the spinal cord are named for him.

Walker, A. Earl (b.1907) Contemporary American neurosurgeon (born and educated in Canada). Made contributions to cerebellar and cerebral cortical physiology, anatomy and physiology of the thalamus, and various clinical topics.

Wallenberg, Adolf (1862–1949) German physician. Described the lateral medullary syndrome.

Waller, Augustus Volney (1816–1870) English physician and physiologist. Described the degenerative changes in the distal portion of a sectioned peripheral nerve, known as wallerian degeneration.

Warwick, Roger (b. 1912) Contemporary British anatomist. Among other contributions, described the organization of the oculomotor nucleus with respect to the ocular muscles that it supplies.

Weber, Sir Hermann David (1823–1918) English physician. Described the midbrain lesion causing hemiparesis and ocular paralysis.

Weigert, Karl (1843–1905) German pathologist. Introduced several staining methods, including a stain for myelin and therefore for white matter in sections of nervous tissue.

Wiesel, Torsten Nils (b. 1924) Contemporary Swedish neurobiologist who, with D.H. Hubel, discovered columnar organization of the visual cortex of the monkey.

Wernicke, Carl (1848–1905) German neuropsychiatrist. Made a special study of disorders in the use of language. Wernicke's sensory language area and Wernicke's aphasia are named for him.

Westphal, Karl Friedrich Otto (1833–1890) German neurologist. Among other contributions to neurology, described the Edinger–Westphal nucleus in the oculomotor complex.

Willis, Thomas (1621–1675) English physician. One of the dominant figures in English medicine of the 17th century and one of the founders of the Royal Society. Among numerous contributions to the anatomy of the brain, described the arterial circle that bears his name.

Wilson, Samuel Alexander Kinnier (1878–1937) British neurologist. Described hepatolenticular degeneration, known as Wilson's disease.

Wrisberg, Heinrich August (1739–1808) German anatomist. Among other contributions to anatomy, described the sensory root of the facial nerve (nervus intermedius of Wrisberg).

Glossary of Neuroanatomical Terms

Abducens. L. *ab*, from + *ducens*, leading. The sixth cranial (abducens) nerve supplies the muscle that moves the direction of gaze away from the midline.

Adiadochokinesia. *a*, neg. + Gr. *diadochos*, succeeding + *kinēsis*, movement. Inability to perform rapidly alternating movements. Also called dysdiadochokinesia.

Agnosia. *a*, neg. + Gr. *gnōsis*, knowledge. Lack of ability to recognize the significance of sensory stimuli (auditory, visual, tactile, etc. agnosia).

Agraphia. *a*, neg. + Gr. *graphō*, to write. Inability to express thoughts in writing owing to a central lesion.

Akinesia. *a*, neg. + Gr. *kinēsis*, movement. The lack of spontaneous movement, as seen in Parkinson's disease.

Ala cinerea. L. wing + *cinereus*, ashen-hued. Vagal triangle in floor of fourth ventricle.

Alexia. *a*, neg. + Gr. *lexis*, word. Loss of the power to grasp the meaning of written or printed words and sentences.

Allocortex. Gr. *allos*, other + L. *cortex*, bark. The phylogenetically older cerebral cortex, usually consisting of three layers. Includes paleocortex and archicortex.

Alveus. L. trough. The thin layer of white matter covering the ventricular surface of the hippocampus. The name seems quite inappropriate, but has become an accepted part of anatomical terminology.

Amacrine. *a*, neg. + Gr. *makros*, long + *is, inos*, fiber. Amacrine nerve cell of the retina.

Ammon's horn. The hippocampus, which has an outline in cross section suggestive of a ram's horn. Also known as the cornu Ammonis. Ammon was an Egyptian deity with a ram's head.

Amygdala. L. from Gr. *amygdalē*, almond. Amygdala or amygdaloid body in the temporal lobe of the cerebral hemisphere.

Anopsia. *an*, neg. + Gr. *opsis*, vision. A defect of vision.

Antidromic. Gr. *anti*, against + *dromos*, a running. Relating to the propagation of an impulse along an axon in a direction that is the reverse of the normal or usual direction.

Aphasia. *a*, neg. + Gr. *phasis*, speech. A defect of the power of expression by speech or of comprehending spoken or written language.

Apraxia. *a*, neg. + Gr. *prattō*, to do. Inability to carry out purposeful movements in the absence of paralysis.

Arachnoid. Gr. *arachnē*, spider's web + *eidos*, resemblance. The meningeal layer forming the outer boundary of the subarachnoid space.

Archicerebellum. Gr. *archē*, beginning + diminutive of cerebrum. A phylogenetically old part of the cerebellum, functioning in the maintenance of equilibrium. Also spelled archeocerebellum.

Archicortex. Gr. *archē*, beginning + L. *cortex*, bark. Three-layered cortex included in the limbic system; located mainly in the hippocampus and dentate gyrus of the temporal lobe. Also spelled archeocortex.

Area postrema. An area in the caudal part of the floor of the fourth ventricle.

Astereognosis. *a*, neg. + *stereos*, solid + *gnōsis*, knowledge. Loss of ability to recognize objects or to appreciate their form by touching or feeling them.

Astrocyte. Gr. *astron*, star + *kylos*, hollow (cell). A type of neuroglial cell.

Asynergy. *a*, neg. + Gr. *syn*, with + *ergon*, work. Disturbance of the proper association in the contraction of muscles that ensures that the different components of an act follow in proper sequence, at the proper moment, and of the proper degree, so that the act is executed accurately.

Ataxia. *a*, neg. + Gr. *taxis*, order. A loss of power of muscle coordination, with irregularity of muscle action.

Athetosis. Gr. *athetos*, without position or place. An affliction of the nervous system, caused by degenerative changes in the corpus striatum and cerebral cortex, and characterized by bizarre, writhing movements of the fingers and toes, especially.

Autonomic. Gr. *autos*, self + *nomos*, law. Autonomic system; the efferent or motor innervation of viscera.

Autoradiography. Gr. *autos*, self + L. *radius*, ray + Gr. *graphō*, to write. A technique that uses a photographic emulsion to detect the location of radioactive isotopes in tissue sections. Also called radioautography.

Axolemma. Gr. *axōn*, axis + *lemma*, husk. The plasma membrane of an axon.

Axon. Gr. *axōn*, axis. Efferent process of a neuron conducting impulses to other neurons or to muscle fibers (striated and smooth) and gland cells.

Axon hillock. The region of the nerve cell body from which the axon arises; it contains no Nissl material.

Axon reaction. Changes in the cell body of a neuron following damage to its axon.

Axoplasm. Gr. *axōn*, axis + *plasm*, anything formed or molded. The cytoplasm of the axon.

Baroreceptor. Gr. *baros*, weight + *receptor*, receiver. A sensory nerve terminal that is stimulated by changes in pressure, as in the carotid sinus and aortic arch.

Basis pedunculi. The ventral part of the cerebral peduncle of the midbrain on each side, separated from the dorsal part by the substantia nigra. Also called the crus cerebri.

Brachium. L. from Gr. *brachiōn*, arm. As used in the central nervous system, denotes a large bundle of fibers connecting one part with another (*e.g.*, brachia associated with the colliculi of the midbrain).

Bradykinesia. Gr. *brady*, slow + *kinēsis*, movement. Abnormal slowness of movements.

Brain stem. In the mature human brain, denotes the medulla, pons, and midbrain. In descriptions of the embryonic brain the diencephalon is included as well.

Bulb. Referred at one time to the medulla oblongata but, in the context of "corticobulbar tract," refers to the brain stem, in which motor nuclei of cranial nerves are located.

Calamus scriptorius. L. *calamus*, a reed, therefore a reed pen. Refers to an area in the caudal part of the floor of the fourth ventricle, which is shaped somewhat like a pen point.

Calcar. L. spur, used to denote any spur-shaped structure. Calcar avis, an elevation on the medial aspects of the lateral ventricles at the junction of occipital and temporal horns. Also calcarine sulcus of occipital lobe, which is responsible for the calcar avis.

Cauda equina. L. horse's tail. The lumbar and sacral spinal nerve roots in the lower part of the spinal canal.

Caudate nucleus. Part of the corpus striatum, so named because it has a long extension or tail.

Cerebellum. L. diminutive of *cerebrum*, brain. A large part of the brain with motor functions, situated in the posterior cranial fossa.

Cerebrum. L. brain. The principal portion of the brain, including the diencephalon and cerebral hemispheres, but not the brain stem and cerebellum.

Chordotomy. Gr. *chordē*, cord + *tomē*, a cutting. Division of the spinothalamic and spinoreticular tracts for intractable pain (tractotomy). Also spelled cordotomy.

Chorea. L. from Gr. *choros*, a dance. A disorder characterized by irregular, spasmodic, involuntary movements of the limbs or facial muscles. Attributed to degenerative changes in the neostriatum.

Choroid. Gr. *chorion*, a delicate membrane + *eidos*, form. Choroid or vascular coat of the eye; choroid plexuses in the ventricles of the brain. Also spelled chorioid.

Chromatolysis. Gr. *chrōma*, color + *lysis*, dissolution. Dispersal of the Nissl material of neurons following axon section or in viral infections of the nervous system.

Cinerea. L. *cinereus*, ashen-hued, from *cinis*, ash. Refers to gray matter, but limited in usage. Tuber cinereum (ventral portion of the hypothalamus, from which the median eminence and infundibular stem of the neurohypophysis arises); tuberculum cinereum (slight elevation on medulla formed by spinal tract and nucleus of trigeminal nerve); ala cinerea (vagal triangle in floor of fourth ventricle).

Cingulum. L. girdle. A bundle of association fibers in the white matter of the cingulate gyrus on the medial surface of the cerebral hemisphere.

Claustrum. L. a barrier. A thin sheet of gray matter, of unknown function, situated between the lentiform nucleus and the insula.

Colliculus. L. a small elevation or mound. Superior and inferior colliculi comprising the tectum of the midbrain; facial colliculus in the floor of the fourth ventricle.

Commissure. L. a joining together. A bundle of nerve fibers passing from one side to the other in the brain or spinal cord. Strictly, this term should be applied to tracts that connect symmetrical structures (cf. **decussation**).

Corona. L. from Gr. *korōnē*, a crown. Corona radiata (fibers radiating from the internal capsule to various parts of the cerebral cortex).

Corpus callosum. L. body + *callosus*, hard. The main neocortical commissure of the cerebral hemispheres.

Corpus striatum. L. body + *striatus*, furrowed or striped. A mass of gray matter, with motor functions, at the base of each cerebral hemisphere.

Cortex. L. bark. Outer layer of gray matter of the cerebral hemispheres and cerebellum.

Crus. L. leg. The crus cerebri is the ventral part of the cerebral peduncle of the midbrain on each side, separated from the dorsal part by the substantia nigra. Also called the basis pedunculi. Crus of the fornix.

Cuneus. L. wedge. A gyrus on the medial surface of the cerebral hemisphere. Fasciculus cuneatus in the spinal cord and medulla; nucleus cuneatus in the medulla.

Cytosol. Gr. *kytos*, a hollow vessel + solution. The soluble portion of the cytoplasm, excluding all membranous and particulate components.

Decussation. L. *decussatio*, from *decussis*, the number X. The point of crossing of paired tracts. Decussations of the pyramids, medial lemnisci, and superior cerebellar peduncles are examples. A decussation connects asymmetrical parts of the nervous system.

Dendrite. Gr. *dendritēs*, related to a tree. A process of a nerve cell, on which axons of other neurons terminate. Sometimes also used for the peripheral process of a primary sensory neuron, although this has the histological and physiological properties of an axon.

Dentate. L. *dentatus*, toothed. Dentate nucleus of the cerebellum; dentate gyrus in the temporal lobe.

Diencephalon. Gr. *dia*, through + *enkephalos*, brain. Part of the cerebrum, consisting of the thalamus, epithalamus, subthalamus, and hypothalamus. The posterior of the two brain vesicles formed from the prosencephalon of the developing embryo.

Diplopia. Gr. *diplous*, double + *ōps*, eye. Double vision.

Dura. L. *dura*, hard. Dura mater (the thick external layer of the meninges).

Dyskinesia. Gr. *dys*, difficult or disordered + *kinēsis*, movement. Abnormality of motor function, characterized by involuntary, purposeless movements.

Dysmetria. Gr. *dys*, difficult or disordered + *metron*, measure. Disturbance of the power to control the range of movement in muscular action.

Emboliform. Gr. *embolos*, plug + L. *forma*, form. Emboliform nucleus of the cerebellum.

Endoneurium. Gr. *endon*, within + *neuron*, nerve. The delicate connective tissue sheath surrounding an individual nerve fiber of a peripheral nerve. Also called the sheath of Henle.

Engram. Gr. *en*, in + *gramma*, mark. Used in psychology to mean the lasting trace left in the brain by previous experience; a latent memory picture.

Entorhinal. Gr. *entos*, within + *rhis (rhin-)*, nose. The entorhinal area is the anterior part of the parahippocampal gyrus of the temporal lobe adjacent to the uncus. It is included in the lateral olfactory area.

Ependyma. Gr. *ependyma*, an upper garment. Lining epithelium of the ventricles of the brain and central canal of the spinal cord.

Epineurium. Gr. *epi*, upon + *neuron*, nerve. The connective tissue sheath surrounding a peripheral nerve.

Epithalamus. Gr. *epi*, upon + *thalamos*, inner chamber. A region of the diencephalon above the thalamus; includes the pineal gland.

Exteroceptor. L. *exterus*, external + *receptor*, receiver. A sensory receptor that serves to acquaint the individual with his environment (exteroception).

Extrapyramidal system. In broadest terms, consists of all motor parts of the central nervous system except the pyramidal motor system. "Extrapyramidal system" is subject to various interpretations, and is more often used clinically than anatomically.

Falx. L. sickle. Two of the dural partitions in the cranial cavity are the falx cerebri and the small falx cerebelli.

Fasciculus. L. diminutive of *fascis*, bundle. A bundle of nerve fibers.

Fastigial. L. *fastigium*, the top of a gabled roof. Fastigial nucleus of the cerebellum.

Fimbria. L. *fimbriae*, fringe. A band of nerve fibers along the medial edge of the hippocampus, continuing as the fornix.

Forceps. L. a pair of tongs. Used in neurological anatomy for the U-shaped configuration of fibers constituting the anterior and posterior portions of the corpus callosum (forceps frontalis and forceps occipitalis).

Fornix. L. arch. The efferent tract of the hippocampal formation, arching over the thalamus and terminating mainly in the mamillary body of the hypothalamus.

Fovea. L. a pit or depression. Fovea centralis (the depression in the center of the macula lutea of the retina).

Funiculus. L. diminutive of *funis*, cord. An area of white matter that may consist of several functionally different fasciculi, as in the lateral funiculus of white matter of the spinal cord.

Ganglion. Gr. knot or subcutaneous tumor. A swelling composed of nerve cells, as in cerebrospinal and sympathetic ganglia. Also used inappropriately for certain regions of gray matter in the brain (*e.g.*, basal ganglia of the cerebral hemisphere).

Gemmule. L. *gemmula*, diminutive of *gemma*, bud. Minute projections on dendrites of certain neurons, especially pyramidal cells and Purkinje cells, for synaptic contact with other neurons.

Genu. L. *genus*, knee. Anterior end of corpus callosum; genu of facial nerve. Also geniculate ganglion of facial nerve and geniculate nuclei of thalamus.

Glia. Gr. glue. Neuroglia, the interstitial or accessory cells of the central nervous system.

Glioblast. Gr. *glia*, glue + *blastos*, germ. An embryonic neuroglial cell.

Gliosome. Gr. *glia*, glue + *soma*, body. Granules in neuroglial cells, in particular astrocytes.

Globus pallidus. L. a ball + pale. Medial part of lentiform nucleus of corpus striatum. Also globose nuclei of cerebellum.

Glomerulus. Diminutive of L. *glomus*, ball of yarn. Synaptic glomeruli of the olfactory bulb.

Glomus. L. ball of yarn. Applied to various small organs, including the carotid and aortic bodies, and to one of their characteristic cell types.

Glycocalyx. Gr. *glycyx*, sweet + *kalyx*, cup. An outer coating of carbohydrate molecules on the surface of cells.

Gracilis. L. slender. Fasciculus gracilis of the spinal cord and medulla; nucleus gracilis and gracile tubercle of the medulla.

Granule. L. *granulum*, diminutive of *granum*, grain. Used to denote small neurons, such as granule cells of cerebellar cortex and stellate cells of cerebral cortex. Hence granular cell layers of both cortices.

Habenula. L. diminutive of *habena*, strap or rein. A small swelling in the epithalamus, adjacent to the posterior end of the roof of the third ventricle.

Haarscheibe. Ger. *haar*, hair + *scheibe*, disk. A small elevated area of skin that develops in association with specialized hair follicles and serves as a receptor for tactile stimuli.

Hemiballismus. Gr. *hēmi*, half + *ballismos*, jumping. A violent form of motor restlessness involving one side of the body, caused by a destructive lesion involving the subthalamic nucleus.

Hemiplegia. Gr. *hēmi*, half + *plēgē*, a blow or stroke. Paralysis of one side of the body.

Hippocampus. Gr. *hippocampus*, sea horse. A rather inappropriate name given to a gyrus that constitutes an important part of the limbic system; produces an elevation on the floor of the temporal horn of the lateral ventricle.

Homeostasis. Gr. *homois*, like + *stasis*, standing. A tendency toward stability in the internal environment of the organism.

Hydrocephalus. Gr. *hydrōr*, water + *kephalē*, head. Excessive accumulation of cerebrospinal fluid.

Hyperacusis. Gr. *akousis*, a hearing. Abnormal loudness of perceived sounds.

Hypothalamus. Gr. *hypo*, under + *thalamos*, inner chanber. A region of the diencephalon that serves as the main controlling center of the autonomic nervous system.

Indusium. L. a garment, from *induo*, to put on. Indusium griseum, a thin layer of gray matter on the dorsal surface of the corpus callosum (gray tunic).

Infarction. L. *infarcire*, to stuff or fill in. Regional death of tissue due to loss of blood supply.

Infundibulum. L. funnel. Infundibular stem of the neurohypophysis.

Insula. L. island. Cerebral cortex concealed from surface view and lying at the bottom of the lateral sulcus. Also called the island of Reil.

Interoceptor. L. *inter*, between + *receptor*, receiver. One of the sensory end organs within viscera.

Ischemia. Gr. *ischein*, to check + *haimos*, blood. The condition of tissue that is not adequately perfused with oxygenated blood.

Isocortex. Gr. *isos*, equal + L. *cortex*, bark. Cerebral cortex having six layers (neocortex).

Kinesthesia. Gr. *kinēsis*, movement + *aisthēsis*, sensation. The sense of perception of movement.

Koniocortex. Gr. *konis*, dust + L. *cortex*, bark. Areas of cerebral cortex containing large numbers of small neurons; typical of sensory areas.

Lemniscus. Gr. *lēmniskos,* fillet (a ribbon or band). Used to designate a bundle of nerve fibers in the central nervous system (*e.g.,* medial lemniscus and lateral lemniscus).

Lentiform. L. *lens (lent-),* a lentil (lens) + *forma,* shape. Lens-shaped. Lentiform nucleus, a component of the corpus striatum. Also called lenticular nucleus.

Leptomeninges. Gr. *leptos,* slender + *mēninx,* membrane. The arachnoid and pia mater.

Limbus. L. a border. Limbic lobe: a C-shaped configuration of cortex on the medial surface of the cerebral hemisphere, consisting of the septal area and the cingulate and parahippocampal gyri. Limbic system: limbic lobe, hippocampal formation, and portions of the diencephalon, especially the mamillary body and anterior thalamic nuclei.

Limen. L. threshold. Limen insulae: the ventral part of the insula (island of Reil); included in the lateral olfactory area.

Locus ceruleus. L. place + *caeruleus,* dark blue. A small dark spot on each side of the floor of the fourth ventricle; marks the position of a group of nerve cells that contain melanin pigment.

Macroglia. Gr. *makros,* large + *glia,* glue. The larger types of neuroglial cells—namely, astrocytes, oligodendrocytes, and ependymal cells.

Macrosmatic. Gr. *makros,* large + *osmē,* smell. Having the sense of smell strongly or acutely developed.

Macula. L. a spot. Macula lutea: a spot at the posterior pole of the eye, having a yellow color when viewed with red-free light. Maculae sacculi and utriculi: sensory areas in the vestibular portion of the membranous labyrinth.

Mamillary. L. *mammilla,* diminutive of *mamma,* breast (shaped like a nipple). Mamillary bodies: swellings on the ventral surface of the hypothalamus. Also spelled mammillary.

Massa intermedia. A bridge of gray matter connecting the thalami of the two sides across the third ventricle; present in 70% of human brains. Also called the interthalamic adhesion.

Medulla. L. marrow, from *medius,* middle. Medulla spinalis: spinal cord. Medulla oblongata: caudal portion of the brain stem. In current usage, "medulla" refers to the medulla oblongata.

Mesencephalon. Gr. *mesos,* middle + *enkephalos,* brain. The midbrain; the second of the three primary brain vesicles.

Metathalamus. Gr. *meta,* after + *thalamos,* inner chamber. The medial and lateral geniculate bodies (nuclei).

Metencephalon. Gr. *meta,* after + *enkephalos,* brain. Pons and cerebellum; the anterior of the two divisions of the rhombencephalon or posterior primary brain vesicle.

Microglia. Gr. *mikros,* small + *glia,* glue. A type of neuroglial cell.

Microsmatic. Gr. *mikros,* small + *osmē,* smell. Having a sense of smell, but of relatively poor development.

Mimetic. Gr. *mimētikos,* imitative. The muscles of expression, supplied by the facial nerve, are sometimes referred to as mimetic muscles.

Mitral. L. *mitra,* a coif or turban (bishop's miter). Mitral cell of the olfactory bulb.

Mnemonic. Gr. *mnēmē,* memory. Pertaining to memory.

Molecular. L. *molecula,* diminutive of *moles,* mass. Used in neurohistology to denote tissue containing large numbers of fine nerve fibers, and which therefore has a punctate appearance in silver-stained sections. Molecular layers of cerebral and cerebellar cortices.

Myelencephalon. Gr. *myelos,* marrow + *enkephalos,* brain. Medulla oblongata; the posterior of the two divisions of the rhombencephalon or posterior primary brain vesicle.

Myelin. Gr. *myelos,* marrow. The layers of lipid and protein substances composing a sheath around nerve fibers.

Myotrophic. Gr. *mys,* muscle + *trephein,* to nourish. Responsible for maintaining the structural and functional integrity of muscle. (Principally by chemical agents from motor neurons—hence the earlier but ambiguous term "neurotrophic.")

Neocerebellum. Gr. *neos*, new + diminutive of cerebrum. The phylogenetically newest part of the cerebellum, present in mammals and especially well developed in humans. Ensures smooth muscle action in the finer voluntary movements.

Neocortex. Gr. *neos*, new + L. *cortex*, bark. Six-layered cortex, characteristic of mammals and constituting most of the cerebral cortex in humans.

Neostriatum. Gr. *neos*, new + L. *striatus*, striped or grooved. The phylogenetically newer part of the corpus striatum consisting of the caudate nucleus and putamen; the striatum.

Neurite. Gr. *neurites*, of a nerve. The cytoplasmic processes of neurons. The term embraces both axons and dendrites.

Neurobiotaxis. Gr. *neuron*, nerve + *bios*, life + *taxis*, arrangement. The tendency of nerve cells to move during embryological development toward the area from which they receive the most stimuli.

Neuroblast. Gr. *neuron*, a nerve + *blastos*, germ. An embryonic nerve cell.

Neurofibril. Gr. *neuron*, nerve + L. *fibrilla*, diminutive of *fibra*, fiber. Delicate filaments in the cytoplasm of neurons.

Neuroglia. Gr. *neuron*, nerve + *glia*, glue. Accessory or interstitial cells of the central nervous system; includes astrocytes, oligodendrocytes, microglial cells, and ependymal cells.

Neurokeratin. Gr. *neuron*, nerve + *keras* (*kerat-*), horn. Fibrillar material, consisting of proteins, which remains after lipids have been dissolved from myelin sheaths.

Neurolemma. Gr. *neuron*, nerve + *lemma*, husk. The delicate sheath surrounding a peripheral nerve fiber consisting of a series of neurolemma cells or Schwann cells. Also spelled neurilemma.

Neuron. Gr. a nerve. The morphological unit of the nervous system, consisting of the nerve cell body and its processes (dendrites and axon).

Neuropil. Gr. *neuron*, nerve + *pilos*, felt. A complex net of nerve cell processes occupying the intervals between cell bodies in gray matter.

Nociceptive. L. *noceo*, to injure + *capio*, to take. Responsive to injurious stimuli.

Nystagmus. Gr. *nystagmos*, a nodding, from *nystazō*, to be sleepy. An involuntary oscillation of the eyes.

Obex. L. barrier. A small transverse fold overhanging the opening of the fourth ventricle into the central canal of the closed portion of the medulla.

Oligodendrocyte. Gr. *oligos*, few + *dendron*, tree + *kytos*, hollow (cell). A type of neuroglial cell. Forms the myelin sheath in the central nervous system in the same manner as the Schwann cell in peripheral nerves.

Olive. L. *oliva*. Oval bulging of the lateral area of the medulla. Inferior, accessory, and superior olivary nuclei.

Operculum. L. a cover or lid, from *opertus*, to cover. Frontal, parietal, and temporal opercula bound the lateral sulcus of the cerebral hemisphere and conceal the insula.

Pachymeninx. Gr. *pachys*, thick + *mēninx*, membrane. The dura mater.

Paleocerebellum. Gr. *palaios*, ancient + diminutive of cerebrum. A phylogenetically old part of the cerebellum functioning in postural changes and locomotion.

Paleocortex. Gr. *palaios*, ancient + L. *cortex*, bark. Olfactory cortex consisting of three to five layers.

Paleostriatum. Gr. *palaios*, ancient + L. *striatus*, striped or grooved. The phylogenetically older and efferent part of the corpus striatum; the globus pallidus or pallidum.

Pallidum. L. *pallidus*, pale. The globus pallidus of the corpus striatum; medial portion of the lentiform nucleus comprising the paleostriatum.

Pallium. L. cloak. The cerebral cortex with subjacent white matter, but usually used synonymously with cortex.

Paralysis. Gr. *paralyein*, to loosen, dissolve, or weaken. Loss of voluntary action.

Paraplegia. Gr. *para*, beside + *plēgē*, a stroke.

Paralysis of both legs and lower part of trunk.

Parenchyma. Gr. *parenchein,* to pour in beside. The essential and distinctive tissue of an organ. (The name is from an early notion that internal organs contained material poured in by their blood vessels.)

Paresis. Gr. *parienai,* to relax. Partial paralysis.

Perikaryon. Gr. *peri,* around + *karyon,* nut, kernel. The cytoplasm surrounding the nucleus. Sometimes refers to the cell body of a neuron.

Perineurium. Gr. *peri,* around + *neuron,* nerve. The cellular and connective tissue sheath surrounding a bundle of nerve fibers in a peripheral nerve.

Pes. L. foot. Pes hippocampi: the anterior thickened end of the hippocampus.

Pia mater. L. tender mother. The thin innermost layer of the meninges, attached to the surface of the brain and spinal cord; forms the inner boundary of the subarachnoid space.

Pineal. L. *pineus,* relating to the pine. Shaped like a pine cone (pertaining to the pineal gland).

Plexus. L. *plectere,* to plait. An arrangement of interwoven and intercommunicating fibers or vessels that form a network.

Pneumoencephalography. Gr. *neuma,* air + *enkephalos,* brain + *graphō,* to write. The replacement of cerebrospinal fluid by air, followed by x-ray examination (pneumoencephalogram); permits visualization of the ventricles and subarachnoid space. This technique has been replaced by computed tomography (CT scan).

Pons. L. bridge. That part of the brain stem that lies between the medulla and the midbrain; appears to constitute a bridge between the right and left halves of the cerebellum.

Positron. (From *positive electron.*) A subatomic particle with the same mass as an electron and equal but opposite charge. Positrons emitted by radioactive elements combine with electrons, with elimination of matter and emission of x-rays. Detection of

the latter forms the basis of positron emission tomography (PET).

Proprioceptor. L. *proprius,* one's own + *receptor,* receiver. One of the sensory endings in muscles, tendons, and joints; provides information concerning movement and position of body parts (proprioception).

Prosencephalon. Gr. *pros,* before + *enkephalos,* brain. The forebrain, consisting of the telencephalon (cerebral hemispheres) and diencephalon; the anterior primary brain vesicle.

Prosopagnosia. Gr. *prosōpon,* person or face + agnosia *(q.v.).* Inability to recognize previously familiar faces.

Ptosis. Gr. *ptōsis,* a falling. Drooping of the upper eyelid.

Pulvinar. L. a cushioned seat. The posterior projection of the thalamus beneath which the medial and lateral geniculate bodies are situated.

Putamen. L. shell. The larger and lateral part of the lentiform nucleus of the corpus striatum.

Pyramidal system. Corticospinal and corticobulbar tracts. So-called because the corticospinal tracts occupy the fancifully pyramid-shaped area on the ventral surface of the medulla. The term pyramidal tract refers specifically to the corticospinal tract.

Pyriform. L. *pyrum,* pear + *forma,* form. Pyriform area is a region of olfactory cortex consisting of the uncus, limen insulae, and entorhinal area; has a pear-shaped outline in animals with a well-developed olfactory system.

Quadriplegia. L. *quadri,* four + Gr. *plēgē,* stroke. Paralysis affecting the four limbs. Also called tetraplegia.

Raphe. Gr. seam. An anatomical structure in the midline. In the brain, several raphe nuclei of the reticular formation are in the midline of the medulla, pons, and midbrain.

Receptor. L. *receptus,* received. A word used in two different ways in neurobiology: (a) A structure of any size or complexity that collects and usually also edits information about conditions, inside or outside the body. Examples are the eye, the muscle spindle, and the free ending of the peripheral neu-rite of a sensory neuron. (b) A protein mol-ecule embedded in the surface of a cell (or sometimes inside the cell) that specifically binds the molecules of hormones, neuro-transmitters, drugs, or other substances that can change the activity of the cell.

Reticular.   L. *reticularis*, pertaining to or re-sembling a net. Reticular formation of the brain stem.

Rhinal.   Gr. *rhis*, nose, therefore related to the nose. Rhinal sulcus in the temporal lobe indicates the margin of the lateral olfactory area.

Rhinencephalon.   Gr. *rhis (rhin-)*, nose + *en-kephalos*, brain. An obsolete term that re-ferred to components of the olfactory sys-tem. In comparative neurology structures incorporated in the limbic system (espe-cially the hippocampus and dentate gyrus) were included.

Rhombencephalon.   Gr. *rhombos*, a lozenge-shaped figure + *enkephalos*, brain. The pons and cerebellum (metencephalon) and medulla (myelencephalon); the posterior primary brain vesicle.

Roentgenogram.   After Wilhelm Konrad Roentgen (1845–1923), who discovered x-rays, + Gr. *gamma*, a letter or record. A picture made with x-rays; more often called an x-ray or a radiograph.

Rostrum.   L. beak. Recurved portion of the corpus callosum, passing backward from the genu to the lamina terminalis.

Rubro-.   L. *ruber*, red. Pertaining to the red nucleus (nucleus ruber), as in rubrospinal and corticorubral.

Saccadic.   Fr. *saccader*, to jerk. Saccadic or quick movements of the eyes in altering di-rection of gaze.

Satellite.   L. *satteles*, attendant. Satellite cells: flattened cells of ectodermal origin forming a capsule for nerve cell bodies in dorsal root ganglia and sympathetic ganglia. Also satel-ite oligodendrocytes adjacent to nerve cell bodies in the central nervous system.

Septal area.   An area ventral to the genu and rostrum of the corpus callosum on the me-dial aspect of the frontal lobe that is the site of the septal nuclei. It is a component of the limbic system.

Septum pellucidum.   L. partition + transpar-ent. A triangular double membrane separat-ing the frontal horns of the lateral ventricles. Situated in the median plane, it fills in the interval between the corpus callosum and the fornix.

Somatic.   Gr. *somatikos*, bodily. Used in neu-rology to denote the body, exclusive of the viscera (as in somatic efferent neurons sup-plying the skeletal musculature).

Somesthetic.   Gr. *soma*, body + *aisthēsis*, per-ception. The consciousness of having a body. Somesthetic senses are the general senses of pain, temperature, touch, pres-sure, position, movement, and vibration. Also spelled somatesthetic.

Splenium.   Gr. *splēnion*, bandage. The thick-ened posterior extremity of the corpus cal-losum.

Squint.   From Middle English *asquint*, with the eyes askew. See also **strabismus.**

Strabismus.   Gr. *strabismos*, a squinting. A constant lack of parallelism of the visual axes of the eyes. Also known as a **squint.** (This is the only correct usage of the word "squint.")

Stria terminalis.   L. a furrow, groove + bound-ary, limit. A slender strand of fibers running along the medial side of the tail of the cau-date nucleus. Originating in the amygdaloid body, most of the fibers end in the septal area and hypothalamus.

Striatum.   L. *striatus*, furrowed. The phylo-genetically more recent part of the corpus striatum (neostriatum) consisting of the cau-date nucleus and the putamen or lateral por-tion of the lentiform nucleus. In compara-tive anatomy, striatum refers to a region of the brain in fishes, amphibians, and reptiles that is comparable to the corpus striatum of mammals.

Subiculum.   L. diminutive of *subex (subic-)*, a layer. Transitional cortex between that of the parahippocampal gyrus and the hippo-campus.

Substantia gelatinosa.   A column of small neu-rons at the apex of the dorsal gray horn throughout the spinal cord.

Substantia nigra.   A large nucleus with motor functions in the midbrain; many of the con-stituent cells contain dark melanin pigment.

Subthalamus. L. under + Gr. *thalamos*, inner chamber. Region of the diencephalon beneath the thalamus, containing fiber tracts and the subthalamic nucleus.

Synapse. Gr. *synaptō*, to join. The word was introduced by Sherrington in 1897 for the site of contact between neurons, at which site one neuron is excited or inhibited by another neuron.

Syndrome. Gr. *syndrome*, the act of running together or combining. A collection of concurring clinical symptoms and signs. A syndrome is often due to a single disease. However, the word is frequently used incorrectly as a synonym for "disease," even for clinical entities that produce varied and unpredictable symptoms and signs, such as acquired immune deficiency.

Syringomyelia. Gr. *syrinx*, pipe, tube + *myelos*, marrow. A condition characterized by central cavitation of the spinal cord and gliosis around the cavity.

Tanycyte. Gr. *tanyō*, to stretch + *kytos*, hollow (cell). A specialized type of ependymal cell present in the floor of the third ventricle.

Tapetum. L. *tapete*, a carpet. Fibers of the corpus callosum sweeping over the lateral ventricle and forming the lateral wall of its temporal horn.

Tectum. L. roof. Roof of the midbrain consisting of the paired superior and inferior colliculi.

Tegmentum. L. cover, from *tego*, to cover. The dorsal portion of the pons; also the major portion of the cerebral peduncle of the midbrain, lying between the substantia nigra and the tectum.

Tela choroidea. L. a web + Gr. *chorioeidēs*, like a membrane. The vascular connective tissue continuous with that of the pia mater that continues into the core of the choroid plexuses.

Telencephalon. Gr. *telos*, end + *enkephalos*, brain. Cerebral hemispheres; the anterior of the two divisions of the prosencephalon or anterior primary brain vesicle.

Telodendria. Gr. *telos*, end + *dendrion*, tree. The terminal branches of axons.

Tentorium. L. tent. The tentorium cerebelli is a dural partition between the occipital lobes of the cerebral hemispheres and the cerebellum.

Tetraplegia. Gr. *tetra-*, four + *plēgē*, a blow or stroke. Paralysis affecting the four limbs. Also called quadriplegia.

Thalamus. Gr. *thalamos*, an inner chamber; also meant a bridal couch, so that the *pulvinar (q.v.)* was its cushion or pillow. Galen made up the word *thalamus* because he thought the optic tract was a hollow prolongation of the lateral ventricle. Willis was probably the first to use the word in its modern sense.

Tomography. G. *tomos*, cutting + *graphō*, to write. Sectional roentgenography. Computed tomography (CT scan) is a valuable diagnostic technique.

Torcular. L. wine press, from *torquere*, to twist. The confluence of the dural venous sinuses at the internal occipital protuberance was formerly known as the torcular Herophili.

Transducer. L. *transducere*, to lead across. A structure or mechanism for converting one form of energy into another; applied to sensory receptors.

Trapezoid body. Transverse fibers of the auditory pathway situated at the junction of the dorsal and ventral portions of the pons.

Trigeminal. L. born three at a time. The trigeminal nerve (cranial nerve V) has three large branches or divisions.

Trochlear. Gr. *trochileia*, a pulley. The fourth cranial (trochlear) nerve supplies the superior oblique muscle, whose tendon passes through a fibrous ring, the trochlea. This ring changes the direction in which the muscle pulls.

Uncinate. L. hook-shaped. Uncinate fasciculus: association fibers connecting cortex of the ventral surface of the frontal lobe with that of the temporal pole. Also a bundle of fastigiobulbar fibers (uncinate fasciculus of Russell) that curves over the superior cerebellar peduncle in its passage to the inferior cerebellar peduncle.

Uncus. L. a hook. The hooked-back portion of the rostral end of the parahippocampal gyrus of the temporal lobe, constituting a landmark for the lateral olfactory area.

Uvula. L. little grape. A portion of the inferior vermis of the cerebellum.

Vagus. L. wandering. The tenth cranial nerve is so named on account of the wide distribution of its branches in the thorax and abdomen.

Vallecula. L. diminutive of *vallis*, valley. The midline depression on the inferior aspect of the cerebellum.

Velate. L. *velum*, sail, curtain, veil. Velate or protoplasmic astrocytes have flattened processes.

Velum. L. sail, curtain, veil. A membranous structure. The superior and inferior medullary vela forming the roof of the fourth ventricle.

Ventricle. L. *ventriculus*, diminutive of *venter*, belly. Lateral, third, and fourth ventricles of the brain.

Vermis. L. worm. The midline portion of the cerebellum.

Zona incerta. Gray matter in the subthalamus representing a rostral extension of the reticular formation of the brain stem.

Zonula occludens. L. diminutive of *zona*, belt + occluding. Also known as a tight junction. A form of continuous close apposition of the membranes of neighboring cells, impermeable to macromolecules.

Index

The letter *f* after a page number indicates a figure; *t* following a page number indicates tabular material.